BIOCHEMISTRY OF PARASITES

THEODOR VON BRAND

LABORATORY OF PARASITIC DISEASES
NATIONAL INSTITUTES OF HEALTH
U.S. PUBLIC HEALTH SERVICE
BETHESDA, MARYLAND

1966

ACADEMIC PRESS · New York and London

ACADEMIC PRESS INC.
111 Fifth Avenue, New York, New York 10003

United Kingdom Edition published by
ACADEMIC PRESS INC. (LONDON) LTD.
Berkeley Square House, London W.1

LIBRARY OF CONGRESS CATALOG CARD NUMBER: 65-26413

PRINTED IN THE UNITED STATES OF AMERICA

PREFACE

In the preface to "Chemical Physiology of Endoparasitic Animals," which was published in 1952, I pointed out that the physiological aspects of parasitology had been developed since the beginning of this century, and that after a slow start work in the field gathered increasing momentum in the 10 to 15 years preceding publication of the book. This development has continued unabated since, but a certain shift in research emphasis has occurred.

Initially, purely physiological aspects of the general problem, such as nutritional relationships, stood in the foreground of interest of many investigators. Modern workers tend more and more to emphasize purely biochemical topics. Although the present book is based on the 1952 publication, the material had to be rearranged completely in order to do justice to the newer trends. Furthermore, the development of the field has been so rapid and the literature has increased to such an extent that it proved necessary to omit completely certain physiological topics, such as the endocrinological relationships, and to mention others only briefly, such as the growth requirements or water exchanges. On the other hand, many biochemical aspects had to be greatly expanded, for instance the discussion of the carbohydrases, or the intermediate carbohydrate or protein metabolism. Other topics, such as the nucleic acids, are discussed separately for the first time.

It is not surprising then that only very few paragraphs could be taken over without change from the 1952 publication, even though the range of parasites covered, i.e., endoparasitic protozoa, helminths, and arthropods, remained the same. To emphasize the change in research trends and to

characterize the monograph better, its title has been changed to "Biochemistry of Parasites." It is hoped that in this new guise the book will
be accorded the same favorable reception as its predecessor and that it
will prove helpful to graduate students and research workers and will
thus contribute to the further development of parasite biochemistry.

I am indebted to Dr. D. Fairbairn for reading the entire manuscript,
to Drs. E. Bueding and H. J. Saz for reviewing Chapters 2 to 4, to Dr.
P. P. Weinstein for reading Chapters 1 and 8, and to Dr. B. A. Newton
for reading Chapter 7. All reviewers have contributed helpful sugges-
tions, but, since they have not seen the final revision, I alone am responsible for any error that may have remained. I shall be grateful if such
errors are brought to my attention.

January, 1966   THEODOR VON BRAND

CONTENTS

Chapter 3

CARBOHYDRATES II:
METABOLISM OF CARBOHYDRATES

Chapter 4

CARBOHYDRATES III:
HOST-PARASITE CARBOHYDRATE RELATIONSHIPS

Chapter 5

LIPIDS

Chapter 6

PROTEINS

Chapter 7

NUCLEIC ACIDS

Chapter 8

VITAMINS

Chapter 9

RESPIRATION

Chapter 1

INORGANIC SUBSTANCES

I. QUANTITATIVE CONSIDERATIONS

The amount of inorganic material occurring in parasitic trematodes, nematodes, and Acanthocephala varies approximately between 0.6 and 1.1% of the fresh tissues (Table I), but in cestodes frequently much higher values, up to 41% of the dry matter or 19.2% of the fresh tissues, have been observed. This, unquestionably, is a consequence of the enormous number of calcareous corpuscles deposited in many tapeworms. It should be realized that the figures for the ash content are derived almost universally from dry combustion at relatively high temperatures. During this process carbonates are decomposed with a loss of carbon dioxide. This can introduce an appreciable error. In larval and adult *Taenia taeniaeformis,* which are rich in carbonate-containing calcareous corpuscles and therefore constitute an extreme example, the ash obtained by incineration at 650°C has to be multiplied by 1.85 and 1.53, respectively, to compensate for the carbon dioxide loss (von Brand and Bowman, 1961). Another possible source of error, when expressing the ash in per cent of the fresh tissues, is the fact that the water content of some parasites, especially cestodes and Acanthocephala, may rapidly change in an unphysiological way under experimental conditions. The figures assembled in Table I should therefore be considered as approximations rather than as absolute values.

The ash of parasites contains expectedly many elements besides the main inorganic components listed in Table I. Qualitative data, largely gained by emission spectroscopy, are shown in Table II. It is of interest to note that some of the trace elements occur in unusually large amounts in some parasites. Thus, the tissues of *Clonorchis sinensis* contain 38 mg copper per 100 gm dry tissue (Ma, 1963) while the corresponding figure for *Diphyllobothrium latum* is only 3.6 to 4.4 mg (Villako and Hange, 1958). The high copper content of the fluke is explained, at least in part,

1

TABLE I

PERCENTAGE OF INORGANIC SUBSTANCES IN SOME PARASITES[a]

Species	Total ash in % of		Single components in % of dry weight						References
	Fresh weight	Dry weight	Ca	Mg	K	Na	P	Cl	
Trematodes									
Clonorchis sinensis	0.46	5.10							Ma (1963)
Fasciola hepatica	1.14	4.9	0.078	0.019	0.199	0.645	0.532		Weinland and von Brand (1926)
Cestodes									
Cysticercus fasciolaris[b]	8.37	28.5							von Brand and Bowman (1961)
Cysticercus tenuicollis,									
scolex	19.2	41.1							Schopfer (1932)
membranes	0.3	1.2							Schopfer (1932)
Hymenolepis diminuta			0.075	0.061	0.836	0.323			Goodchild et al. (1962)
Raillietina cesticillus	2.36	11.5							Reid (1942)
Schistocephalus solidus, plerocercoids	1.85	5.8							Hopkins (1950)
Taenia taeniaeformis[c]	5.87	27.0							von Brand and Bowman (1961)
Nematodes									
Ascaris lumbricoides ♂	1.08	4.84	0.076	0.012	1.36	0.685	0.343	0.561	Cavier and Savel (1951a)
Ascaris lumbricoides ♀	0.96	4.84	0.076	0.013	1.29	0.824	0.392	0.616	Cavier and Savel (1951a)
Eustrongylides ignotus, larvae	1.1	4.4							von Brand (1938)
Acanthocephala									
Macracanthorhynchus hirudinaceus	0.58	5.0							von Brand (1939)

[a] Further quantitative data on inorganic substances will be found in the papers by Agosin et al. (1957); von Brand (1933); Flury (1912); Hopkins (1960); Rogers and Lazarus (1949a); Schopfer (1932); Smith (1962); Smorodincev and Bebesin (1936a,b); Smorodincev et al. (1933); Wardle (1937a).
[b] Tissue ash (total ash minus calcareous corpuscles): 1.44% of fresh weight.
[c] Tissue ash (total ash minus calcareous corpuscles): 2.40% of fresh weight.

TABLE II

INORGANIC SUBSTANCES, INCLUDING TRACE ELEMENTS IN PARASITES[a]

Species	K	Na	Mg	Ca	Fe	Zn	Cu	Cl	S	P	Si	Al	Pb	Rb	Mo	Mn	Co	Sn	Sb	Cd	As	Li	B
Trematodes																							
Clonorchis sinensis[b]	x	x	x	x	x	x	x			x	x	x	x	x	x	x	-	-	-	-	-	-	-
Cestodes																							
Cysticercus fasciolaris[c]	x	x	x	x					x	x													
Cysticercus cellulosae[d,e]		x	x	x			-			x		-	-			-			-				-
Diphyllobothrium latum[d,f]	x	x	x	x	x		x			x	x	x	x			x		x					x
Spirometra mansonoides Sparganum[d,g]		x	x	x	x		-			x	x	-	-			-		-					-
Taenia saginata[d,h]	x	x	x	x	x		x			x	x	x	-			x		-					-
Taenia taeniaeformis[d,i]	x	x	x	x	x		x			x	x	-	x			x		x					-
Nematodes																							
Ascaris lumbricoides[j]	x	x	x	x	x		-	x	x	x	x	x				-							

[a] KEY: x = element present; - = element not demonstrable; blank spaces = no information available.
[b] Ma (1963).
[c] Salisbury and Anderson (1939).
[d] Isolated calcareous corpuscles.
[e] von Brand et al. (1965).
[f] von Brand et al. (1965).
[g] von Brand et al. (1965).
[h] von Brand et al. (1965).
[i] von Brand et al. (1965).
[j] Flury (1912); Smorodincev and Bebesin (1936a); Cavier and Savel (1951a).

3

by its having a powerful copper-containing enzyme, polyphenol oxidase. On the other hand, *Clonorchis* does not show detectable amounts of cobalt, while 14 μg% was found in the fish tapeworm. The relatively high cobalt content of *Diphyllobothrium* is undoubtedly due to its ability to absorb large quantities of vitamin B_{12} from the host's intestine (Brante and Ernberg, 1957; Nyberg, 1958a; Nyberg *et al.*, 1961b). Substantial amounts of cobalt (0.075 to 0.227 on Co-deficient diet, 0.200–0.891 parts per million dry weight on Co-supplemented host diet) have also been reported for *Haemonchus contortus* (Threlkeld *et al.*, 1956).

Little is known about host-induced variations in inorganic substances which undoubtedly do occur. Significant in this respect is probably the observation that the freezing point depression of -2 to $-2.41°C$ found in cestodes and nematodes of marine fishes is considerably lower than that of the fresh-water trout parasite *Eubothrium crassum* with $-0.933°C$ (Schopfer, 1932) or that of various helminths of terrestrial vertebrates with values ranging from -0.6 to $-1.1°C$ (Vialli, 1923, 1926; Schopfer, 1927, 1932). It must be kept in mind, however, that in a worm extract, substances other than ash material can contribute to the freezing point depression. Cestodes from selachians, for instance, contain very large amounts of urea, constituting 3.7% of the dry material in *Calliobothrium* (Read *et al.*, 1959).

Some data cautioning against generalizations have been obtained from the fluids of some parasites (Table III). The relatively low chloride concentration in the body fluid of ascarids, reported as early as 1865 by Marcet, is especially interesting. Here, chlorides are quantitatively not of prime importance to the total molecular solute concentration, contributing only between 12 (Schopfer, 1932) and 36% (Duval and Courtois, 1928). The latter investigators found bicarbonates of significance in this respect, reporting 58 ml of total carbon dioxide in 100 ml body fluid. Chlorides, bicarbonates, and amino nitrogen (60 mg/100 ml fluid) accounted for 68% of the total molecular concentration in the case of *Parascaris*. In the fluid of larval tapeworms, on the other hand, the chlorides account for a much higher proportion of the total molecular concentration, e.g., 66.8% in the case of *Cysticercus tenuicollis* (Schopfer, 1932). The hemocele fluid of *Gastrophilus* larvae resembles that of ascarids in respect to low chloride content, accounting for only 7% of the total base. Here, organic acids play a prominent role (22%), as shown by Levenbook (1950).

The other components listed in Table III require little comment with the exception of the uncommonly high sulfur concentration found by Mazzocco (1923) in *Echinococcus*. Schopfer (1932) assumes Mazzocco's value to be in error and a reinvestigation appears desirable.

TABLE III

INORGANIC CONSTITUENTS OF SOME PARASITIC FLUIDS[a,b]

| Species | Material | Inorganic components in mmole per liter | | | | | | | | | | | References |
		K	Na	Mg	Ca	Fe	Zn	Cu	Cl	S	P	Si	
Cysticercus tenuicollis	Cyst fluid	x	x	2.1	1.2				120	2.0	1.9		Schopfer (1925, 1926b, 1932)
Echinococcus granulosus	Cyst fluid	9.6	171	1.5	0.9	x			115	44	4.0	x	Mazzocco (1923)
Ascaris lumbricoides	Body fluid	23.5	119	4.95		0.13	0.14	0.02	55		12.0		Rogers (1945)
Ascaris lumbricoides	Body fluid	24.6	129	4.9	5.9				52.7		17.0		Hobson *et al.* (1952b)
Gastrophilus intestinalis	Body fluid	11.5	175	4.7	2.8		0.14	0.09	15	3.0	2.2		Levenbook (1950)

[a] Further quantitative data will be found in the papers by Cavier and Savel (1951b); Codounis and Polydorides (1936); Duval and Courtois (1928); Flury (1912); Ishizaki *et al.* (1957); Kutsumi *et al.* (1957); Lemaire and Ribére (1935); Moniez (1880); Rogers and Lazarus (1949a); Schopfer (1924, 1926a).

[b] Key: x = element present; blank spaces = no information available.

II. FORMED INORGANIC DEPOSITS

The calcareous corpuscles, though missing or rare in a few tapeworm species, are a major and characteristic constituent of most cestodes. Their weight has been reported as 4.1% of the fresh tissues in the case of *Taenia marginata,* while the corresponding figures for larval and adult *Taenia taeniaeformis* are 6.93 and 3.15% (von Brand, 1933; von Brand *et al.,* 1960). In the latter form no gradient along the adult strobila exists, apparently indicating that the deposition of corpuscles parallels closely the formation of new living tissues.

The calcareous corpuscles of cestodes consist of a protein base into which are incorporated such substances as glycogen, mucopolysaccharides, lipids, and alkaline phosphatase (Chowdhuri *et al.,* 1955, 1962; von Brand *et al.,* 1960). The major inorganic components of the corpuscles are always calcium, magnesium, and carbon dioxide. Phosphorus occurs in fairly large amounts in most species studied, but is found only in traces in the corpuscles of *Cysticercus cellulosae.* Minor constituents are aluminum, boron, copper, iron, lead, manganese, silicon, sodium, and tin, all or some of which have been reported for all species studied (von Brand *et al.,* 1965). The corpuscles isolated from intestinal stages seem to contain a larger variety of these minor elements than the larval stages from tissues; the former are probably exposed to a greater variety of exogenous compounds than the latter. The corpuscles are amorphous *in situ.* Their inorganic components can, however, readily be brought to crystallization by treatment with KOH or by heat. What minerals are formed depends on the type of treatment and the species of tapeworm (Table IV). The formation of different minerals in different species, despite uniform treatment, is a curious phenomenon. The ratio of elements present may be of importance.

Nothing definite is known about the calcification mechanism of the corpuscles. *In vivo* experiments have shown (Desser, 1963) that *Echinococcus multilocularis* accumulates calcium rapidly, 8-month-old cysts containing up to 23 times more calcium than the blood plasma of the host. While in this case no differentiation between total body calcium and calcium segregated in the corpuscles has been made, it has been proven that P^{32} present in the environment rapidly appears in the corpuscles of *Cysticercus fasciolaris.* Isolated corpuscles of this worm incorporate phosphorus with a Q_{10} of only slightly higher than 1, indicating that physical processes are predominantly involved. Whether the same relationships prevail when corpuscles are located within the living body is problematical and the question is not open to a ready experimental approach (von Brand and Weinbach, 1965).

TABLE IV

CRYSTALLIZATION PATTERNS OF CALCAREOUS CORPUSCLES[a]

Species	Isolation by means of KOH		Isolation by means of ethylenediamine			
	Treatment		Treatment (18 hours)			
	None	None	300°C	450°C	600°C	950°C
Cysticercus cellulosae	Brucite, calcium carbonate	Amorphous, trace of calcite	Dolomite	Calcite, magnesium oxide	Calcite, calcium oxide, magnesium oxide	Calcium oxide, magnesium oxide
Spirometra mansonoides, larvae	Brucite, calcium carbonate, hydroxyapatite	Amorphous	Dolomite	Hydroxyapatite, calcite, magnesium oxide	Hydroxyapatite, calcium oxide, magnesium oxide	Hydroxyapatite, calcium oxide, magnesium oxide
Taenia saginata	Brucite, hydroxyapatite	Amorphous	Dolomite	Hydroxyapatite, trace of calcite, magnesium oxide	Hydroxyapatite, whitlockite, magnesium oxide	Whitlockite, magnesium oxide
Diphyllobothrium latum	Brucite, hydroxyapatite	Amorphous	Amorphous	Hydroxyapatite	Hydroxyapatite, trace of whitlockite, magnesium oxide	Whitlockite, calcium–magnesium–orthophosphate, magnesium oxide

[a] Data from Epprecht *et al.* (1950); von Brand *et al.* (1960); Trautz (1960); D. B. Scott *et al.* (1962); von Brand *et al.* (1965).

Insofar as the biological significance of the corpuscles is concerned, the view has been expressed (von Brand, 1933; Lagachev, 1951) that they may serve as buffer reserve to neutralize acids originating within the body from anaerobic or aerobic fermentations or acids encountered by the worms in the environment. This view recently received some experimental support from the observation (von Brand *et al.,* 1960; von Brand and Bowman, 1961) that the amount of calcareous material decreases significantly upon *in vitro* incubation of worms, especially if the surroundings are slightly acid. It is, however, probable that calcareous corpuscles also can fulfill other functions. Von Brand and Weinbach (1965) assume on the basis of studies on the incorporation into and the release of phosphorus from the corpuscles that the latter may serve as phosphate reserve. Timofeyev (1964), on the contrary, considers the corpuscles as waste products, though conceding that they may act as buffer.

Concretions morphologically somewhat similar to the calcareous corpuscles of cestodes occur within the excretory system, especially the excretory bladder of several trematodes (Claparède, 1858; Fraipont, 1880, 1881). Recent histochemical and electron-microscopic studies of the corpuscles occurring in *Acanthoparyphium spinulosum* (Martin and Bils, 1964) indicate a remarkable morphological similarity to the calcareous corpuscles of cestodes. The excretory concretions of trematodes consist chiefly of calcium carbonate and a trace of phosphate.

Inorganic deposits are found in the form of small, red-brown, weakly birefringent crystals in the intestinal cells of many parasitic nematodes. Originally described as end products of hemoglobin decomposition (Askanazy, 1896; Looss, 1905; Fauré-Fremiet, 1913a) or as zymogen granules (von Kemnitz, 1912), their inorganic nature was established by Quack (1913) and Chitwood and Chitwood (1938), who found the granules to consist essentially of calcium sulfate. However, Rogers (1940) and D. T. Clark (1956) could not confirm this finding; according to their observations the sphaerocrystals do not contain gypsum, but they consist of β-zinc sulfide. Clark (1956) speculates that a desulfhydrogenase may produce H_2S from sulfur-containing amino acids of ingested blood. The sulfur ions of the ionized H_2S would then precipitate zinc ions as zinc sulfide. It is, of course, possible that the cell inclusions in the nematodes' intestines are not uniform and that some of the above contradictions could be related to various authors having studied different types of granules.

The hyaline spheres of the *Parascaris equorum* oocytes were originally described as consisting of calcium phosphate (Fauré-Fremiet, 1913b; Panijel, 1951). It was, however, later established that they contain but little phosphorus and large amounts of nitrogen and that they are actually of a proteinaceous nature (Fauré-Fremiet et al., 1954).

Granules giving positive iron reaction occur in the intestinal cells of some nematodes and trematodes. The derivation of these granules is obscure and Hsü (1938a,b,c) was unable to correlate their occurrence with the amount of blood ingested by the parasites.

While no causal connection between breakdown of hemoglobin and deposition of corpusculate inorganic material has been established as yet for parasitic worms, such evidence has been presented in fairly definite form for the pupae of *Gastrophilus intestinalis*. Beaumont (1948) found that the hemoglobin of the red organ is completely destroyed during pupation and that an unusually large amount of granules giving iron reactions is then deposited within the intestinal cells. Their exact chemical composition has, however, not yet been established. It may also be mentioned that iron-positive granules have been found in the oenocytes of the larvae (Dinulescu, 1932).

III. PATHOLOGICAL AND EXPERIMENTAL INORGANIC DEPOSITS

Pathological calcium deposits are frequently found in organisms which have harbored parasites for a long time; they often involve host tissues. One well-known example is the *Trichinella* capsule, which begins calcifying about 7 months after infection (Theman, 1956). Another example is the hardening of the enlarged bile ducts in old *Fasciola* infections. According to X-ray diffraction analysis (Epprecht et al., 1950), only hydroxyapatite is deposited in the walls of the bile ducts. No calcite, aragonite, or vaterite was found. However, since the material had been treated, prior to analysis, with hot 10% KOH, these negative results may be artifacts. Calcification of the host tissues does in general not appear to damage the parasite. Living *Trichinella* larvae can readily be isolated from even heavily calcified capsules. Parasites themselves may also be found calcified; calcified filarial worms, for instance, have often been observed. Apparently calcium salts are deposited in the worms only after their death. This has been pointed out by Boehm (1908) for *Trichinella* larvae and by Otto and von Brand (1941) for *Capillaria hepatica* specimens. According to Oda (1959), the calcification of *Schistosoma japonicum* eggs begins about 40 days after their death.

Experimentally, the calcification phenomena can be speeded up considerably by administration of excessive doses of irradiated ergosterol or parathormone, while calcium preparations require longer administration. Almost invariably these experimental calcifications are confined to host tissues, e.g., the *Trichinella* cyst. Always, nonparasitized tissues of the host (kidney, coronaries and others) are at least as susceptible as the parasite-connected structures, thus excluding artificial calcification as a possible therapeutic measure. Parasites usually remain uncalcified, as long as they are alive. The only possible exceptions are some doubtful calcium reactions within schistosome eggs or the *Trichinella* larvae of a single rat (von Brand *et al.,* 1933, 1938; Wantland, 1934, 1936; Wantland *et al.,* 1936; Otto and von Brand, 1941; Theman, 1956).

A related question is whether the presence of parasites modifies the reactions of the host to calcifying doses of irradiated ergosterol derivatives. Differences in response exist which may be related to the host species, the parasite species, the age of the host, the type of ergosterol derivative used, or some unrecognized factor. Thus, von Brand and Holtz (1933) found canary birds infected with *Plasmodium praecox* somewhat more susceptible to the pathological calcification than uninfected ones, while the opposite is true in chickens infected with *Plasmodium gallinaceum* (Mercado and von Brand, 1964). Rats infected with *Plasmodium berghei* are definitely less subject to pathological calcification than uninfected ones and, curiously, different patterns in calcification of the stomach exist between both groups (Mercado and von Brand, 1962). In similar experiments with rats infected with two species of African trypanosomes a comparable decrease in over-all incidence of calcification rate (10 organs) was observed, but it did not occur in uninfected animals stressed by exposure to cold or by injections of cortisone. In view of these findings (Mercado and von Brand, 1965) it appears justified to assume a specific role of parasites in decreasing the susceptibility of host tissues to abnormal calcification.

While there is as yet no reliable way to achieve calcium deposition within the body of parasites by means of ergosterol, the experimental formation of different types of inorganic deposits has been described. Von Kemnitz (1912) found in the lateral lines of *Ascaris* structures superficially similar to calcareous corpuscles of cestodes upon injection of calcium hydroxide. Iron deposits can be achieved by feeding parasites iron saccharate or iron lactate. In *Opalina ranarum* Kedrowsky (1931) found the iron after such treatment within the so-called segregation apparatus, a structure of doubtful morphological identity, whereas in *Ascaris* the iron was exclusively adsorbed by the Golgi apparatus of the intestinal cells (Hirsch and Bretschneider, 1937).

IV. INTIMATE DISTRIBUTION OF ASH CONSTITUENTS

Very little is known about the intimate localization of inorganic substances within the tissues of parasites, aside from the relatively large scale inorganic deposits mentioned in the two preceding sections. Essentially, two procedures have been used: microincineration and, more recently, autoradiography. The former procedure has been applied predominantly to protozoa, the latter to helminths. G. H. Scott and Horning (1932) and Horning and Scott (1933) found ash deposits in the myonemes, cilia, and basal granules of *Opalina* and *Nyctotherus*. The nuclei of the opalinids were practically ash-free, while the nuclear apparatus of *Nyctotherus* was rich in inorganic material. Dense deposits consisting chiefly of calcium oxide were found in the "vegetative granules" of *Opalina,* while in *Nyctotherus* ash probably rich in sodium formed a fine network throughout the cytoplasm. In the cytopharynx of *Nyctotherus* crystals containing silica were observed and the wall of the food vacuoles was rich in inorganic material, the ash consisting in this latter case of variable proportions of calcium and iron. MacLennan and Murer (1934) incinerated several *Trichonympha* species and found most of the mineral ash, consisting chiefly of calcium compounds, in the neuromotor system, the regions of active absorption, the nucleus, and some cytoplasmic granules. The chromatin was especially rich in iron. Kruszynski (1951) demonstrated in *Plasmodium gallinaceum* by microincineration potassium, sodium, calcium, and phosphorus. In *Plasmodium berghei* Kruszynski (1952) found calcium, which is missing, at least insofar as microincineration demonstrates, in the erythrocytes of the host, implying that the parasite gained it from the blood plasma of the host.

Insofar as autoradiography is concerned, Bélanger (1960) found undetermined frog lung trematodes to take up very rapidly, *in situ,* $S^{35}O_4$ and to deposit sulfur under the hypodermis at the level of the peripheral musculature. In later experiments Burton (1963) observed a somewhat slower uptake of radiosulfate by *Haematoloechus medioplexus*. According to his findings the radioactive sulfur is deposited only in the parenchyma. Pantelouris and Gresson (1960) injected Fe^{59} (as ferric chloride solution or as a component of labeled hemoglobin) into the gut of *Fasciola hepatica,* which were then maintained for periods up to 5 days in the abdominal cavity of mice. The iron accumulated in the intestinal and cuticular epithelium, the myoblasts, and the cells forming the walls of the excretory tubules. In subsequent studies Pantelouris and Hale (1962) demonstrated by histochemical tests and microincineration that in the absence of recent administration iron occurs essentially in the same tissues as after recent feeding, with the exception of the now iron-free cuticle. The distribution of vitamin C coincides exactly with that of iron. It may be important by maintaining the iron in a diffusible form (ferric hydroxide-ferrous ascorbate), thus making its excretion possible. This may be significant to a parasite living in an organ as rich in iron as the liver. When *Fasciola* is kept in solutions containing radioactive sulfate, activity can be demonstrated by autoradiography primarily in the vitellarian cells where it may have been bound by the phenols which are abundant in this site (Pantelouris, 1964). When sulfur-labeled methionine is given, considerable activity is found in the gut cells, but also in the vitellaria, the latter cells acquiring the sulfate after the methionine had been metabolized in the gut cells (Pantelouris, 1964).

V. UPTAKE AND METABOLIC FATE OF INORGANIC SUBSTANCES

Very little is known about the mechanism of uptake of inorganic substances by parasites. Mulvey (1960) investigated the uptake and release of radioactive sodium, phosphorus, and iron by the blood-stream form of *Trypanosoma equiperdum*. He reports that both involve active processes when the parasites are maintained in glucose-containing media, but only diffusion in glucose-free environments. Mulvey (1960) used relatively long incubation periods; in view of the rapid death of African trypanosomes in sugar-free surroundings, it can be surmised that he was dealing with dead membranes when he employed glucose-free media.

Cautious interpretation of such findings is indicated by some experiences of Read (1950) with *Hymenolepis diminuta*. He found apparent differences, depending upon the availability or nonavailability of sugar, in the absorption rate of radiophosphate. If trace amounts of P^{32} were given to infected rats, marked accumulation in the worms occurred only if the phosphorus had been given without sugar. In the presence of glucose the radioactive level of the worms stayed low, probably because most of the phosphate was absorbed by the host before reaching the worms. This follows from the fact that upon feeding of larger amounts of phosphate to the rats no corresponding absorption difference by the worms was found. When phosphate was injected intraperitoneally into the hosts, a slow but steady uptake occurred in the worms, considered as an exchange of ions between host tissues and gut contents. Daugherty (1957) concluded that $Na^{22}Cl$ enters *Hymenolepis diminuta* only by diffusion, since he observed only a doubling of the absorption rate between 4 and 38°C.

Similarly, Rogers and Lazarus (1949a) observed a gradual accumulation of phosphate in the tissues of *Nippostrongylus muris* when the host animals were injected intramuscularly with P^{32}. Esserman and Sambell (1951) reported uptake of P^{32} by *Trichostrongylus* spp. and *Oesophagostomum columbianum* after sheep had been dosed intravenously with phosphate. These observations are interpreted as active feeding by the worms on host tissues. In view of the similar behavior of tapeworms mentioned above, this interpretation would seem to require further experimental support. Perhaps the fate of phosphate within the host plays the decisive role. At any rate, another nematode, *Ascaridia galli,* does not accumulate phosphate when it is administered intravenously to chickens. Evidently, there can be no question that tissue parasites and their physiological equivalents (gut-inhabiting bloodsuckers) are capable of acquiring phosphate from host tissues or fluids. It has been demonstrated by McCoy *et al.* (1941) that P^{32} is deposited in and after some time again lost from encapsulated larvae of *Trichinella spiralis.* This phosphate exchange proceeds in the larvae at an appreciably slower rate than in the muscles of the host. It was, however, not decided whether in the case of the larvae a true metabolic exchange or simply a diffusion of phosphate ions occurred. Rapid phosphate accumulation by the bloodsucker *Haemonchus contortus* after both intra-abomasal and intravenous injections of the sheep has been described by Esserman and Sambell (1951).

It is not surprising, in view of their feeding habits, that intestinal nematodes should absorb P^{32} much faster when it is given orally to the host than when administered either intramuscularly or intravenously. However, differences in absorption rates between parasite species exist. Thus, Rogers and Lazarus (1949a) found peak values in *Ascaridia galli* from 20 to 60 minutes after dosing the host, while in the case of *Nippostrongylus muris* maximal values were reached only after 90 to 120 minutes.

There is no clear-cut indication that phosphorus enters the body of nematodes to an appreciable extent through the cuticle, but it is clear from observations of Rogers and Lazarus (1949a) that it is absorbed via the intestinal canal. If normal and ligatured *Ascaris lumbricoides* are exposed for a minimum of 1 hour and a maximum of 20 hours to P^{32} *in vitro,* radioautographs prepared from ligatured worms show only very small amounts of P^{32} in the cuticle and the lateral lines, while unligatured worms have always appreciable amounts in the intestinal tissues.

Indirect indications exist that a well-developed phosphorus metabolism exists in practically all adult parasitic worms. This seems to follow from the enormous production of sexual products which, of course, contain, especially in the case of eggs, the normal complement of phosphorylated compounds. One *Ascaris* female thus passes about 0.49 gm of eggs daily, corresponding to 0.046 gm of dry tissue (Fairbairn, 1957), or approximately 5% of the entire dry matter found in the worm itself. Another example is the small *Haemonchus contortus,* which produces daily about 5000 eggs containing 2.9 μg phosphorus (Martin and Ross, 1934).

Inorganic phosphate absorbed by parasites is generally rapidly incorporated into organic compounds. A fairly slow turnover rate of phosphorus was reported by Moraczewski and Kelsey (1948) for *Trypanosoma equiperdum* kept *in vitro,* less than 4% appearing within 90 minutes in the acid-soluble fraction and, in most instances, less than 1% in the phospholipid, nucleic acid, and phosphoprotein fractions. However, a much higher activity of the last three fractions was found *in vivo,* and it seems obvious that the organisms were capable of synthesizing organic phosphorus compounds from the inorganic phosphate of the blood plasma. A rapid and pronounced phosphate incorporation into phospholipids, nucleic acids, and especially into a fraction extractable with cold trichloracetic acid (intermediates of glucose metabolism, adenosine triphosphate (ATP), inorganic phosphates), but a much smaller one into the phosphoprotein fraction was reported by Cantrell and Genazzani (1955) for the same organism. No significant differences existed in these respects between a normal and an arsenic-resistant strain. On the contrary, the age of the infection appears important in determining the amount of phosphate absorbed by a unit number of *Trypanosoma equiperdum,* flagellates derived from an old infection accumulating less than those from a young one (Cantrell, 1953). Characteristic inclusion bodies of many trypanosomes are the volutin granules, which probably consist of ribonucleic acid (RNA) (van den Berghe, 1942, 1946; Ormerod, 1958; von Brand *et al.,* 1959). It can be presumed that they account for a rather large fraction of the absorbed phosphate.

Phosphorus metabolism has been used in the case of *Plasmodium gallinaceum* as a yardstick of growth and development *in vitro,* making use of the marked incorporation of P^{32} into nucleic acids, especially deoxyribonucleic acid (DNA) (Clarke, 1952a,b). Lewert (1952) did phosphorus analyses on erythrocytes infected with *Plasmodium gallinaceum* and found an increase in total phosphorus as compared to non-infected cells. It was due primarily to an increase in RNA and lipid phosphorus, with smaller increases observed in DNA and acid-soluble phosphorus. These findings are not necessarily in contradiction to those of Clarke (1952a,b), who measured the rate of incorporation while Lewert (1952) studied the absolute amounts after growth. Whitfeld (1953), finally, investigated the uptake of P^{32} into *Plasmodium berghei* after injecting the compound intraperitoneally into mice. The lipid fraction had the highest P^{32} content, but relatively large amounts were also found in the DNA, RNA, and acid-soluble fractions. The phosphoprotein fraction showed but little activity. Whitfeld (1953), however, determined only the total phosphorus content of the various fractions and he emphasizes that the sequence of specific activities might conceivably be quite different.

A curious phosphorus-containing compound, 2-aminoethane phosphonic acid [$C_2H_8NPO_3$: $H_2NCH_2PO(OH)_2$], has been isolated from unspecified genera of rumen protozoa (Horiguchi and Kandatsu, 1959).

Compounds like this one with a C-P bond hitherto have been seldom known to occur in living organisms.

In helminths, as in protozoa, phosphorus taken from the environment is incorporated into many organic compounds. The first observation pointing in this direction is Fischer's (1924) finding of the liberation of phosphoric acid during incubation of *Parascaris* muscle pulp. It was probably derived from organic compounds, presumably largely those involved in the carbohydrate metabolism. Phosphorus-containing compounds, such as phospholipids, nucleic acids, or phosphorylating enzymes occur generally in parasitic worms and will be discussed at appropriate places in subsequent chapters. Here, only some compounds will be discussed briefly which are important to several of the metabolic categories described later on.

Adenosine triphosphate (ATP) plays a key role in many metabolic reactions and can be assumed to be universally distributed. It has been demonstrated first by Rogers and Lazarus (1949b) in *Ascaris* muscle in amounts corresponding to about one third of those encountered in flies or frogs. Further evidence has been presented for its presence in *Ascaris* by Chin and Bueding (1954) and Ichii *et al.* (1958). These latter investigators report that the ATP level of 100–130 mg% in the body wall of *Ascaris* is fairly well preserved *in vitro* for about 3 days, but that later on it falls to about half that value. ATP amounts of approximately 1.5 μmole/gm wet weight have been found in *Trichuris vulpis* (Bueding *et al.*, 1960) and 1.9 μmole/gm in *Hymenolepis diminuta* (Campbell, 1963). Qualitative data on the occurrence of ATP in some other species of nematodes have been presented by Jones *et al.* (1955, 1957).

Only traces of phosphagen seem to occur in *Ascaris* (Rogers and Lazarus, 1949b; Jones *et al.*, 1957), while the filariform larvae and the adult parasitic females of *Strongyloides ratti* and *Trichuris vulpis* contained "labile phosphorus" in appreciable quantities; it may have been arginine phosphate (Jones *et al.*, 1957).

Enzymes hydrolyzing esters of phosphoric acid, phosphatases, are widely distributed and play an important role in many metabolic processes. They can be divided into three classes: pyrophosphatases, phosphomonoesterases, and phosphodiesterases. Inorganic pyrophosphatases, enzymes catalyzing the hydrolytic cleavage of inorganic pyrophosphate, have been reported from six species of nematodes, two tapeworms, and the acanthocephalan *Macracanthorhynchus hirudinaceus* by Marsh and Kelley (1958). In *Ascaris* the crude enzyme was shown to occur, with only slight variations in activity, in body wall, intestine, ovaries, testes, and sperms. The corresponding enzyme of *Ascaridia galli* has been partially purified (Marsh and Kelley, 1959). It has remarkable temperature relationships: it is completely heat-stable up to 50°C, the activity decreases then markedly up to 75°C, but at still higher temperature this apparent inactivation is largely reversed. After 10 minutes' exposure to 99°C 48% of the original activity is still present. The enzyme requires for activity divalent ions with best activation achieved with Mg^{++} and Zn^{++}. When the former activator is used the pH optimum is 6.8 to 7.2, while a pH optimum of 6.2 to 6.5 is found when Zn^{++} is employed; K_m of the enzyme is 6.4×10^{-4}.

Another pyrophosphatase, adenosinetriphosphatase, has been identified in *Trypanosoma equiperdum* and *Trypanosoma hippicum* by Chen (1948) and Harvey (1949), respectively. It seems not to be present in significant amounts in *Plasmodium gallinaceum* (Speck and Evans, 1945). An adenosinetriphosphatase-like enzyme has been found by Rogers and Lazarus (1949b) in *Ascaris* muscle. When the enzyme was inhibited, compounds hydrolyzing like ATP and glucose-6-phosphate accumulated.

Many studies have been done concerning the occurrence of phosphomonoesterases in parasites. The distribution of acid and alkaline phosphatase has been studied frequently by means of histochemical procedures. These are, of course, important to establish the exact localization of the enzymes, thus providing clues to their possible biological significance. They do, however, tend to hide the fact that the terms "acid and alkaline phosphatase" are group names and do not designate well-defined entities. First some biochemical data will be reviewed and then the histochemical evidence.

An alkaline phosphatase with a pH optimum of 9.8 and only slight response to Mg^{++} activation has been found in *Trypanosoma hippicum* by Harvey (1949). It splits α- and β-glycerophosphates. In *Schistosoma mansoni* there is evidence for at least two acid phosphatases which differ in their pH optima, substrate specificity, response to such inhibitors as berryllium, and thermostability (Nimmo-Smith and Standen, 1963). In the female worms higher activity per unit protein was found than in the males; this difference was most pronounced in respect to the alkaline phosphatase which was found in addition to the acid enzymes. There was some indication that the alkaline phosphatase activity was due to more than one enzyme, but no definite data proving this assumption have yet come to light. Pennoit-DeCooman and van Grembergen (1942) found in *Fasciola hepatica* an acid phosphatase which was activated by Mg^{++} and which was insensitive to NaF. More recently, Ma (1963) separated the acid phosphatase of *Clonorchis sinensis* electrophoretically into three isozymes with different pH optima and Michaelis constants.

Insofar as cestodes are concerned, Pennoit-DeCooman and van

Grembergen (1942, 1947) found in adult *Moniezia* a phosphatase with a pH optimum of about 8 which was not activated by Mg^{++}, but was inhibited by NaF. Erasmus (1957b), on the other hand, found in *Moniezia expansa* at least three different phosphatases: an acid enzyme with a pH optimum of 5.0–6.0 which can be inhibited by NaF, but not by KCN, a phosphatase with an optimum pH of 7.0–8.0 which is uninfluenced by either NaF or KCN, and finally an alkaline phosphatase with a pH optimum of 10–11 which is not affected by NaF, but is inhibited by KCN. In *Hymenolepis diminuta* Phifer (1960) found an alkaline phosphatase with a pH optimum of 9.5 and a Michaelis constant of 3.2×10^{-3} M, which is not inhibited by phloridzin. Thus, while differences between various tapeworm species seem probable, the interesting question whether differences exist between developmental stages of one species is not resolved. Pennoit-DeCooman and van Grembergen (1947) report two quite different pH optima for the single phosphatase found by them in the larval and the adult *Taenia pisiformis,* respectively. However, in contrast to these findings, Erasmus (1957a) has demonstrated the presence of both an acid and an alkaline phosphatase in both stages of the same species. There were only minor differences in pH optima between the enzymes of the larva and the adult worm.

The histochemical localization of phosphatases has been studied for many species of parasitic flatworms. Thus, data are available for *Schistosoma mansoni* (Dusanic, 1959; Lewert and Dusanic, 1961; Robinson, 1961; Nimmo-Smith and Standen, 1963), *Paragonimus ohirai* and *P. westermani* (Yamao, 1952b; Yokogawa and Yoshimura, 1957; Yoshimura and Yokogawa, 1958; Hamada, 1959), *Fasciola hepatica* (Yamao and Saito, 1952; Tarazona Vilas, 1958), and other flukes (Yamao, 1952a; Takagi, 1962). It is impossible to go into detail here and to show any of the differences described for various species, or to point out some contradictions between the findings of different authors in respect to one species or another. In general terms, it can be stated that phosphatase activity is often marked in sites where absorption can be expected to occur, such as the intestinal epithelium or the cuticle, a finding frequently interpreted as indicating a connection between phosphatases and sugar absorption. In other cases, however, it would appear that the enzymes might be involved in excretory processes. A marked alkaline phosphatase activity has thus been reported for the excretory organ of *Paragonimus westermani* (Yamao, 1952b; Yoshimura and Yokogawa, 1958; Hamada, 1959) a lighter one for that of *Clonorchis sinensis* (Takagi, 1962) and *Fasciola hepatica* (Yamao and Saito, 1952). In the daughter sporocyst of an unnamed gorgoderid trematode, alkaline phosphatase in relatively high concentration was found in the walls of the capillaries leading from the flame cells (Coil, 1958). In the cercariae of *Posthodiplostomum minimum* the enzyme is limited to the excretory bladder (Bogitsh, 1963), while in those of *Schistosoma mansoni* it occurs both in the nephridia and other organs (Dusanic, 1959).

In cestodes and Acanthocephala all nutritive material is absorbed through the cuticle. There is again some presumptive evidence, but no proof, for a causal connection between localization of phosphatases and absorption. In cestodes strong phosphatase reaction is given by the cuticle (Rogers, 1947; Lefevere, 1952; Yamao, 1952d,e; Marzullo *et al.,* 1957b; Erasmus, 1957a,b; Tarazona Vilas, 1958; Kilejian *et al.,* 1961; Waitz, 1963), while internal organs, such as vitellaria, testes, ovaries, or excretory organs usually give lighter, if any, reaction. The distribution of alkaline phosphatase was studied in all three orders of Acanthocephala by Bullock (1949, 1958). The enzymatic reaction was most pronounced, in the majority of species examined, in the outer layer of the subcuticula, while its middle layer and most internal organs were enzyme-free. In some species, such as several Neoechinorhynchidae and *Leptorhynchoides thecatus,* no enzyme was demonstrable in the cuticle. Proboscis and lemnisci were usually without enzyme, but some exceptions were found, e.g., *Fessisentis vancleavei.*

The histochemical phosphatase distribution in nematodes has been examined primarily for *Ascaris lumbricoides* and *Parascaris equorum* and in less detail for some other species (Rogers, 1947; Yamao, 1951a,b, 1952c, 1957; Marzullo *et al.,* 1957a). The enzymatic activity is very pronounced, in most cases, in the intestinal cells, again suggesting a connection between absorption and phosphatases. Other organs, such as lateral lines, testes, and others contain usually smaller amounts.

The occurrence of alkaline and acid phosphatase in protozoa has often been reported. In trichomonads the alkaline enzyme reaction is usually most pronounced in the axostyle, an organ of polysaccharide storage, while the acid phosphatase is commonly distributed throughout the body, including the nucleus (Nomura, 1956, 1957; Gerzeli, 1959). The latter phosphatase is localized exclusively in the parabasal apparatus of *Trichonympha turkestanica* (El Mofty, 1957). In blood-stream trypanosomes the occurrence of phosphatases appears to be sporadic (Gerzeli, 1955), but both alkaline and acid phosphatase have been found regularly in the culture forms of *Trypanosoma ranarum* (Lehmann, 1963). In *Entamoeba histolytica* alkaline phosphatase has been reported for both nucleus and endoplasm (Hara *et al.,* 1954), while in *Opalina carolinensis* the enzyme is localized almost exclusively in mitochondria (Hunter, 1957).

As to sporozoa, phosphatases have been observed in coccidia (Gill and Ray, 1954a,b; Ray and Gill, 1954; Tsunoda and Ichikawa, 1955; Das Gupta, 1961), haemogregarines (Gerzeli, 1954a), *Toxoplasma* (Gerzeli, 1954b) and malaria parasites of various species (Das Gupta, 1961). Because of the complicated life cycle of most sporozoa differences in localization of enzymes can be expected between various stages and it is not surprising that this facet of the problem should have received some attention. As an example Das Gupta's (1961) study of alkaline phosphatase of *Plasmodium gallinaceum* may be briefly summarized. Ookinetes were essentially negative, showing only a few positive granules. Similarly, young oocysts gave only a faint reaction, but a marked one was found in older oocysts. Sporozoites and early exoerythrocytic schizonts were practically negative, while exoerythrocytic merozoites were strongly positive. Erythrocytic stages and male gametes, finally, were completely negative.

VI. INFLUENCE OF ENVIRONMENTAL INORGANIC SUBSTANCES

Although *Ascaris* is always able to maintain the chloride concentration of its body fluid below that of the medium, Hobson *et al.* (1952a) have shown that the concentration varies to some extent with that of the environment. If the worm is immersed in various dilutions of sea water, the difference between internal and external chloride concentration is smallest in 20% sea water. If the chloride concentration of the perivisceral fluid is first raised by immersion of the worms into 30% sea water and they are then transferred to an isotonic salt solution in which half the chloride has been replaced by nitrate, both normal and ligatured specimens reduce the chloride content of their body fluid below that of the medium. It appears that *Ascaris* can regulate the chloride concentration of its body fluid to some extent. The mechanism by which it can maintain it below that of the environment is an active process of chloride excretion which takes place against a concentration gradient. Experiments with ligatured worms, eviscerated cylinders of body wall, and isolated cuticle showed that this mechanism is bound to the intact body wall; the isolated cuticle is freely permeable to chloride (Hobson *et al.*, 1952a). However, external conditions have apparently some influence on the movements of chloride. According to Rogers (1945) more chloride enters the body of *Ascaris* in media lacking phosphate than in those containing this salt. It is at present not clear whether other nematodes possess similar regulatory mechanisms. In the case of *Hammerschmidtiella diesingi* there appears to exist no active method of osmoregulation. There appear to be indications that this cockroach parasite can take ions from hypertonic solutions (Lee, 1960).

The sodium concentration of *Ascaris* body fluid seems not to vary appreciably with that of the external medium, nor is there a definite correlation between the potassium content of external and internal mediums. However, when worms are transferred from intestinal contents to saline media, a drop in potassium concentration of the body fluid occurs. Calcium and magnesium concentrations are quite constant and are not affected by concentration variations of the external medium (Hobson *et al.*, 1952b).

In larval cestodes relationships between external and internal inorganic substances differ from those reviewed above for *Ascaris*. The chloride content of *Cysticercus tenuicollis* fluid is somewhat higher than that of its normal environment. Schopfer (1932) found an approximate equilibrium between external and internal chlorides at an external sodium chloride concentration of 0.87 %. In more dilute solutions salt diffused out from the cystic fluid while in higher concentrations this flow was reversed. The diffusion from the outside towards the inside proceeded at a much slower rate than the reverse process. Schopfer (1932) considers it possible that the differences in sodium chloride concentration between the host's blood plasma and the *Cysticercus* fluid may be due to a Donnan equilibrium, but whether such a relatively simple physicochemical concept is sufficient to explain a rather complex biological phenomenon remains to be seen; a search for active transport mechanisms seems not to have been done in this case.

It is worth noting in this connection that considerable differences in permeability to inorganic substances exist between different cyst membranes of larval cestodes. Schopfer (1932) demonstrated that the pericystic membrane of *Cysticercus tenuicollis* rather readily allows the passage of various iron salts but is less permeable to copper sulfate. The vesicular membrane, on the other hand, is entirely impermeable to the salts used as long as the parasites are alive, but becomes permeable upon death. Identical results were obtained in every case regardless of whether the salts were placed on the outside or inside of the respective membranes. Schwabe (1959) found that the laminated membrane of the *Echinococcus* cyst is readily permeable to calcium, potassium, and sodium chloride. However, potassium and CN ions in hypertonic media seem to have an effect on permeability; they cause withdrawal of the germinal membrane from the laminated one. The complexity of the situation is evidently considerable. Acetylcholine, physostigmine, and iodoacetate seem to antagonize this potassium effect, preventing the withdrawal of the germinal membrane. It is possible (Schwabe, 1959) that cholinesterase functions in osmotic regulation of the hydatid cyst.

In many of the early studies (e.g., Weinland, 1901b; Harnisch, 1933; von Brand, 1934; Krueger, 1936; Oesterlin, 1937; and many others) parasitic worms used for experimental purposes were maintained in sodium chloride solutions considered to be of physiological concentration (usually varying between 0.7 and 1.1% NaCl) and the same simple medium has been employed even in recent years for some specialized studies (e.g., Haskins and Weinstein, 1957). Realization of a possible beneficial influence of ion antagonism, so well-known for vertebrate tissues and organs, led soon to the use of so-called balanced salt solutions, such as Ringer's and Tyrode's and their innumerable variants (e.g., Slater, 1925; Weinland and von Brand, 1926; von Brand, 1933; Toryu, 1936; Fenwick, 1938; Stannard et al., 1938; Cavier and Savel, 1953, and others). While such solutions are quite satisfactory for many purposes, especially short-term experiments, it must be realized that their ionic composition had been worked out to meet the requirements of vertebrate tissues which do not necessarily coincide with those of a parasite.

It is not surprising then that for many types of experiments, especially for studies involving maintenance in vitro over long periods or true culture, special salt solutions have been developed; examples are shown in Table V. It should be noted that the solutions of inorganic salts used in cultivation studies constitute only one part of the complete media; the others are made up of many organic compounds which are often ill-defined, such as chick embryo mince, liver extract, or similar complex ingredients. They may well provide trace minerals not contained in the inorganic moiety of the media. The composition of the complex salines used in recent years has been arrived at usually by empirical methods and does not necessarily indicate that all the salts used are actually required by the parasites.

Only in a few instances have the actual requirements in regard to inorganic substances been studied. Citri (1954) lists the following ions as essential for the growth of *Trypanosoma cruzi* in culture: Na^+, K^+, Fe^{++}, Mg^{++}, Cl^-, PO_4^{3-}. Trager (1955) emphasizes that a high potassium content of the medium is required, in addition to Na^+, Ca^{++}, Mg^{++}, Mn^{++}, Cl^-, PO_4^{3-}, HCO_3^-, SO_4^{--} for a successful extracellular maintenance of *Plasmodium lophurae*. It would not be surprising if this high potassium requirement would be encountered in many intracellular parasites. Curiously, high potassium rather than sodium concentration seems also to benefit *Entodinium caudatum* (Coleman, 1960), a ciliate which, of course, does not live intracellularly, while the optimal K^+ concentrations for cultures of *Trypanosoma gambiense* are close to that found in human serum (Sardou and Ruffié, 1964). On the other hand, erythrocytic forms of *Plasmodium berghei*, separated from the host cell, show a much more vigorous metabolism when the K^+/Na^+ ratio corresponds to that of the erythrocytes rather than the blood serum (Bowman et al., 1960). How-

TABLE V

INORGANIC CONSTITUENTS (GM/LITER) OF SALINE SOLUTIONS USED IN MAINTAINING SOME PARASITES *in vitro*

Species	NaCl	KCl	CaCl₂	MgCl₂	MgSO₄	Na₂HPO₄	NaH₂PO₄	KH₂PO₄	NaHCO₃	Na₂CO₃	Na-acetate	NH₄Cl	References
Protozoa													
Leishmania tarentolae[a]	2.0		0.026		0.49	1.25		0.50					Trager (1957)
Plasmodium hexamerium	5.83	0.41	0.68	0.095		0.242		0.057		1.48			Nydegger and Manwell (1962)
Strigomonas oncopelti[b]	9.0	0.42		0.047		0.20		0.08				5.0	Newton (1956)
Trichonympha spp.	1.0		0.1		0.1			0.1	1.0[c]				Gutierrez (1956)
Helminths													
Ascaris lumbricoides	8.18	0.20	0.20		0.048								Epps *et al.* (1950)
Fasciola hepatica	7.0	0.3	0.1		0.3	0.5			1.5				Dawes (1954)
Schistosoma mansoni	6.8	0.4	0.2		0.2		0.14		2.2		0.05		Senft and Senft (1962)
Taenia crassiceps	8.0	0.4	0.14		0.04	0.08		0.047	0.35				Taylor (1963)

[a] Medium also contains small amounts of ZnSO₄, FeSO₄, MnSO₄, CuSO₄, CoSO₄, H₃BO₃.
[b] Medium also contains small amounts of ZnSO₄, FeSO₄, MnSO₄, CuSO₄, MgSO₄.
[c] Added when gassed with 95 % N₂ + 5 % CO₂.

ever, normal *in vitro* development of male gametocytes of *Plasmodium gallinaceum* requires only Na^+, Cl^-, and HCO_3^-; the absence of Mg^{++}, Ca^{++}, K^+, SO_4^{--} or PO_4^{3-} proved to be immaterial (Bishop and McConnachie, 1960). Trace elements may well be of greater importance than is sometimes, usually tacitly, assumed. Thus, Sugden and Oxford (1952) found that the ash from an ethanolic precipitate of whole grass juice extended the *in vitro* life of holotrich rumen ciliates. They are of the opinion that this effect is probably due to a trace element, possibly Ti, Mo, Cr, Co, or V, but not Zn, Fe, Sn, Sr, Mn, Cu, or Ni.

The importance of inorganic substances to intestinal parasites at least is also demonstrated by the influence on helminths of mineral deficiencies in the host's diet. Ackert and Gaafar (1949) found that a phosphorus-deficient diet reduces the number of *Ascaridia galli* able to establish themselves in chickens. Low calcium diet had an analogous effect, but magnesium deficiency did not influence the worms materially (Gaafar and Ackert, 1952). Threlkeld *et al.* (1956) report that the ability of *Haemonchus contortus* to establish itself in sheep depends upon the presence of sufficient cobalt in the host's diet.

Richard *et al.* (1954) did experiments with lambs whose diet was supplemented with trace minerals and which received one infective dose of *Haemonchus contortus*. The dietary supplement increased the resistance of the host to the deleterious effects of the infection. However, if the salt mixture administered contained cobalt, the worms matured more rapidly than in the absence of this trace mineral and they produced a significantly larger number of eggs. Shumard *et al.* (1956) subsequently made experiments with pasture lambs which first received an initial infection with *Haemonchus contortus* and were then exposed to repeated natural infections on the pasture, where they also contracted infections with other species of nematodes. The lambs receiving trace-mineralized salt (NaCl 96.0, Fe 0.30, Mn 0.150, Co 0.010, Cu 0.060, I 0.007) lost most blood and showed the highest mortality rate. The worms harbored by this group of lambs also produced the greatest number of eggs. The addition of dicalcium phosphate to the diet, in addition to the trace-mineralized salt mixture, did offer some protection against the ill effects of the infection as indicated by a good weight gain. The supplement, however, did not prevent the development of rather severe anemia. Emerick *et al.* (1957) reached similar conclusions concerning the influence of trace-mineralized salt and dicalcium phosphate on the resistance of grazing lambs against *Haemonchus* infection.

Environmental inorganic substances can be of importance to parasites in various respects. Evidently, they represent the source of the inorganic material found in the organisms. Then their quantity determines largely the osmotic concentration of the medium. Finally, inorganic substances present in the surroundings of a parasite can be beneficial when they form a balanced ionic solution, an aspect of the problem touched upon previously. On the other hand, they can be harmful if a serious ionic imbalance exists, or if one of the inorganic constituents of the medium is toxic.

A detailed description of the osmotic relationships of parasites is outside the scope of this presentation; only a few of the relevant observations can be mentioned. The failure of most parasitic protozoa to show a contractile vacuole is usually explained by the assumption that they are primarily osmoregulatory organelles which are not needed by organisms living in surroundings with high molecular concentrations. It is in this connection of special interest that *Vahlkampfia calkensis,* a parasite of the digestive tract of oysters, which does not normally possess a contractile vacuole, develops one when transferred to an agar medium made up with tap or distilled water (Hogue, 1923). *Crithidia fasciculata* has a contractile vacuole-like structure the output of which increases as the solute concentration in the external medium decreases (Cosgrove and Kessel, 1958). The parasitic ciliates have retained contractile vacuoles, perhaps because here the excretion of metabolites plays a larger role than in other forms, but they usually pulsate slowly. In some cases, at least, a correlation between the frequency of pulsation and the concentration of the medium has been established (Wertheim, 1934). However, some protozoa, as, for instance, *Balantidium,* seem to possess an active defense mechanism against uncontrolled water influx which is effective only over a limited range of dilutions (Eisenberg-Hamburg, 1929). *Diplodinium* spp. survive better in media containing 0.5 to 0.7% NaCl as principal salt, than at 0.4 or 0.8% (Hungate, 1942), indicating only very limited osmotic resistance. Curiously, culture forms of *Trypanosoma gambiense* develop best in media containing 1.4% NaCl which is almost twice the concentration found in serum (Sardou and Ruffié, 1963).

In parasitic worms definite connections between concentration of the external medium and water elimination have also been established. A few examples may illustrate the types of observation available. Herfs (1922) observed that the bladder of an undetermined cercaria pulsated about twice as fast in fresh water as in Ringer's solution. Weinstein (1952) found an inverse relation between pulsation rate of the excretory ampulla of the filariform larvae of *Nippostrongylus muris* and *Ancylostoma caninum* and the sodium chloride concentration of the medium. Curiously, in sucrose solutions the pulsation rate of the *Nippostrongylus* ampulla was independent of the concentration between 4.5 and 8.5% sucrose, indicating that the environmental compound providing the osmotic concentration can have influence on the rate of water influx or excretion. These relationships have been reviewed recently by Weinstein (1960).

Some parasitic worms are surprisingly resistant to changes in environmental osmotic concentrations. The plerocercoids of *Diphyllobothrium latum* survive for at least 48 hours in 1.7 M NaCl solution, but only 5 and 2.5 hours, respectively, in 2.6 and 3.4 M solutions (Birkeland, 1932). Most other helminths are less tolerant, but still show some resistance to variations in external molecular concentration. Thus, Stephenson (1945, 1947) found only small differences in survival time of *Fasciola hepatica* in solutions containing NaCl in concentrations varying between 58 and 230 mM and Bueding (1950) observed no marked differences in metabolic activity of *Schistosoma mansoni* in media containing between 68 and 137 mM NaCl.

A frequently used tool to determine the osmotic relationships of helminths is to immerse them into hypo- or hypertonic salt solutions and to study the resulting weight changes. They are quite pronounced as the older experiments of Schopfer (1929, 1932) on *Cysticercus tenuicollis,* or those of Wardle (1937b) on *Moniezia expansa* showed. Newer experiments of Read *et al.* (1959) on *Calliobothrium verticillatum* showed weight and chloride changes depending upon the concentration of the medium. The latter's NaCl concentration varied between 180 and 260 mM and contained in addition to NaCl standard amounts of KCl, MgCl$_2$, and CaCl$_2$. For accurate studies the medium also has to contain urea, in this case, since the tissues of *Calliobothrium* contain urea in amounts accounting for 3.7% of the solids which they readily lose during incubation in urea-free solutions. When the worms are incubated in 190mM NaCl + standard salts, an inverse relationship between chloride content of the worms' tissues and urea content of the medium (range tested: 0.1 to 200 mM) exists. Another complicating factor is that the permeability to urea and water is affected by deletion of calcium from the external saline.

Variations in osmotic concentration of physiological significance to parasitic flatworms undoubtedly occur also *in vivo*. Characteristic in this respect is probably the observation of Hopkins and Hutchinson (1960) that variations in water content of *Taenia taeniaeformis* isolated from different cats are about twice those encountered in single tapeworms from a multiple infection. These authors also indicate that physiologically damaged cyclophyllidean cestodes rapidly imbibe water. According to them this explains the low values for dry substance (about 9 to 12%) reported in the older literature (e.g. Weinland, 1901a; Smorodincev and Bebesin, 1936a,b; von Brand, 1933; and others), while they usually found 20 to 25% solids.

The Acanthocephala, just as the flatworms, are quite sensitive to changes in osmotic pressure. Anyone working with these worms is familiar with the fact that they are flat and ribbonlike in isotonic or hypertonic solutions, while they rapidly swell up becoming round and turgid in hypotonic solutions (e.g. Van Cleave and Ross, 1944). For *Neoechinorhynchus emydis* the most suitable molecular concentration for maintenance *in vitro* is 0.5 to 0.7% NaCl (Gettier, 1942), while Dunagan (1962) finds a Tyrode's solution with 0.9% NaCl satisfactory for several species of *Neoechinorhynchus*.

Roundworms are on the whole more resistant to variations in environmental osmotic concentration than flatworms or Acanthocephala. Thus Davey (1938) found approximately equal survival of *Ostertagia* in media having osmotic concentrations equivalent to the range of 0.4 to 1.3% NaCl, while the optimum for *Ascaris lumbricoides* is about 1% NaCl, with only very limited survival in concentrations ranging from 3 to 5% NaCl (Cavier and Savel, 1952, 1953). The larvae of *Ascaris* seem less tolerant; their optimal survival was found in a Tyrode's solution of about 142 mM (Fenwick, 1939). More resistant are the larvae of *Haemonchus contortus* which survive about equally well in balanced salines ranging in concentration from 40 to 120 mM (Stoll, 1940). The most resistant nematode larva so far studied seems to be that of *Eustrongylides ignotus*. Von Brand and Simpson (1942) reported that it survives for several months in media containing, besides organic components, NaCl concentrations varying from 0.5 to 1.0%, while the worms lived for up to 16 days in the presence of 3% NaCl.

The osmotic relationships of parasitic worms resemble in principle those reported for free-living invertebrates, especially aquatic animals. On the whole, their osmotic and ionic regulation seems to be less developed than in many of the latter. For details concerning the free-living organisms the reader is referred to Beadle (1957).

The relative toxicity of various ions to parasites has been studied only a few times and contradictions between various authors exist. Thus, Wendel (1943) found phosphate so toxic to *Plasmodium knowlesi* as to be contraindicated for pH control, a finding not substantiated by the work of McKee *et al.* (1946). Certainly no generalizations are possible at the present time. For instance, potassium markedly stimulates the metabolic rate of larval *Eustrongylides ignotus* (von Brand, 1943) and of adult *Schistosoma mansoni* (Bueding, 1950), but decreases that of *Litomosoides carinii* (Bueding, 1949). The stimulatory influence of various ions on the oxygen consumption of *Eustrongylides ignotus* is as follows:

Cations: Na = or slightly $<$ Mg $<$ Ca = NH$_4$ $<$ K
Anions :   Cl = or slightly $<$ SO$_4$ $<$ NO$_2$ = NO$_3$ $<$ PO$_4$

Of the various salts tested only $NaNO_2$ and to a lesser degree KCl were definitely toxic (von Brand, 1943). For *Neoechinorhynchus emydis* magnesium and potassium proved toxic; while calcium was fairly innocuous, it did not allow quite as long *in vitro* survival as sodium, when all salts were tested as chlorides in concentrations isotonic to a 0.5% NaCl solution (Gettier, 1942).

VII. SOME EXPERIMENTAL USES OF RADIOACTIVE INORGANIC SUBSTANCES

Some data on the use of radioactive inorganic substances in experiments with parasites (phosphorus, sulfate, iron) have been summarized in previous sections. In this section a different type of experiment is reviewed, experiments in which organic substances tagged with some radioactive inorganic compound have been used for experimental purposes.

This procedure has in recent years brought considerable advances in our knowledge of the mechanism underlying parasitic anemias. It has long been recognized that hookworm anemia is due primarily to the loss of blood sustained by the host in consequence of the blood-sucking activities of the worms (review of literature in Foy and Nelson, 1963), rather than to hypothetical toxins produced by them. An exact determination of the amount of blood withdrawn by the parasites is then of obvious fundamental importance in understanding the pathogenesis of the anemia. This was recognized early and Wells (1931) and Nishi (1933) studied the blood-sucking activities of *Ancylostoma caninum* over short periods, extrapolating their findings to a 24-hour period. In this way, blood losses of up to 0.84 ml/worm/day were arrived at. It was soon postulated that this was a somewhat unlikely maximal value (Foster and Landsberg, 1934), but even in the recent literature the high value of 0.4 ml blood/worm/day is reported for human hookworms (Soprunov, 1963). Clarification of the problem has been achieved in recent years by labeling erythrocytes with Fe^{59} or Cr^{51} to study blood losses. The relevant experiments of Gerritsen *et al.* (1954), Roche *et al.* (1957a,b; 1959), Foy *et al.* (1958), Tasker (1960), and Layrisse *et al.* (1961) leave little doubt that the amount of blood sucked by human hookworms is considerably smaller than originally assumed. *Necator americanus* withdraws on an average 0.03 ml blood daily (Roche *et al.,* 1957a). However, there seems to exist a negative correlation between the number of worms present and the amount of blood sucked daily by the individual worms. In light infections one *Necator* sucks about 0.12 ml blood (Tasker, 1960). Specific differences occur also. *Ancylostoma duodenale* can cause a two to three times higher blood loss than *Necator* (Foy *et al.,* 1958; Foy and Kondi,

1960). Similarly, recent studies by C. H. Clark *et al.* (1961) with radio-chromium showed that the mean blood loss caused by *Ancylostoma caninum* is around 0.07 ml/worm/day, while that due to *Haemonchus contortus* averages 0.049 ml (C. H. Clark *et al.* 1962) or 0.08 ml (Baker *et al.* 1959). It should be emphasized that these newer values, although considerably smaller than those found in the early studies, are still large enough to account for the iron-deficiency anemia of hookworm disease.

Chromium-tagging of erythrocytes (Pearson, 1963) helped elucidate the question of food habits of the liver fluke, *Fasciola hepatica*. Pearson's (1963) study, supplementing earlier similar work of Jennings *et al.* (1955, 1956) with P^{32}-tagged erythrocytes, led to the conclusion that the worms suck relatively large amounts of blood. In 2 hours unwashed flukes engorged an average of 0.058 ml, but in saline-washed flukes, who readily regurgitated part of the intestinal contents, the value found was 0.027 ml. Pearson (1963) emphasized that his data cannot be extrapolated to 24 hours because in flukes a feeding cycle of ingestion, absorption, and regurgitation must exist. It is nevertheless obvious that the host loses so much blood as to account readily for the anemia characteristic of fasciolosis.

The anemia caused by *Diphyllobothrium latum* is of a different type and origin than the hookworm anemia; it is a pernicious-type anemia. Older theories to account for its origin, such as production of a toxin by the worm or a hemolytic action of fatty constituents of the worm body, have today only historical interest. They have been superseded by the view that the tapeworm anemia is due to a vitamin B_{12} deficiency, a view developed primarily by von Bonsdorff and his school (review of literature in von Bonsdorff, 1956, and Palva, 1962).

Beginning with Nyberg's (1956) experiments Co^{60}-labeled vitamin B_{12} has played an important role in elucidating the relevant relationships. It has been established that the tapeworm readily absorbs the labeled vitamin *in vitro* (Brante and Ernberg, 1957, 1958), 1 meter of fresh worm (corresponding to about 1 gm of dry material) incorporating in 1 hour about 0.2 μg B_{12}. These authors believed that the worm absorbed the free vitamin, but that this assimilation is prevented when the vitamin is bound to the intrinsic factor. Nyberg (1958b, 1960b) also observed rapid uptake of the labeled vitamin by the worm, but he established that *Diphyllobothrium* can split the B_{12}-binding capacity of the intrinsic factor. Part of the discrepancy between Brante and Ernberg's (1957) and Nyberg's (1960b) findings is explained by the fact that the former used hog intrinsic factor, while the latter employed human material. Nyberg *et al.* (1961b) showed subsequently that the kinetics of the splitting of the B_{12}-gastric juice complex resembles an enzymatic reaction and can be explained on the basis of the Michaelis-Menten equation. However, the factor responsible for it is ultrafiltrable and gives no evidence of having a protein nature; it is hence questionable whether an enzyme is really involved.

Diphyllobothrium takes up Co^{60}-B_{12} also *in vivo;* it does this to such an extent that visualization in autoradiographs is possible (von Bonsdorff *et al.* 1960; Scudamore *et al.* 1961) and this "robbery" may bring about a vitamin B_{12} deficiency in its host. It develops when the B_{12} concentration in blood serum drops below the critical level of about 100 $\mu\mu g/ml$ (von Bonsdorff, 1958). However, because the vitamin B_{12} pool of the human body is large and the vitamin absorption from the food, though impaired, is not completely inhibited, a manifest vitamin deficiency with ensuing anemia develops only in a minority of an infected population. Actually, a level below 100$\mu\mu g/ml$ serum is found in a surprisingly high percentage of tapeworm carriers, namely, more than 50% according to Nyberg *et al.* (1961a). Palva (1962) reports a similar value. Evidently a whole complex of factors must exist in the right combination to elicit the picture of pernicious anemia. One of the factors involved is the location of the worm within the intestine. The vitamin absorption by the host is especially impaired if the worm is located high in the intestine (von Bonsdorff, 1947a,b) and the urinary excretion of the vitamin (Schilling test) is greatly reduced (Nyberg, 1960a; Palva, 1962). Other factors apparently contributing toward the anemic condition becoming manifest are: large amounts of worm material within the intestine, inadequate supply of vitamin B_{12} in the diet, a decrease in secretion of the intrinsic factor, and stress conditions, such as pregnancy, febrile diseases, thyrotoxicosis, and probably others (von Bonsdorff, 1958).

It should be noted that *Diphyllobothrium* absorbs Co^{60} only if it is bound to vitamin B_{12}; labeled cobalt chloride is not taken up (Nyberg, 1958b). Other intestinal worms absorb, if any, only very small amounts of labeled vitamin B_{12}. This has been shown by Nyberg (1958b) for *Taenia saginata* and by Scudamore *et al* (1961). These latter investigators also find by far the greatest uptake in the case of *Diphyllobothrium latum,* with *Taenia saginata* and *Ascaris lumbricoides* consuming at most traces, while no uptake at all could be observed when *Necator americanus* or *Trichuris trichiura* was used. However, more recently Zam *et al.* (1963) report the uptake of rather large amounts of Co^{60}-B_{12} by *Ascaris lumbricoides,* the maximum occurring at pH 6.4 and males consuming somewhat larger amounts than females. In the latter an inverse relationship between size and μg B_{12} absorbed/gm wet weight worm was found. *Ascaris* cannot absorb or split the vitamin B_{12}-intrinsic factor complex, differing in this latter respect from *Diphyllobothrium.*

Organic substances labeled with some inorganic compound have been used also in connection with other parasitological problems. Examples are the use of I^{131}-tagged albumin to study the distribution and turnover of albumin in calves infected with nematodes (Cornelius et al. 1962), or the use of S^{35}-methionine to study the metabolic fate of this amino acid in the erythrocytic form of *Plasmodium knowlesi* (Fulton and Grant, 1956). These studies are more profitably discussed in the section dealing with proteins.

VIII. HOST INORGANIC SUBSTANCES IN PARASITIC INFECTIONS

The potassium level of the blood plasma is increased in many protozoan infections. This has been reported especially for the febrile periods of human malaria (Pinelli, 1929; Andriadse, 1929; Zwemer et al. 1940), for avian malaria (Velick and Scudder, 1940), simian malaria (Zwemer et al. 1940; McKee et al. 1946), for the later stages of trypanosomiasis (Zwemer and Culbertson, 1939; Ikejiani, 1946a,b; Mazzetti and Mele, 1961), and for bartonellosis (Kessler and Zwemer, 1944). The sources from which the potassium is derived are probably not uniform. A certain fraction undoubtedly comes from destroyed erythrocytes. In malaria, changes in permeability of the membranes of nonparasitized erythrocytes lead to a potassium leakage into the plasma (Overman, 1948, Overman et al. 1949). It is probable, however, that these two factors alone are insufficient to explain the potassium increase established for the blood plasma. It is probable that another source must be sought in damaged body cells other than red cells. There are strong indications that in malaria the adrenal cortex, perhaps owing to anoxia, may be involved in this release of potassium (Zwemer et al. 1940; Maegraith, 1948).

It has been assumed that the potassium accumulation together with shifts in other ions may lead to severe metabolic disturbances since an excess of potassium is very toxic and it has been incriminated as responsible for death in malaria (Overman, 1947) and trypanosomiasis (Zwemer and Culbertson, 1939). This latter view cannot, however, be accepted since in malaria the potassium accumulation is well below the fatal level (Maegraith, 1948), and trypanosome-infected rats die at the same rate regardless of whether they have been made resistant to potassium prior to infection or not (Scheff and Thatcher, 1949).

Concomitant with the drop in potassium, the sodium and chlorine content of the erythrocytes increases in malaria (Overman, 1948), while the sodium content of the blood plasma is lowered, at least during the paroxysms (Flosi, 1944; Overman et al. 1949). A similar lowering of the serum sodium level has also been reported during trypanosomiasis of the guinea pig (Mazzetti and Mele, 1961).

The plasma chlorine content, on the other hand, is usually normal during malaria; significant reductions have been observed only in cases with renal involvment (Lahille, 1915; Wakeman, 1929; Miyahara, 1936; Ross, 1932; Fairley and Bromfield, 1934). No significant changes in blood chlorine seem to occur in *Leishmania* infections (Stein and Wertheimer, 1942), or in trypanosomiasis (Linton, 1930; Hudson, 1944), but a lowering of the chlorine content of the cerebrospinal fluid has been reported from human sleeping sickness cases (Sicé, 1930). In chickens infected with *Eimeria tenella,* on the contrary, a marked rise in blood chlorine has been observed (Waxler, 1941). The excess chlorine was in this case apparently derived from the tissues where a small decrease was found. Corresponding changes could be induced by artificial hemorrhage.

The inorganic blood phosphate has been found approximately normal in uncomplicated malaria, but increased in blackwater fever (Ross 1932; Wats and Das Gupta, 1934; Fairley and Bromfield, 1934). Lowered inorganic phosphate has, on the other hand, been described for human patients during paroxysms (Gall and Steinberg, 1947), and the inorganic phosphate of both red cells and plasma is lowered in simian malaria (McKee *et al.* 1946). Alkaline phosphatase level of the liver of rats infected with *Plasmodium berghei* is essentially normal (Chatterji and Sen Gupta, 1957). The serum phosphate level of guinea pigs infected with *Trypanosoma brucei* is normal (Mazzetti and Mele, 1961), and the alkaline phosphatase level of the liver of mice infected with *Trypanosoma evansi,* though somewhat variable, is essentially normal (Chatterji, 1960), but in the liver of hamsters infected with *Leishmania donovani* it is somewhat increased (Chatterji and Sen Gupta, 1959).

Normal blood calcium values have been reported from experimental leishmaniasis (Stein and Wertheimer, 1942), trypanosomiasis (Mazzetti and Mele, 1961), and malaria (Ross, 1932; Fairley and Bromfield, 1934; Wats and Das Gupta, 1934). It must be assumed, however, that erythrocytes infected with *Plasmodium berghei* remove calcium from the plasma. This is inferred from the fact that normal red cells contain but little calcium, but that the calcium content, as evidenced by microincineration, increases during the course of development (Kruszynski, 1952).

Hardly anything is known about the behavior of other ions during protozoan infections. No significant changes in blood magnesium have been observed in malaria (Gall and Steinberg, 1947). Somewhat low serum iron values have been found, though not regularly, in infantile visceral leishmaniasis (Cacioppo, 1947).

Changes in the inorganic blood constituents occurring as a consequence of helminthic infections have been described repeatedly and are summarized in Table VI. In general, these changes are not very pronounced and they have not yet been connected with any specific pathological process or with any specific biological activity of the parasites.

Shearer and Stewart (1933) studied the mineral metabolism of young lambs infected with intestinal nematodes. They found a normal potassium and sodium balance, but an abnormally low phosphorus and calcium retention. The calcium balance was in some cases even negative, leading to the assumption of probable interference with skeletal growth. However, Andrews (1938) was unable to confirm these results. He emphasized that the mineral content of bones of normal and infected lambs did not show significant differences.

Very definite fluctuations of abnormal magnitude in phosphorus and calcium metabolism occur during trichinosis. According to Roger's (1942) observations the excretion of inorganic phosphorus falls off markedly during the initial stages of the infection, but rises to two or three times the normal level about 4 weeks after infection. The assimilation of calcium is decreased shortly after infection; it then rises, to fall off again about 3 weeks after infection. Histochemical studies (Bullock, 1953) showed that 4 to 5 days after a *Trichinella* larva invades a muscle fiber, alkaline phosphatase activity appears there and remains for the duration of the infection. Even calcification of the capsule does not change the activity or distribution of the enzyme, but the question whether it plays a role in the calcification process could not be elucidated. In contrast, the alkaline phosphatase activity of jejunal villi of rats infected with *Nippostrongylus muris* is greatly reduced (Symons and Fairbairn, 1963).

Other observations of Symons (1960a,b,c) and Symons and Fairbairn (1962) on the pathology of the rat jejunum parasitized by this nematode are also very interesting. The sodium and chlorine content of the mucosal tissues is increased both on fresh and dry weight basis, but the potassium increase is demonstrable only on a dry weight basis. While in the jejunum of uninfected rats an absorption of water, sodium, and chloride takes place from isotonic saline solutions, a net influx into the lumen is encountered in infected rats. Experiments with hyper- and hypotonic solutions and perfusion experiments with $NaCl^{24}$ or deuterated water showed that actually the influx into the tissues remains unaffected, but that the efflux out of the tissues is deranged. In the distal ileum, that is a location relatively far away from the site of the parasites, the rates of net flux of water and chlorine are not affected, but the rate of sodium absorption is increased.

Practically nothing is known about disturbances in the mineral metabolism of invertebrates due to parasitism. The only relevant data come from

TABLE VI

CHANGES IN INORGANIC CONSTITUENTS OF THE BLOOD PLASMA OR BLOOD SERUM DURING INFECTIONS WITH HELMINTHS[a]

Host	Parasite	K	Na	Ca	P	S	Cl	Fe	Mg	Cu	References
Man	*Schistosoma mansoni*			n	n		n				Pons (1937)
Rabbit	*Schistosoma japonicum*			d	i	i					Hiromoto (1939)
Rabbit	*Clonorchis sinensis*			d	i	i					Shigenobu (1932)
Cattle, buffalo, sheep	*Fasciola hepatica*			d	n		i		d or i		Balian (1940); Usuelli and Balian (1938); Osman and Georgi (1960); Sinclair (1960); Haiba *et al.* (1964)
Sheep	*Dicrocoelium dendriticum*	v		d	d						Begovic *et al.* (1960)
Man	*Diphyllobothrium latum*							v			Becker (1926); Hirvonen (1941)
Man, dog, guinea pig	*Trichinella spiralis*			n or i	n or i		n				Pierce *et al.* (1939); Hartman *et al.* (1940); Beahm and Jorgensen (1941); Carrick (1944).
Man	Hookworms	i	i								Villela and Teixeira (1929)
Sheep[b]	*Haemonchus contortus*	n	n	n	n						Weir *et al* (1948); Evans *et al.* (1963)
Sheep	*Trichostrongylus colubriformis*			n or d	n or d						Franklin *et al.* (1946)
Calves	*Haemonchus placei* and other nematodes									d	Bremner (1959)
Sheep	*Haemonchus contortus* and other nematodes							i		v	Baker *et al.* (1959)

[a] KEY: n = normal; d = decreased; i = increased; v = variable; blank spaces = no information available.

[b] K increased in erythrocytes, Na decreased.

Drilhon (1936), who found normal sodium and potassium levels in the hemolymph of *Carcinus maenas* infected with *Sacculina,* but rather marked increases in calcium and magnesium amounts. He points out that these changes are somewhat similar to those occurring in normal crabs at the time of molting.

REFERENCES

Ackert, J. E., and Gaafar, S. M. (1949). *J. Parasitol.* **35,** Sect. 2, 11.

Agosin, M., Brand, T. von, Rivera, G. F., and McMahon, P. (1957). *Exptl. Parasitol.* **6,** 37–51.

Andrews, J. S. (1938). *J. Agr. Res.* **57,** 349–362.

Andriadse, N. (1929). *Nachr. Trop. Med. (Tiflis).* **2,** *704* [not seen, quoted in Maegraith (1948)].

Askanazy, M. (1896). *Deut. Arch. Klin. Med.* **57,** 104–117.

Baker, N. F., Cook, E. F., Douglas, J. R., and Cornelius, C. E. (1959). *J. Parasitol.* **45,** 643–651.

Balian, B. (1940). *Nuova Vet.* **18,** No. 6, 14–22, and No. 7, 10–16.

Beadle, L. C. (1957). *Ann. Rev. Physiol.* **19,** 329–358.

Beahm, E. H., and Jorgensen, M. N. (1941). *Proc. Soc. Exptl. Biol. Med.* **47,** 294–299.

Beaumont, A. (1948). *Compt. Rend. Soc. Biol.* **142,** 1369–1371.

Becker, G. (1926). *Acta Soc. Med. Fennicae Duodecim* **7,** No. 9, 1–8.

Begovic, S., Cankovic, M., Cuperlovic, N., Delic, S., Kucic, D., and Rukavina, J. (1960). *Vet. Sarajewo* **9,** 9–28.

Bélanger, L. F. (1960). *Can. J. Zool.* **38,** 226–227.

Berghe, L. van den (1942). *Acta Biol. Belg.* **2,** 464–467.

Berghe, L. van den (1946). *J. Parasitol.* **32,** 465–466.

Birkeland, I. W. (1932). *Medicine* **11,** 1–139.

Bishop, A., and McConnachie, E. W. (1960). *Parasitology* **50,** 431–448.

Boehm, J. (1908). *Z. Fleisch- u. Milchhyg.* **18,** 319–324.

Bogitsh, B. J. (1963). *Exptl. Parasitol.* **14,** 193–202.

Bonsdorff, B. von (1947a). *Acta Med. Scand.* **129,** 142–155.

Bonsdorff, B. von (1947b). *Acta Med. Scand.* **129,** 213–233.

Bonsdorff, B. von (1956). *Exptl. Parasitol.* **5,** 207–230.

Bonsdorff, B. von (1958). *Proc. 6th Intern. Congr. Trop. Med. Malaria, Lisbon 1958* Vol. 2, pp. 541–551. Imprensa Portuguesa, Portugal.

Bonsdorff, B. von, Nyberg, W., and Grasbeck, R. (1960). *Acta Haematol.* **24,** 15–19.

Bowman, I. B. R., Grant, P. T., and Kermack, W. O. (1960). *Exptl. Parasitol.* **9,** 131–136.

Brand, T. von (1933). *Z. Vergleich. Physiol.* **18,** 562–596.

Brand, T. von (1934). *Z. Vergleich. Physiol.* **21,** 220–235.

Brand, T. von (1938). *J. Parasitol.* **24,** 445–451.

Brand, T. von (1939). *J. Parasitol.* **25,** 329–342.

Brand, T. von (1943). *Biol. Bull.* **84,** 148–156.

Brand, T. von, and Bowman, I. B. R. (1961). *Exptl. Parasitol.* **11,** 276–297.

Brand, T. von, and Holtz, F. (1933). *Arch Schiffs- u. Tropen-Hyg.* **37**, 535–541.

Brand, T. von, and Simpson, W. F. (1942). *Proc. Soc. Exptl. Biol. Med.* **49**, 245–248.

Brand, T. von, and Weinbach, E. C. (1965). *Comp. Biochem. Physiol.* **14**, 11–20.

Brand, T. von, Holtz, F., and Vogel, H. (1933). *Z. Parasitenk.* **6**, 308–322.

Brand, T. von, Otto, G. F., and Abrams, E. (1938). *Am. J. Hyg.* **27**, 461–470.

Brand, T. von, McMahon, P., Tobie, E. J., Thompson, M. J., and Mosettig, E. (1959). *Exptl. Parasitol.* **8**, 171–181.

Brand, T. von, Mercado, T. I., Nylen, M. U., and Scott, D. R. (1960). *Exptl. Parasitol.* **9**, 205–214.

Brand, T. von, Scott, D. B., Nylen, M. U., and Pugh, M. H. (1965). *Exptl. Parasitol.* **16**, 382–391.

Brante, G., and Ernberg, T. (1957). *Scand. J. Clin. Lab. Invest.* **9**, 313–314.

Brante, G., and Ernberg, T. (1958). *Acta Med. Scand.* **160**, 91–98.

Bremner, K. C. (1959). *Australian J. Agr. Res.* **10**, 471–485.

Bueding, E. (1949). *J. Exptl. Med.* **89**, 107–130.

Bueding, E. (1950). *J. Gen Physiol.* **33**, 475–495.

Bueding, E., Kmetec, E., Swartzwelder, C., Abadie, S. H., and Saz, H. J. (1960). *Biochem. Pharmacol.* **5**, 311–322.

Bullock, W. L. (1949). *J. Morphol.* **84**, 185–200.

Bullock, W. L. (1953). *Exptl. Parasitol.* **2**, 150–162.

Bullock, W. L. (1958). *Exptl. Parasitol.* **7**, 51–68.

Burton, P. R. (1963). *J. Parasitol.* **49**, 121–122.

Cacioppo, F. (1947). *Boll. Soc. Ital. Biol. Sper.* **23**, 150–152.

Campbell, J. W. (1963). *Comp. Biochem. Physiol.* **8**, 181–185.

Cantrell, W. (1953). *J. Infect. Diseases* **93**, 219–221.

Cantrell, W., and Genazzani, E. (1955). *Arch. Ital. Sci. Farmacol.* [3] **5**, 234–238.

Carrick, L. (1944). *Am. J. Clin. Pathol.* **14**, 24–27.

Cavier, R., and Savel, J. (1951a). *Bull. Soc. Chim. Biol.* **33**, 447–454.

Cavier, R., and Savel, J. (1951b). *Bull. Soc. Chim. Biol.* **33**, 455–460.

Cavier, R., and Savel, J. (1952). *Compt. Rend.* **234**, 1216–1218.

Cavier, R., and Savel, J. (1953). *Ann. Sci. Nat. (Paris), Zool.* [11] **15**, 57–70.

Chatterji, A. (1960). *Bull. Calcutta Sch. Trop. Med.* **8**, 119–121.

Chatterji, A., and Sen Gupta, P. C. (1957). *Bull. Calcutta Sch. Trop. Med.* **5**, 169–170.

Chatterji, A., and Sen Gupta, P. C. (1959). *Bull. Calcutta Sch. Trop. Med.* **7**, 97–99.

Chen, G. (1948). *J. Infect. Diseases* **82**, 226–230.

Chin, C. H., and Bueding, E. (1954). *Biochim. Biophys. Acta* **13**, 331–337.

Chitwood, B. G., and Chitwood, M. B. (1938). *Proc. Helminthol Soc. Wash., D.C.* **5**, 16–18.

Chowdhuri, A. B., Das Gupta, B., Ray, H. N., and Bhadhuri, V. N. (1955). *Bull. Calcutta Sch. Trop. Med.* **3**, 52 [not seen, quoted in Chowdhuri *et al.* (1962)].

Chowdhuri, A. B., Das Gupta, B., and Ray, H. N. (1962). *Parasitology* **52**, 153–157.

Citri, N., (1954). Thesis, Hebrew University of Jerusalem.

Claparède, E. (1858). *Z. Wiss. Zool.* **9**, 99–105.

Clark, C. H., Kling, J. M., Woodley, C. H., and Sharp, N. (1961). *Am. J. Vet. Res.* **22**, 370–373.

Clark, C. H., Kiesel, G. K., and Goby, C. H. (1962). *Am. J. Vet. Res.* **23**, 977–980.

Clark, D. T. (1956). *J. Parasitol.* **42**, 77–80.

Clarke, D. H. (1952a). *J. Exptl. Med.* **96**, 439–450.

Clarke, D. H. (1952b). *J. Exptl. Med.* **96**, 451–463.

Codounis, A., and Polydorides, J. (1936). *Proc. 3rd Intern. Congr. Comp. Pathol., Athens, 1936* Vol. 2, pp. 195–202. Eleftheroudakis, Athens, Greece.

Coil, W. H. (1958). *Proc. Helminthol Soc. Wash., D.C.* **25**, 137–138.
Coleman, G. S. (1960). *J. Gen. Microbiol.* **22**, 555–563.
Cornelius, C. E., Baker, N. F., Kaneko, J. J., and Douglas, J. R. (1962). *Am. J. Vet. Res.* **23**, 837–842.
Cosgrove, W. B., and Kessel, R. G. (1958). *J. Protozool.* **5**, 296–298.
Dasgupta, B. (1961). *Acta Soc. Zool. Bohemoslov.* **25**, 16–21.
Daugherty, J. W. (1957). *Exptl. Parasitol.* **6**, 60–67.
Davey, D. G. (1938). *Parasitology* **30**, 278–295.
Dawes, B. (1954). *Nature* **174**, 654.
Desser, S. S. (1963). *Can. J. Zool.* **41**, 1055–1059.
Dinulescu, G. (1932). *Ann. Sci. Nat. (Paris), Zool.* [10] **15**, 1–183.
Drilhon, A. (1936). *Compt. Rend.* **202**, 981–982.
Dunagan, T. T. (1962). *Proc. Helminthol. Soc. Wash., D.C.* **29**, 131–135.
Dusanic, D. G. (1959). *J. Infect. Diseases* **105**, 1–8.
Duval, M., and Courtois, A. (1928). *Compt. Rend. Soc. Biol.* **99**, 1952–1953.
Eisenberg-Hamburg, E. (1929). *Arch. Protistenk.* **68**, 451–470.
El Mofty, M. M. (1957). *Nature* **180**, 1367.
Emerick, R. J., Bemrick, W. J., Pope, A. L., Hoekstra, W. G., and Phillips, P. H. (1957). *J. Animal Sci.* **16**, 937–942.
Epprecht, W., Schinz, H. R., and Vogel, H. (1950). *Experientia* **6**, 187.
Epps, W., Weiner, M., and Bueding, E. (1950). *J. Infect. Diseases* **87**, 149–151.
Erasmus, D. A. (1957a). *Parasitology* **47**, 70–80.
Erasmus, D. A. (1957b). *Parasitology* **47**, 81–91.
Esserman, H. B., and Sambell, P. M. (1951). *Australian J. Sci. Res.* **B4**, 575–580.
Evans, J. V., Blunt, M. H., and Southcott, W. H. (1963). *Australian J. Agr. Res.* **14**, 549–558.
Fairbairn, D. (1957). *Exptl. Parasitol.* **6**, 491–554.
Fairley, N. H., and Bromfield, R. J. (1933). *Trans. Roy. Soc. Trop. Med. Hyg.* **27**, 289–314.
Fairley, N. H., and Bromfield, R. J. (1934). *Trans. Roy Soc. Trop. Med. Hyg.* **28**, 307–334.
Fauré-Fremiet, E. (1913a). *Compt. Rend. Soc. Biol.* **74**, 567–569.
Fauré-Fremiet, E. (1913b). *Arch. Anat. Microscop.* **15**, 435–757.
Fauré-Fremiet, E., Ebel, J. P., and Colas, J. (1954). *Exptl. Cell Res.* **7**, 153–168.
Fenwick, D. W. (1938). *Proc. Zool. Soc. London* **A108**, Part I, 85–100.
Fenwick, D. W. (1939). *J. Helminthol.* **17**, 211–228.
Fischer, A. (1924). *Biochem. Z.* **144**, 224–228.
Flosi, A. Z. (1944). *Rev. Clin. São Paulo* **16**, 1–6.
Flury, F. (1912). *Arch Exptl. Pathol. Pharmakol.* **67**, 275–392.
Foster, A. O., and Landsberg, J. W. (1934). *Am. J. Hyg.* **20**, 259–290.
Foy, H., and Kondi, A. (1960). *Trans. Roy. Soc. Trop. Med. Hyg.* **54**, 419–433.
Foy, H., and Nelson, G. S. (1963). *Exptl. Parasitol.* **14**, 240–262.
Foy, H., Kondi, A., and Austin, W. H. (1958). *East African Med. J.* **35**, 607–615.
Fraipont, J. (1880). *Arch. Biol (Paris)* **1**, 415–456.
Fraipont, J. (1881). *Arch. Biol. (Paris)* **2**, 1–40.
Franklin, M. C., Gordon, H. McL., and Macgregor, C. H. (1946). *J. Council Sci. Ind. Res.* **19**, 46–60.
Fulton, J. D., and Grant, P. T. (1956). *Biochem. J.* **63**, 274–282.
Gaafar, S. M., and Ackert, J. E. (1952). *J. Parasitol* **38**, Suppl., 17.
Gall. E. A., and Steinberg, A. (1947). *J. Lab. Clin. Med.* **32**, 508–525.
Gerritsen, T., Heinz, H. J., and Stafford, G. H. (1954). *Science* **119**, 412–413.
Gerzeli, G. (1954a). *Riv. Istochim.* **1**, 91–94.
Gerzeli, G. (1954b). *Riv. Istochim.* **1**, 205–210.

Gerzeli, G. (1955). *Riv. Parassitol.* **16,** 209–215.

Gerzeli, G. (1959). *Acta Histochim.* **8,** 191–198.

Gettier, A. (1942). *Proc. Helminthol. Soc. Wash., D.C.* **9,** 75–78.

Gill, B. S., and Ray, H. N. (1954a). *Indian J. Vet Sci. Animal Husbandry* **24,** 223–228.

Gill, B. S., and Ray, H. N. (1954b). *Indian J. Vet. Sci. Animal Husbandry* **24,** 239–244.

Goodchild, C. G., Dennis, E. S., and Moore, J. D. (1962). *Exptl. Parasitol.* **12,** 107–113.

Gutierrez, J. (1956). *J. Protozool.* **3,** 39–42.

Haiba, M. H., EL-Rawii, K. A., and Osman, H. G. (1964). *Z. Parasitenk.* **23,** 527–531.

Hamada, M. (1959). *Shikoku Acta Med.* **14,** 165–186.

Hara, K.. Oka, S., Sawada, T., and Fuse, M. (1954). *Gunma J. Med. Sci.* **3,** 249–265.

Harnisch, O. (1933). *Z. Vergleich. Physiol.* **19,** 310–348.

Hartman, E., Foote, M., and Pierce, H. B. (1940). *Am. J. Hyg.* **31,** Sect. D, 74–75.

Harvey, S. C. (1949). *J. Biol. Chem.* **179,** 435–453.

Haskins, W. T., and Weinstein, P. P. (1957). *J. Parasitol.* **43,** 19–24.

Herfs, A. (1922). *Arch. Protistenk.* **44,** 227–260.

Hiromoto, T. (1939). *Mitt. Med. Ges. Okayama* **51,** 1637 (German summary).

Hirsch, G. C., and Bretschneider, L. H. (1937). *Protoplasma* **29,** 9–30.

Hirvonen, M. (1941). *Acta Med. Scand.* **108,** 63–72.

Hobson, A. D., Stephenson, W., and Beadle, L. C. (1952a). *J. Exptl. Biol.* **29,** 1–21.

Hobson, A. D., Stephenson, W., and Eden, A. (1952b). *J. Exptl. Biol.* **29,** 22–29.

Hogue, M. J. (1923). *J. Elisha Mitchell Sci. Soc.* **39,** 49–55.

Hopkins, C. A. (1950). *J. Parasitol.* **36,** 384–390.

Hopkins, C. A. (1960). *Exptl. Parasitol.* **9,** 159–166.

Hopkins, C. A., and Hutchinson, W. M. (1960). *Exptl. Parasitol.* **9,** 257–263.

Horiguchi, M., and Kandatsu, M. (1959). *Nature* **184,** 901–902.

Horning, E. S., and Scott, G. H. (1933). *J. Morphol.* **54,** 389–397.

Hsü, H. F. (1938a). *Bull. Fan Mem. Inst. Biol. (Peking) Zool.* **8,** 121–132.

Hsü, H. F. (1938b). *Bull. Fan Mem. Inst. Biol. (Peking) Zool.* **8,** 347–366.

Hsü, H. F. (1938c). *Bull. Fan Mem. Inst. Biol. (Peking) Zool.* **8,** 403–406.

Hudson, J. R. (1944). *J. Comp. Pathol. Therap.* **54,** 108–119.

Hungate, R. E. (1942). *Biol. Bull.* **83,** 303–319.

Hunter, N. W. (1957). *Trans. Am. Microscop. Soc.* **76,** 36–45.

Ichii, S., Sugiura, K., and Matsumoto, K. (1958). *Kiseichugaku Zasshi* **7,** 661–665.

Ikejiani, O. (1946a). *J. Parasitol.* **32,** 374–378.

Ikejiani, O. (1946b). *J. Parasitol.* **32,** 379–382.

Ishizaki, T., Kutsumi, H., and Kubota, H. (1957). *Japan. J. Parasitol.* **6,** 107–110.

Jennings, F. W., Mulligan, W., and Urquhart, G. M. (1955). *Trans. Roy. Soc. Trop. Med. Hyg.* **49,** 305.

Jennings, F. W., Mulligan, W., and Urquhart, G. M. (1956). *Exptl. Parasitol.* **5,** 458–468.

Jones, C. A., Swartzwelder, C., and Abadie, S. H. (1955). *J. Parasitol.* **41,** Sect. 2, 48.

Jones, C. A., Swartzwelder, C., and Abadie, S. H. (1957). *Am. J. Trop. Med. Hyg.* **6,** 385–386.

Kedrowsky, B. (1931). *Z. Zellforsch. Mikroskop. Anat.* **13,** 1–81.

Kemnitz, G. von (1912). *Arch. Zellforsch.* **7,** 463–603.

Kessier, W. R., and Zwemer, R. L. (1944). *J. Infect. Diseases* **75,** 134–137.

Kilejian, A., Schinazi, L. A., and Schwabe, C. W. (1961). *J. Parasitol.* **47,** 181–188.

Krueger, F. (1936). *Zool. Jahrb., Abt. Allgem. Zool. Physiol.* **57,** 1–56.

Kruszynski, J. (1951). *Ann. Trop. Med. Parasitol.* **45,** 85–91.

Kruszynski, J. (1952). *Ann. Trop. Med. Parasitol.* **46,** 117–120.

Kutsumi, H., Ishizaki, T., and Kubota, H. (1957). *Japan. J. Parasitol.* **6,** 107–110.

Lagachev, Y. D. (1951). *Dokl. Akad. Nauk SSSR* **80,** 693–695.

Lahille, A. (1915). *Bull. Mem. Soc. Med. Hop. Paris* **31**, 905–917.

Layrisse, M., Paz, M., Blumenfeld, N., and Roche, M. (1961). *Blood* **18**, 61–72.

Lee, D. L. (1960). *Parasitology* **50**, 241–246.

Lefevere. S. (1952). *Mededel. Koninkl. Belg. Inst. Natuurwet.* **28**, No. 167, 1–4.

Lenmann, D. L. (1963). *J. Protozool.* **10**, 399–400.

Lemaire, G., and Ribère, R. (1935). *Compt. Rend. Soc. Biol.* **118**, 1578–1579.

Levenbook, L. (1950). *Biochem. J.* **47**, 336–346.

Lewert, R. M. (1952). *J. Infect. Diseases* **91**, 125–144.

Lewert, R. M., and Dusanic, D. G. (1961). *J. Infect. Diseases* **109**, 85–89.

Linton, R. W. (1930). *J. Exptl. Med.* **52**, 103–111.

Looss, A. (1905). *Records Sch. Med. Cairo* **3**, 1–158.

Ma, L. (1963). *J. Parasitol.* **49**, 197–203.

McCoy, O. R., Downing, V. F., and Van Voorhis, S. N. (1941). *J. Parasitol.* **27**, 53–58.

McKee, R. W., Ormsbee, R. A., Anfinsen, C. B., Geiman, Q. M., and Ball, E. G. (1946). *J. Exptl. Med.* **84**, 569–582.

MacLennan, R. F., and Murer, H. K. (1934). *J. Morphol.* **56**, 231–239.

Maegraith, B. G. (1948). "Pathological Processes in Malaria and Blackwater Fever." Thomas, Springfield, Illinois.

Marcet, W. H. (1865). *Proc. Roy. Soc.* **14**, 69–70.

Marsh, C. L., and Kelley, G. W. (1958). *Exptl. Parasitol.* **7**, 366–373.

Marsh, C. L., and Kelley, G. W. (1959). *Exptl. Parasitol.* **8**, 274–285.

Martin, C. J., and Ross, I. C. (1934). *J. Helminthol.* **12**, 137–142.

Martin, W. E., and Bils, R. F. (1964). *J. Parasitol.* **50**, 337–344.

Marzullo, F., Squadrini, F., and Taparelli, F. (1957a). *Boll. Soc. Med. Chir. Modena* **57**, 84–88.

Marzullo, F., Squadrini, F., and Taparelli, F. (1957b). *Boll. Soc. Med. Chir. Modena* **57**, 327–331.

Mazzetti, M., and Mele, G. (1961). *Arch. Ital. Sci. Med. Trop. Parassitol.* **42**, 65–72.

Mazzocco, P. (1923). *Compt. Rend. Soc. Biol.* **88**, 342–343.

Mercado, T. I., and Brand, T. von (1962). *J. Parasitol.* **48**, 215–222.

Mercado, T. I., and Brand, T. von (1964). *Poultry Sci.* **43**, 222–232.

Mercado, T. I., and Brand, T. von (1965). In preparation.

Miyahara, H. (1936). *J. Formosan Med. Assoc.* **35**, 1092 [not seen, quoted in Maegraith (1948)].

Moniez, R. L. (1880). Thesis, University of Lille.

Moraczewski, S. A., and Kelsey, F. E. (1948). *J. Infect. Diseases* **82**, 45–51.

Mulvey, P. F. (1960). *J. Infect. Diseases* **107**, 155–159.

Newton, B. A. (1956). *Nature* **177**, 279–280.

Nimmo-Smith, R. H., and Standen, O. D. (1963). *Exptl. Parasitol.* **13**, 305–322.

Nishi, M. (1933). *J. Formosan Med. Assoc.* **32**, 677–691.

Nomura, H. (1956). *Keio Igaku* **33**, 241–247.

Nomura, H. (1957). *Keio Igaku* **34**, 131–140.

Nyberg, W. (1956). *Proc. 5th Congr. Eur. Soc. Hematol., Freiburg, 1955* pp. 58–60. Springer, Berlin [not seen, quoted in Nyberg (1958a)].

Nyberg, W. (1958a). *Acta Haematol.* **19**, 90–98.

Nyberg, W. (1958b). *Exptl. Parasitol.* **7**, 178–190.

Nyberg, W. (1960a). *Acta Med. Scand.* **167**, 185–187.

Nyberg, W. (1960b). *Acta Med. Scand.* **167**, 189–192.

Nyberg, W., Grasbeck, R., Saarni, M., and Bonsdorff, B. von (1961a). *Am. J. Clin. Nutr.* **9**, 606–612.

Nyberg, W., Saarni, M., Gothoni, G., and Järventie, G. (1961b). *Acta Med. Scand.* **170**, 257–262.

Nydegger, L., and Manwell, R. D. (1962). *J. Parasitol.* **48**, 142–147.

Oda, T. (1959). *J. Kurume Med. Assoc.* **22**, 185–236.

Oesterlin, M. (1937). *Z. Vergleich. Physiol.* **25**, 88–91.

Ormerod, W. E. (1958). *J. Gen. Microbiol.* **19**, 271–288.

Osman, H. G., and Georgi, B. N. (1960). *J. Chem. UAR* **3**, 159–164.

Otto, G. F., and Brand, T. von (1941). *Am. J. Hyg.* **34**, Sect. D, 13–17.

Overman, R. R. (1947). *Federation Proc.* **6**, 174–175.

Overman, R. R. (1948). *Am. J. Physiol.* **152**, 113–121.

Overman, R. R., Hill, T. S., and Wong, Y. T. (1949). *J. Natl. Malaria Soc.* **8**, 14–31.

Palva, I. (1962). *Acta Med. Scand.* **171**, Suppl. 374.

Panijel, J. (1951). "Métabolisme des nucléoproteines dans la gamétogénèse et la fécondation," pp. 80 and 162. Hermann, Paris [not seen, quoted in Fauré-Fremiet *et al.* (1954)].

Pantelouris, E. M. (1964). *Life Sciences* **3**, 1–5.

Pantelouris, E. M., and Gresson, R. A. R. (1960). *Parasitology* **50**, 165–169.

Pantelouris, E. M., and Hale, P. A. (1962). *Res. Vet. Sci.* **3**, 300–303.

Pearson, I. G. (1963). *Exptl. Parasitol.* **13**, 186–193.

Pennoit-DeCooman, E., and Grembergen, G. van (1942). *Verhandel. Koninkl. Vlaam. Acad. Wetenschap. Belg., Kl. Wetenschap.* **4**, No. 6, 7–77.

Pennoit-DeCooman, E., and Grembergen, E. van (1947). *Natuurw. Tijdschr. (Belg).* **29**, 9–12.

Phifer, K. (1960). *J. Parasitol.* **46**, 145–153.

Pierce, H. B., Hartman, E., Simcox, W. J., Aitken, T., Meservey, A. B., and Farnham, W. B. (1939). *Am. J. Hyg.* **29**, Sect. D, 75–81.

Pinelli, L. (1929). *Riv. Malariol.* **8**, 310–314.

Pons, J. A. (1937). *Puerto Rico J. Public Health. Trop. Med.* **13**, 171–254.

Quack, M. (1913). *Arch. Zellforsch.* **11**, 1–50.

Ray, H. N., and Gill, B. S. (1954). *Ann. Trop. Med. Parasitol.* **48**, 8–10.

Read, C. P. (1950). *J. Parasitol.* **36**, 34–40.

Read, C. P., Douglas, L. T., and Simmons, J. E. (1959). *Exptl. Parasitol.* **8**, 58–75.

Reid, W. M. (1942). *J. Parasitol.* **28**, 319–340.

Richard, R. M., Shumard, R. F., Pope, A. L., Phillips, P. H., Herrick, C. A., and Bohstedt, G. (1954). *J. Animal Sci.* **13**, 694–705.

Robinson, D. L. H. (1961). *Nature* **191**, 473–474.

Roche, M., Perez-Gimenez, M. E., Layrisse, M., and Di Prisco, E. (1957a). *J. Clin. Invest.* **36**, 1183–1192.

Roche, M., Perez-Gimenez, M. E., Layrisse, M., and Di Prisco, E. (1957b). *Am. J. Digest. Diseases* [N.S.] **2**, 265–277.

Roche, M., Perez-Gimenez, M. E., and Levy, A. (1959). *J. Lab. Clin. Med.* **54**, 4–52.

Rogers, W. P. (1940). *J. Helminthol.* **18**, 103–116.

Rogers, W. P. (1942). *J. Helminthol.* **20**, 139–158.

Rogers, W. P. (1945). *Parasitology* **36**, 211–218.

Rogers, W. P. (1947). *Nature* **159**, 374.

Rogers, W. P., and Lazarus, M. (1949a). *Parasitology* **39**, 245–250.

Rogers, W. P., and Lazarus, M. (1949b). *Parasitology* **39**, 302–314.

Ross, G. R. (1932). *Mem. London Sch. Hyg. Trop. Med.* **6**, 1–262.

Salisbury, L. F., and Anderson, R. J. (1939). *J. Biol. Chem.* **129**, 505–517.

Sardou, R., and Ruffié, J. (1963). *Compt. Rend.* **256**, 4533–4535.

Sardou, R., and Ruffié, J. (1964). *Compt. Rend.* **258**, 1322–1323.

Scheff, G., and Thatcher, J. S. (1949). *J. Parasitol.* **35,** 35–40.

Schopfer, W. H. (1924). *Actes Soc. Helv. Sci. Nat.* **105,** Aarau 188–189.

Schopfer, W. H. (1925). *Actes. Soc. Helv. Sci. Nat.* **106,** Aarau 157–158.

Schopfer, W. H. (1926a). *Parasitology* **18,** 277–282.

Schopfer, W. H. (1926b). *Compt. Rend. Soc. Phys. Hist. Nat. Geneve* **43,** 64–67.

Schopfer, W. H. (1927). *Compt. Rend. Soc. Phys. Hist. Nat. Geneve* **44,** 4–7.

Schopfer, W. H. (1929). *Rev. Suisse Zool.* **36,** 221–228.

Schopfer, W. H. (1932). *Rev. Suisse Zool.* **39,** 59–194.

Schwabe, C. W. (1959). *Am. J. Trop. Med. Hyg.* **8,** 20–28.

Scott, D. B., Nylen, M. U., Brand, T. von, and Pugh, M. H. (1962). *Exptl. Parasitol.* **12,** 445–458.

Scott, G. H., and Horning, E. S. (1932). *J. Morphol.* **53,** 381–388.

Scudamore, H., Thompson, J. H., and Owen, C. A. (1961). *J. Lab. Clin. Med.* **57,** 240–246.

Senft, A. W., and Senft, D. G. (1962). *J. Parasitol.* **48,** 551–554.

Shearer, G. D., and Stewart, J. (1933). *Univ. Cambridge, Inst. Animal Pathol. Rept. Director* **3,** 87–97.

Shigenobu, T. (1932). *Mitt. Med. Ges. Okayama* **44,** 1099–1112.

Shumard, R. F., Emerick, R. J., Bemrick, W. E., Herrick, C. A., Pope, A. L., and Phillips, P. H. (1956). *Am. J. Vet. Res.* **17,** 252–255.

Sicé, A. (1930). *Bull. Soc. Pathol. Exotique* **23,** 640–650.

Sinclair, K. B. (1960). *Vet. Record* **72,** 506.

Slater, W. K. (1925). *Biochem. J.* **19,** 604–610.

Smith, M. H. (1962). *Comp. Biochem. Physiol.* **6,** 165–168.

Smorodincev, I., and Bebesin, K. W. (1936a). *J. Biochem.* **23,** 19–20.

Smorodincev, I., and Bebesin, K. W. (1936b). *J. Biochem.* **23,** 21–22.

Smorodincev, I., and Bebesin, K. W. (1936c). *J. Biochem.* **23,** 23–25.

Smorodincev, I., Bebesin, K. W., and Pawlowa, P. I. (1933). *Biochem. Z.* **261,** 176–178.

Soprunov, F. F. (1963). *Med. Parazitol. i Parazitarn. Bolezni* **32,** 159–163 [only abstract seen, *Helminthol. Abst.* **33,** 348, (1964)].

Speck, J. F., and Evans, E. A. (1945). *J. Biol. Chem.* **164,** 71–96.

Stannard, J. N., McCoy, O. R., and Latchford, W. B. (1938). *Am. J. Hyg.* **27,** 666–682.

Stein, L., and Wertheimer, E. (1942). *Ann. Trop. Med. Parasitol.* **36,** 17–37.

Stephenson, W. (1945). *Nature* **155,** 240.

Stephenson, W. (1947). *Parasitology* **38,** 116–122.

Stoll, N. R. (1940). *Growth* **4,** 383–406.

Sugden, B., and Oxford, A. E. (1952). *J. Gen. Microbiol.* **7,** 145–153.

Symons, L. E. A. (1960a). *Australian J. Biol. Sci.* **13,** 163–170.

Symons, L. E. A. (1960b). *Australian J. Biol. Sci.* **13,** 171–179.

Symons, L. E. A. (1960c). *Australian J. Biol. Sci.* **14,** 165–171.

Symons, L. E. A., and Fairbairn, D. (1962). *Federation Proc.* **21,** 913–918.

Symons, L. E. A., and Fairbairn, D. (1963). *Exptl. Parasitol.* **13,** 284–304.

Takagi, K. (1962). *Tokushima J. Exptl. Med.* **9,** 60–66.

Tarazona Vilas, J. M. (1958). *Rev. Iberica Parasitol.* **18,** 233–242.

Tasker, P. W. G. (1960). *Trans Roy. Soc. Trop. Med. Hyg.* **55,** 36–39.

Taylor, A. E. R. (1963). *Exptl. Parasitol.* **14,** 304–310.

Theman, H. (1956). *Z. Parasitenk.* **17,** 300–329.

Threlkeld, W. L., Price, N. O., and Linkous, W. N. (1956). *Am. J. Vet. Res.* **17,** 246–251.

Timofeyev, V. A. (1964). *Dokl. Akad. Nauk SSSR* **156,** 1244–1247.

Toryu, W. (1936). *Sci. Rept. Tohoku Imp. Univ., Fourth Ser.* **10,** 687–696.

Trager, W. (1955). *Proc. 11th Conf. Protein Metabolism, New Brunswick 1955* pp. 3–14. Rutgers Univ. Press, New Brunswick, New Jersey.

Trager, W. (1957). *J. Protozool.* **4**, 269–276.

Trautz, O. R. (1960). *Ann. N.Y. Acad. Sci.* **85**, 145–160.

Tsunoda, K., and Ichikawa, O. (1955). *Govt. Expt. Sta. Animal Hyg., Expt. Rept.* **29**, 73–82.

Usuelli, F., and Balian, B. (1938). *Boll. Soc. Ital. Biol. Sper.* **13**, 45–46.

van den Berghe, L., *see* Berghe, L. van den.

Van Cleave, H. J., and Ross, E. L. (1944). *J. Parasitol.* **30**, 369–372.

Velick, S. F., and Scudder, J. (1940). *Am. J. Hyg.* **31**, Sect. C, 92–94.

Vialli, M. (1923). *Rend. Ist. Lombardo Sci.* **56**, 935–938.

Vialli, M. (1926). *Arch. Fisiol.* **23**, 577–596.

Villako, K., and Hange, L. (1958). *Vitamine Hormone* **8**, 31–33.

Villela, G. G., and Teixeira, J. C. (1929). *Mem. Inst. Oswaldo Cruz* Suppl. **6**, 62–68.

von Bonsdorff, B., *see* Bonsdorff, B. von.

von Brand, T., *see* Brand, T. von.

von Kemnitz, G., *see* Kemnitz, G. von.

Waitz, J. A. (1963). *J. Parasitol.* **49**, 73–80.

Wakeman, A. M. (1929). *W. African Med. J.* **2**, 169.

Wantland, W. W. (1934). *Proc. Soc. Exptl. Biol. Med.* **32**, 438–444.

Wantland, W. W. (1936). *J. Parasitol.* **22**, 537.

Wantland, W. W., Hausen, C., and Feeney, R. E. (1936). *J. Parasitol.* **22**, 538.

Wardle, R. A. (1937a). *Manitoba Essays* 60th Anniv. Commem. Vol., 338–364.

Wardle, R. A. (1937b). *Can. J. Res.* **D15**, 117–126.

Wats, R. C., and Das Gupta, B. M. (1934). *Indian J. Med. Res.* **21**, 475–481.

Waxler, S. H. (1941). *Am. J. Physiol.* **134**, 19–25.

Weinland, E. (1901a). *Z. Biol.* **41**, 69–74.

Weinland, E. (1901b). *Z. Biol.* **42**, 55–90.

Weinland, E., and Brand, T. von (1926). *Z. Vergleich. Physiol.* **4**, 212–285.

Weinstein, P. P. (1952). *Exptl. Parasitol.* **1**, 363–376.

Weinstein, P. P. (1960). *In* "Host Influence on Parasite Physiology" (L. A. Stauber, ed.), pp. 65–92. Rutgers Univ. Press, New Brunswick, New Jersey.

Weir, W. C., Bahler, T. L., Pope, A. L., Phillips, P. H., Herrick, C. A., and Bohstedt, G. (1948). *J. Animal Sci.* **7**, 466–474.

Wells, H. S. (1931). *J. Parasitol.* **17**, 167–182.

Wendel, W. B. (1943). *J. Biol. Chem.* **148**, 21–34.

Wertheim, P. (1934). *Zool. Anz.* **106**, 20–24.

Whitfeld, P. R. (1953). *Australian J. Biol. Sci.* **6**, 591–596.

Yamao, Y. (1951a). *Zool. Mag. Tokyo* **60**, 101–105.

Yamao, Y. (1951b). *Zool. Mag. Tokyo* **60**, 168–172.

Yamao, Y. (1952a). *J. Coll. Arts Sci., Chiba Univ., Nat. Sci. Ser.* **1**, 9–13.

Yamao, Y. (1952b). *Jikken Seibutsugaku Ho* **2**, 159–162.

Yamao, Y. (1952c). *Zool. Mag. Tokyo* **61**, 184–190.

Yamao, Y. (1952d). *Dobutsugaku Zasshi* **61**, 254–260.

Yamao, Y. (1952e). *Dobutsugaku Zasshi* **61**, 290–294.

Yamao, Y. (1957). *J. Coll. Arts Sci., Chiba Univ., Nat. Sci. Ser.* **2**, 212–224.

Yamao, Y., and Saito, A. (1952). *Jikken Seibutsugaku Ho* **2**, 153–158.

Yokogawa, M., and Yoshimura, H. (1957). *Kiseichugaku Zasshi* **6**, 546–554.

Yoshimura, H., and Yokogawa, M. (1958). *Kiseichugaku Zasshi* **7**, 363–369.

Zam, S. G., Martin, W. E., and Thomas, L. J. (1963). *J. Parasitol.* **49**, 190–196.

Zwemer, R. L., and Culbertson, J. T. (1939). *Am. J. Hyg.* **29**, Sect. C, 7–12.

Zwemer, R. L., Sims, E. A. H., and Coggeshall, L. T. (1940). *Am. J. Trop Med.* **20**, 701.

Chapter 2

CARBOHYDRATES I: DISTRIBUTION AND NATURE OF CARBOHYDRATES

I. INTRODUCTORY REMARKS

It has been known for more than a 100 years (Claude Bernard, 1859) that parasitic worms contain polysaccharides; Weinland's classical work (Weinland, 1901a,b) demonstrated at the turn of the century that the metabolism of intestinal worms is characterized by the fermentation of carbohydrate. Following the work of these and other pioneers (such as Bunge, 1883, 1889, who was the first to demonstrate acid production by a parasitic worm), many investigators have studied some phase of the carbohydrate relationships of parasites. This is no coincidence. It very soon became obvious that many endoparasites have a pronounced carbohydrate metabolism.

All forms living in anaerobic or semianaerobic habitats (such as the intestine or the bile ducts) and having no special means of securing oxygen, utilize carbohydrate primarily because it is the best source of anaerobic energy. Intermediately oxidized carbon atoms of carbohydrate

$$(\text{H}-\overset{\displaystyle |}{\underset{\displaystyle |}{\text{C}}}-\text{OH})$$

are ideally suited for anoxidative processes which essentially are oxidation-reduction processes (Hellerman, 1947; Hungate, 1955). Parasites living in oxygen-rich surroundings, such as the blood, could, theoretically, derive most of their energy from the oxidation of fats or proteins, but carbohydrate metabolism nevertheless predominates in such forms as trypanosomes or schistosomes. No definite reason for this specialization has been recognized as yet.

43

It is interesting to note that almost all hitherto studied parasites do not completely oxidize sugar to carbon dioxide or water. This, of course, is a necessary consequence of lack of oxygen when organisms live in anaerobic habitats, but it happens also even if oxygen is plentiful. In other words, most endoparasites are characterized by the prevalence of anaerobic or aerobic fermentations. The only exception reported so far is *Plasmodium lophurae,* which apparently does not show aerobic fermentations (Wendel, 1946). It is obvious that both anaerobic and aerobic fermentations are very uneconomical since the large amount of energy contained in the end products of fermentation remain unutilized by the parasites. From the parasite's standpoint this is no handicap, since they practically always live in surroundings with a surplus of readily available food. From the host's standpoint the inefficient utilization of food may be more serious, since some of the organic end products may be toxic. On the other hand, however, the host may be able to utilize at least some of the end products of the parasites' metabolism. Harvey (1949) has pointed out that the pyruvic acid produced by pathogenic trypanosomes is probably metabolized further by the host and this point has definitely been proven subsequently by Grant and Fulton (1957) and Coleman and von Brand (1957). The most extreme examples in this direction are the termites, which have become dependent for survival upon the metabolic end products of their intestinal fauna (Cleveland, 1925).

In discussing aerobic fermentations, a clear distinction has to be made between two points: first, the intracellular mechanisms involved, and second, the reasons for their widespread occurrence among endoparasites. In respect to the first point, quite evidently a parallel exists with malignant tumors. With them a variety of mechanisms has been incriminated without an agreement having been reached by the various workers involved (for a recent discussion see Boxer and Devlin, 1961). It is probable that no single mechanism can explain all facts known about the aerobic fermentations of parasites. In some forms, such as the bloodstream forms of the pathogenic African trypanosomes, missing enzymes (e.g., Marshall, 1948) prevent complete oxidation of carbohydrate. Other parasites, such as the malaria plasmodia, have a full complement of enzymes, but a differential activity of various enzymes of the glycolytic chain seem to lead to a piling up and final excretion of partially oxidized compounds (e.g., McKee *et al.,* 1946). Finally, in cases such as *Trypanosoma cruzi,* which excretes large amounts of succinic acid (Ryley, 1956) despite possessing potent mechanisms of metabolizing that particular acid (Agosin and von Brand, 1955; Seaman, 1956), one has to postulate the existence of regulatory mechanisms which restrict for unknown reasons the activity of certain enzymes (von Brand, 1963).

Why aerobic fermentations are common to most parasites is a very puzzling question which hardly can be answered authoritatively at present. Read (1961) alone has tentatively expressed a definite view. He points out that the elimination of some enzymatic steps from the sequence normally involved in sugar utilization may represent a thermodynamic advantage which could have led to positive selection. This is an interesting view, which, however, would seem to require more support. It should not be overlooked that fermentations are uneconomical not only from a caloric standpoint, but they may, in some respects, impose even increased energy demands on an organism. Thus, the processes of food intake and excretion of partially oxidized compounds often involve active transport mechanisms which require energy; these processes, however, are of necessity much more pronounced in animals subsisting by means of fermentations (be they aerobic or anaerobic) than in animals oxidizing their food materials completely.

II. DISTRIBUTION OF LOW-MOLECULAR WEIGHT CARBOHYDRATES

Little is known about the distribution of simple sugars in parasitic protozoa. Very small amounts of glucose (0.06% of dry weight) and trehalose (<0.05%) have been found in the culture form of *Trypanosoma cruzi* by Fairbairn (1958b). Glucosamine (0.1 to 1.0 μg/mg protein) has been observed in hydrolyzed trypanosomes (Williamson and Desowitz, 1961) and a hexosamine tentatively identified as glucosamine occurs in relatively large amount in *Entamoeba histolytica* (Loran et al., 1956).

More information is available for parasitic worms. However, the glucose values found in the older and much of the newer literature (e.g., Foster, 1865; Weinland, 1901b; Schulte, 1917; von Brand, 1934; Salisbury and Anderson, 1939; Daugherty and Taylor, 1956; Goodchild and Vilar-Alvarez, 1962) have been obtained by rather unspecific chemical methods which tend to give too high values. Reliable are the data obtained with the help of a specific enzyme, glucose oxidase; those reported by Fairbairn (1958b) are summarized in Table VII. They show the great variations occurring between different species. However, the complete absence of glucose in *Taenia taeniaeformis,* as reported by Fairbairn (1958b), must have been due to an exceptional worm. In more recent experiments von Brand et al. (1964) found in the tissues of this tapeworm species glucose amounts varying around 100 μg/100 mg fresh weight when newly isolated worms were analyzed. After *in vitro* incubation for 2 hours in the presence of glucose the glucose concentration of the tissues rose to 200–300 μg/100 mg. Nothing is known about the distribution of free glucose in the tissues of tapeworms; Goodchild (1961), however,

TABLE VII

GLUCOSE AND TREHALOSE CONTENT OF SOME HELMINTHS[a]

Species	Glucose (%) of tissue solids	Trehalose (%) of tissue solids
Trematodes		
Fasciola hepatica	–	0.11
Cestodes		
Hymenolepis diminuta	0.19	0.22
Moniezia expansa	0.06	Traces
Raillietina cesticillus	0.14	0.10
Taenia taeniaeformis	None	None
Acanthocephala		
Moniliformis dubius	3.0	2.3
Nematodes		
Ascaridia galli	0.78	0.38
Ascaris lumbricoides,		
hemolymph	0.07	4.0
Heterakis gallinae	0.43	0.10
Litomosoides carinii	0.01	0.06
Porrocaecum decipiens,		
larva	0.16	2.18
Trichinella spiralis,		
larva	0.04	1.76
Trichuris ovis	0.09	0.48
Uncinaria stenocephala	0.77	0.91

[a] From Fairbairn (1958b).

briefly reports indications that the glucose is not evenly distributed along the strobila of *Hymenolepis diminuta*.

It can be expected that the use of specific enzymatic methods for the determinations of single sugars, such as glucose or galactose, will find increased use. When working with previously nonanalyzed material, these procedures should be employed, at least initially, in conjunction with a total carbohydrate method. If there is a pronounced discrepancy between the results given by both methods, a search should be made for sugars other than that determined by the enzyme. It should be recalled in this connection that glucose is not always the predominant sugar. In the blood of the *Gastrophilus* larva, for instance, fructose is the prevalent hexose (Levenbook, 1950) and trehalose, the occurrence of which will be mentioned below, escapes both the enzymatic method and methods relying on the reducing power of sugars.

Reducing sugars, customarily expressed as glucose, but as a rule not identified as such, occur in the body fluids of parasitic worms. Their concentration is usually low, as emphasized by Fairbairn and Passey (1957) and Fairbairn (1960) for nematodes. Thus "glucose" has been found to account for 0.15% of the fresh weight of the body fluid of *Parascaris* (Fauré-Fremiet, 1913), 0.22% of that of *Ascaris* (Rogers, 1945), and 0.05% in the case of the female *Macracanthorhynchus* (von Brand, 1940). But Fairbairn (1958b) found with the glucose oxidase method only 0.07% of the dry substance of the *Ascaris* hemolymph to consist of glucose. Reducing sugars have also been found regularly in the fluids of larval tapeworm cysts. In *Echinococcus granulosus* the data vary between 0.03 and 0.04% (Mazzocco, 1923; Lemaire and Ribère, 1935), but in liver hydatids somewhat higher values, up to 0.1% have been observed (Codounis and Polydorides, 1936). In *Cysticercus fasciolaris* fluid 0.14% has been found (Schopfer, 1932).

The nonreducing disaccharide trehalose is widely distributed in helminths (Table VII); it is found in greater amounts than glucose in several species. Surprisingly high concentrations, 2.18% and 2.30% of the dry substance, have been reported for larval *Porrocaecum decipiens* and *Moniliformis dubius* (Fairbairn, 1958b; Laurie, 1959), respectively, while the hitherto studied cestodes contain relatively little trehalose. Fairbairn *et al.* (1961) state thus that *Hymenolepis diminuta* does apparently not contain larger amounts. The highest trehalose value so far reported, 7.9% of the tissue solids, has been found in unembryonated, decoated eggs of *Ascaris lumbricoides* by Fairbairn and Passey (1957). During embryonation Passey and Fairbairn (1957) and Fairbairn (1957) observed an initial decrease of both trehalose and glycogen which was followed by a resynthesis of both carbohydrates. In embryonated eggs the original levels of both were approximately regained. In the infective eggs trehalose was found almost exclusively in the perivitelline fluid where the surprisingly high concentration of 13.7% was reached, while glycogen was encountered only in the embryo proper (Fairbairn and Passey, 1957).

In adult *Ascaris,* all tissues studied by Fairbairn and Passey (1957) contained trehalose. It is especially remarkable that in testis and seminal vesicle trehalose accounts for a very high percentage of the total carbohydrates (Table VIII). More recently Harpur (1963) reports trehalose values of $1.11 \pm 0.35\%$ of the fresh tissue weight for the muscles of female *Ascaris lumbricoides* and $0.27 \pm 0.13\%$ for the ovaries.

Simple sugars occur in the bodies of parasites not only as free sugars, but also polymerized as polysaccharides (see below), or as constituents of such compounds as glycoproteins or glycolipids. The sugar component

TABLE VIII

ALKALI-STABLE CARBOHYDRATES (IN % OF FRESH TISSUE WEIGHT)
OF *Ascaris Lumbricoides* [a]

Tissue	Total carbohydrate	Glycogen	Trehalose
Hemolymph			
Male	1.40	0.88	0.52
Female	1.17	0.40	0.77
Intestine			
Male	0.32	0.29	0.03
Female	0.84	0.70	0.14
Muscle			
Male	14.2	13.6	0.60
Female	17.2	15.4	1.80
Integument			
Male	0.76	0.72	0.04
Female	0.75	0.61	0.14
Ovaries	8.4	7.6	0.80
Uteri	3.5	2.0	1.5
Testis	1.27	0.26	1.01
Seminal vesicle	1.60	0.48	1.12

[a] After Fairbairn and Passey (1957).

of the former seems not to have been specifically identified as yet; it may well be, in many cases at least, glucose. A little more is known about the simple sugars occurring in glycolipids. Thus galactose has been isolated from the cerebroside fraction of *Cysticercus fasciolaris* (Lesuk and Anderson, 1941) and *Moniezia expansa* (Kent *et al.,* 1948). Of great interest is the elucidation of the nature of the carbohydrate moiety of the ascarosides, structural lipids described from *Ascaris* and *Parascaris*. It is a sugar which previously had not been observed in nature. It received the name ascarylose and has been identified as 3,6-dideoxy-L-arabinohexose (3,6-dideoxy-L-mannose) by Fouquey *et al.* (1957, 1958a,b, 1959). This sugar is the optical antipode of tyvelose which has been found in the endotoxin of *Salmonella typhi.* The configurations of tyvelose and ascarylose are shown in Fig. 1.

III.   CHEMISTRY OF RESERVE POLYSACCHARIDES

The reserve polysaccharides identified so far in parasites are polymers of D-glucopyranose. They appear essentially under two distinct forms: amylopectin and glycogen.

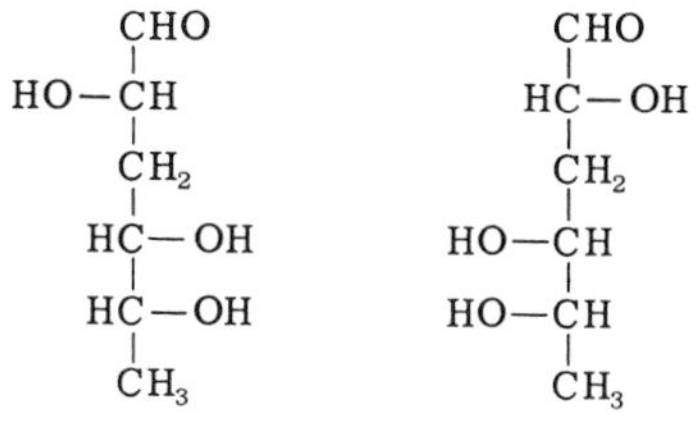

```
        CHO                      CHO
         |                        |
   HO—CH                    HC—OH
         |                        |
        CH₂                      CH₂
         |                        |
     HC—OH                  HO—CH
         |                        |
     HC—OH                  HO—CH
         |                        |
        CH₃                      CH₃

     Tyvelose                 Ascarylose
```

Fig. 1.   Configuration of tyvelose and ascarylose. (After Fouquey *et al.*, 1959.)

It has been established in recent years that the polysaccharide known originally as paraglycogen really consists of amylopectin, at least insofar as some species of rumen ciliates and ciliates parasitizing the horse's intestine are concerned. It should be recalled that the term paraglycogen had been coined originally by Buetschli (1885) for the polysaccharide granules of gregarines and that it was later extended, with questionable justification, to other protozoan polysaccharides, mainly on the grounds of solubility characteristics different from true glycogen. Whether future research will identify the storage polysaccharide of gregarines and coccidia with amylopectin is at present an open question. The old experiments of Panzer (1913) indicate that the polysaccharide of the coccidium *Goussia gadi,* in contrast to that of gregarines, is readily water-soluble.

Masson and Oxford (1951) were the first to point out that the iodine-polysaccharide complex of the polysaccharide granules isolated from rumen ciliates resembled that of starch rather than that of glycogen. Isolation of larger polysaccharide quantities in pure form from the holotrich sheep ciliates *Isotricha* and *Dasytricha* (Forsyth and Hirst, 1953), the oligotrich sheep parasite *Entodinium* (Eadie *et al.,* 1963), and the oligotrich horse ciliate *Cycloposthium* (Forsyth *et al.,* 1953) allowed chemical analysis. The polysaccharide isolated from holotrich ciliates consisted of chains of 22α-1,4-D-glucose units, that from *Entodinium* of 19 such units and that of *Cycloposthium* of 23. These chains are linked together by C_1-C_6 bonds, forming highly branched polysaccharides. The blue value with iodine is very low and the Nussenbaum test for amylose is negative, facts indicating that the substances do not contain a linear component, but consonant with the idea that they are amylopectins. This view is further supported by the observation of Mould and Thomas (1958) that the so-called R enzyme readily attacks the protozoan polysaccharides and genuine amylopectin, while it is more or less inactive with glycogen as substrate. After being degraded partially by the R enzyme the blue value of the protozoan polysaccharides markedly increases. The β-amylolysis value varies about between 51 and 58%, but the degradation to maltose, where tested, rises to about 101% when the polysaccharides are exposed to the simultaneous action of β-amylase and the R enzyme. In view of this evidence it appears justified to abandon the old term paraglycogen and to substitute for it the term amylopectin insofar at least as the above protozoa are concerned.

The most widely distributed reserve polysaccharide of parasites is unquestionably glycogen. It has been reported from parasitic protozoa, mesozoa (Nouvel, 1929, 1931), helminths, and arthropods. Glycogen is a highly branched homopolysaccharide containing only glucose units, linked to each other in α-1,4' and α-1,6' bonds, arranged in a branched, treelike structure; the ratio of 1,4' to 1,6' bonds varies between 12 and 15. Glycogen is extremely polydisperse with average molecular weights, depending upon the tissue and species, varying between 5 and over 200 million. It is readily water-soluble, gives red-brown to yellow-brown colors with iodine and is rapidly attacked by amylase. Its heat of combustion has been determined for the *Ascaris* glycogen; the relevant values reported by Emery and Benedict (1911) and Schulte (1917) are 4212 and 4125 cal/gm respectively.

Those parasite glycogens that have been studied to some extent by physicochemical or chemical methods (Table IX) show some differences among themselves or as compared to typical vertebrate glycogens. Some of these differences are that the *Ascaris* glycogen, in common with glycogens isolated from free-living invertebrates, has iodine-staining properties slightly different from those shown by vertebrate glycogens (Kjölberg *et al.*, 1963), or that the degree of branching and the average location of the branching sites vary. The *Trichomonas gallinae* polysaccharide is thus more branched than other protozoan glycogens (Manners and Ryley, 1955).

The most significant recent development has been the recognition that the mode of isolation of the polysaccharides is of the utmost importance in determining the molecular weight of the isolates. In all the older procedures alkali, trichloracetic acid, or hot water is used and this leads to a drastic reduction in the molecular weights of the isolated products (Orrell and Bueding, 1958, 1964; Bueding and Orrell, 1961). A comparison of the molecular weights shown in Table IX illustrates this point; Fig. 2 does so even more clearly. In the light of these new results it is justified to look upon the older ones with caution, since the drastic isolation procedures do introduce changes which justifiably can be considered as artifacts. Glycogens isolated from various sources with cold water show definite differences and a considerably higher degree of polydispersity,

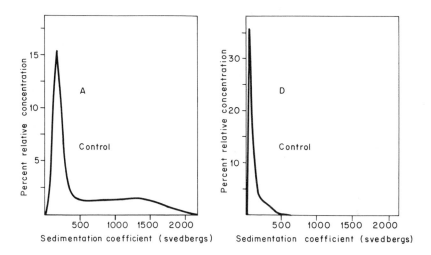

Fig. 2. Sedimentation coefficient distribution of glycogen extracted from *Fasciola hepatica* by means of cold water (A) and KOH (D). (After Bueding and Orrell, 1961.)

that is, broader molecular weight range, than samples purified by one of the classic, more drastic procedures (Bueding, 1962). In respect to species differences it may be mentioned that the *Ascaris lumbricoides* glycogen is divided essentially equally between two varieties, one with an average molecular weight of 450 million, the other one of only about 50 million. In *Fasciola hepatica,* on the other hand, approximately 30% of the polysaccharide forms a continuation from the light-molecular-weight variety to fractions with very high molecular weights. In *Hymenolepis diminuta,* finally, approximately 30% of the material isolated is represented by polysaccharide with very high molecular weight, which is clearly separated from a variety with lower molecular weight (Bueding, 1962).

The differences reported for various helminth glycogens are remarkable, especially in contrast to the fact that marked similarities in properties exist between glycogens isolated from different families of cestodes (E. Bueding, personal communication, 1965).

When *Fasciola* is starved for 24 hours *in vitro,* the heavy polysaccharide component (sedimentation coefficient above 1300 S) decreases from 13.2% of the total material isolated to 5.2%, but it rapidly rises again upon refeeding of the flukes. Whether the heavy component is utilized and resynthesized preferentially, or whether interconversions between the heavy and light fractions are involved, is at present not known (Bueding and Orrell, 1961). Recent experiments with *Hyme-*

TABLE IX

SOME PROPERTIES OF PARASITE GLYCOGENS

Glycogen isolated from	$[\alpha]_D$	Average chain length	β-Amylolysis limit (%)	Average molecular weight	References
Flagellates					
Trichomonas foetus	+196 to +199	15	60	3×10^6	Feinberg and Morgan (1953); Manners and Ryley (1955)
Trichomonas gallinae	+197	9	51	$3-4 \times 10^6$	Manners and Ryley (1955)
Trematodes					
Fasciola hepatica	+201.2			$<1-2 \times 10^{8\,a}$	Oesterlin and von Brand (1934); Bueding and Orrell (1961)
Cestodes					
Moniezia expansa	+187 to +194				Weinland (1901a); Oesterlin and von Brand (1934); Abdel-Akher and Smith (1951)
Acanthocephala					
Macracanthorhynchus hirudinaceus	+187.5				von Brand and Saurwein (1942)
Moniliformis dubius	+197				Laurie (1959)

Nematodes

Ascaris lumbricoides	+189 to +196	11–13	38–50	0.7×10^6–18×10^6; 5×10^7–$4.5 \times 10^{8\,a}$	Weinland (1901a); Baldwin and King (1942); Bell (1944, 1948); Bell *et al.* (1948); Halsall *et al.* (1947); Abdel-Akher and Smith (1951); Kjölberg *et al.* (1951); Orrell and Bueding (1963); Bueding (1962); Manners and Wright (1961)

Arthropods

Gastrophilus intestinalis, larvae	+192.6				von Kemnitz (1916)

[a] Molecular weight upon cold water isolation; all other figures for glycogens isolated with more drastic procedures.

nolepis diminuta (Colucci *et al.*, 1964, 1965), involving analysis of the heavy and light glycogen fractions after exposure of the worms to U C^{14}-glucose seem to indicate metabolic differences between these fractions.

Glycogen is frequently stated to occur in two physical states in organisms: As lyoglycogen (trichloracetic-extractable, "free glycogen") and desmoglycogen (combined with proteins or other cell components, extractable only after alkali treatment). This type of heterogeneity has been described by Monteoliva and Guevara (1958) for the *Ascaridia galli* polysaccharide. Its desmoglycogen yielded only glucose upon acid hydrolysis, while, surprisingly, some mannose was found besides glucose as constituent of the lyoglycogen. Whether perhaps in this case a mixture of two discrete polysaccharides was present will have to be decided by a reinvestigation. Probably unrelated to desmoglycogen are the various protein-glycogen complexes described from tapeworms. Kent and Macheboeuf (1947) isolated from *Moniezia expansa* two such fractions which were electrophoretically homogeneous. One, baerine, contained 60% glycogen; the other, moniezine, 11%. An even greater variety of similar protein-carbohydrate complexes has later been found in *Hymenolepis diminuta* (Kent, 1957a) and *Raillietina cesticillus* (Kent, 1957b). In both worms four main fractions were encountered, of which at least one could be subdivided into two components by electrophoresis and ammonium sulfate fractionation. Three of the main fractions were protein-carbohydrate complexes with carbohydrate content varying between 12 and 61%. The fourth fraction, however, appears to be a nucleoprotein-carbohydrate complex with a carbohydrate content of 2 and 12.8% in *Raillietina* and *Hymenolepis*, respectively. It is very probable that polysaccharide-protein complexes (though not necessarily glycogen-protein compounds) are widely distributed. Some with antigenic properties will be discussed below. Here the mucoid secretions of many cercariae, studied by Kruidenier (1953a,b), Lewert and Lee (1954), Stirewalt and Evans (1960), Bogitsh (1963), and Ortigoza and Hall (1963), may be mentioned. They have been studied only histochemically and the polysaccharide component has not been characterized as yet.

IV. QUANTITATIVE AND QUALITATIVE ASPECTS OF RESERVE CARBOHYDRATES

Few quantitative data are available for parasitic protozoa. It has been established that very large amounts of polysaccharides are deposited in many species of rumen ciliates. Masson and Oxford (1951) found in *Isotricha* 70% of the dry substance to consist of amylopectin and Abou

Akkada and Howard (1960) observed 64% in *Entodinium,* while Eadie *et al.* (1963) reported only 6 to 7% in the same organism. Perhaps the state of nutrition differed in the two sets of experiments. As will be mentioned later, these ciliates have a very high rate of carbohydrate metabolism and during starvation rapidly deplete their polysaccharide stores. Quite high glycogen values, ranging usually from 10 to 30% of the dried material, with the extremes lying around 5%, on the one hand, and 55%, on the other, have been found in *Trichomonas foetus* and *Trichomonas gallinae* (Feinberg and Morgan, 1953; Manners and Ryley, 1955). On the other side of the scale are protozoa very poor in reserve carbohydrate, or even lacking it completely. Thus, in the blood-stream form of trypanosomes no glycogen is demonstrable histochemically (Krijgsman, 1936; Gerzeli, 1955), but some polysaccharide has been found in several *Trypanoplasma* species (Keysselitz, 1906; Schindera, 1922); in cultured *Strigomonas oncopelti* Ryley (1955) found 2.5 to 2.8% of the dried tissues to consist of a substance that could be isolated with the methods used for isolation of glycogen. Caution as to interpretation of its nature is indicated, as it seems not to be used in endogenous metabolism. Also very poor in glycogen are malaria parasites. They appear glycogen-free in histochemical tests (Lillie, 1947; Das Gupta, 1960), but Christophers and Fulton (1938) found in *Plasmodium knowlesi* by chemical procedure small amounts of glycogen (0.022–0.057% of the fresh material).

The relatively extensive literature dealing with the histochemical demonstration of glycogen or amylopectin (usually described as "paraglycogen") in a variety of parasitic protozoa can be reviewed only briefly and without attempt at completeness. In trophozoites of parasitic amoebas polysaccharide, at least part of it glycogen, is spread throughout the body without specific localization, while in young *Entamoeba* cysts, and especially in *Iodamoeba* cysts, the polysaccharide is deposited in well-defined vacuoles (Kuenen and Swellengrebel, 1913, 1917; Dobell, 1919; Dobell and O'Connor, 1921; Morita, 1938; von Brand, 1932; Armer, 1944; Lillie, 1947; Hara *et al.,* 1954; Hallman *et al.,* 1955). In trichomonads the polysaccharide may be distributed throughout the body, as occurs frequently in *Trichomonas foetus* or *Trichomonas vaginalis* (Stewart, 1938; Gerzeli, 1959), but often it is found located preferentially along the axostyle, as shown for various species by Nomura (1957a,b), or the cytosome, as observed by Wantland *et al.* (1962). Much glycogen deposition along the axostyle has also been described for the termite flagellate *Joenia annectens* (Lavette, 1960).

As to sporozoa, polysaccharide in relatively large amounts occurs in mature asexual stages of *Eimeria* spp., in late macrogametocytes, and in oocysts, while no polysaccharides, or at most small amounts, are observed in young schizonts, microgametocytes, and other stages (Gill and Ray, 1954a; Tsunoda and Ichikawa, 1955; Patillo and Becker, 1955; Scholtyseck, 1964). In *Barrouxia schneideri* the female gametocytes contain much larger polysaccharide stores than the male gametocytes. In the latter the polysaccharide is deposited in form of much finer granules than in the former (Canning, 1963). In gregarines the "paraglycogen" granules have been known since Buetschli's (1885) account; they occur primarily within the deutomerite (Giovannola, 1934). Positive polysaccharide reactions have also been reported for hemogregarines (Gerzeli, 1954a), *Hepatozoon* spp. and *Theileria parva* (Das Gupta, 1960), *Sarcocystis tenella* (Ludvik, 1958) and *Toxoplasma* where it has been found both in extracellular stages (Gerzeli, 1954b) and, in especially high concentration, in cysts (Lillie, 1947; Das Gupta and Kulasiri, 1959).

Polysaccharide in the form of more or less distinct granules can be demonstrated histochemically in many parasitic ciliates. Smaller or larger stores have thus been described for *Nyctotherus* spp. (Armer, 1944; Lom, 1955; Dutta, 1958), *Balantidium* spp. (Lom, 1955; Dutta, 1959), many Astomata (Lom, 1960), but especially for rumen and related ciliates. In the oligotrich forms, such as *Entodinium, Ophryoscolex,* or *Thoracodinium,* the polysaccharide is found largely in, though not exclusively confined to the complicated skeletal plates, while in holotrich species, such as *Isotricha* or *Dasytricha,* the amylopectin granules are distributed throughout the body which they often fill to such an extent as to obscure any morphological detail (Schulze, 1924; Trier, 1926; Weineck, 1931; Westphal, 1934; Hungate, 1943; Oxford, 1951; Sugden and Oxford, 1952; Eadie and Oxford, 1955; Latteur, 1958).

The glycogen content of a relatively large number of helminths has been determined quantitatively, but few such data are available for endoparasitic arthropods. A survey of Table X makes it likely that a certain correlation between habitat and glycogen exists, at least in broad outlines. The parasites living in oxygen-poor habitats or in habitats with periodic oxygen deficiencies (e.g., stomach) regularly have a high glycogen content. Apparent exceptions, such as *Ancylostoma caninum,* can be explained by the assumption that as bloodsuckers they are not forced to lead a predominantly anaerobic life in nature. No clear-cut correlation exists in the case of parasites living in environments with moderate or high oxygen tensions, such as the tissue parasites. Some, like the filariae, usually have but little glycogen, but others, such as *Cysticercus fasciolaris* or larval *Eustrongylides ignotus,* contain as much glycogen as the large intestinal helminths. The subsequent fate of the worms may be the determining factor. The adult *Taenia taeniaeformis* can be assumed to lead a predominantly anaerobic life, but whether an analogous assumption can be made for the adult *Eustrongylides* is an open question. Another factor potentially important in relating glycogen levels of helminths to pecularities in the habitat is the fact that tissue helminths usually have continuous access to carbohydrate, while this will be the case only intermittently in the intestine.

Sexual differences in glycogen content have been described for several species. The females of *Schistosoma mansoni* (Bueding and Koletsky, 1950; Robinson, 1956), of *Macracanthorhynchus hirudinaceus* (von Brand, 1940), and of *Moniliformis dubius* (Graff and Allen, 1963) contain less glycogen than the males. In nematodes the data are contradictory. According to Smorodincev and Bebesin (1936), Cavier and Savel (1951), Toryu (1933), and Reid (1944), the females of *Ascaris, Parascaris,* and *Ascaridia* store more glycogen than the males, but von Brand (1957) and Ro (1939) found more glycogen in male than female *Ascaris.*

Little is known about seasonal variations in glycogen content. They do not seem to occur in parasites of warm-blooded hosts which live the year round under uniform conditions. As to parasites of cold-blooded hosts, Hopkins (1950) did not observe seasonal variations in the plerocercoids of *Schistocephalus solidus,* but Dunagan (1963) mentions the occurrence of such variations in the case of *Neoechinorhynchus* spp. of turtles. He has, however, not yet published the details of his observations. As to protozoa, Dubosq and Grasse (1933) found glycogen in *Cryptobia helicis* only during the winter, but not during the summer. Similarly, Sukhanova (1963) observed the highest glycogen concentration in *Opalia ranarum* during fall and winter.

Meager are also the data concerning the possibility of diurnal variations in glycogen content. Read and Rothman (1958) found in *Moniliformis* isolated from their hosts at 11 P.M. almost twice as much glycogen as in worms isolated at 2 P.M. On the other hand, Dunagan (1963) observed no similar diurnal cycle in *Neoechinorhynchus* spp.

It cannot be doubted, however, that the physiological state of the host frequently has a profound influence on the glycogen content of its parasites, especially intestinal parasites. Thus, starvation of the host reduces the polysaccharide stores drastically in *Raillietina cesticillus* (Reid, 1942), *Hymenolepis diminuta* (Read, 1949; Goodchild, 1961), and *Moniliformis dubius* (Read and Rothman, 1958). Round worms may be less sensitive. According to an old observation of Weinland (1901b), ascarids expelled from a dog after 4 days' starvation still showed the relatively high value of 1.8% glycogen. The polysaccharide content of

TABLE X

GLYCOGEN CONTENT OF PARASITIC WORMS AND ARTHROPODS[a]

Species	Glycogen in per cent of		Habitat	Availability of significant amounts of oxygen	References
	Fresh weight	Dry weight			
Trematodes					
Fasciola hepatica	3.1–3.7	15–21	Bile ducts	No	Flury and Leeb (1926); Weinland and von Brand (1926); Mansour (1959)
Gastrothylax crumenifer	6.5		Stomach	Variable	Goil (1957)
Haplometra cylindracea	1.5		Lung	Yes	Dawes and Muller (1957)
Paramphistomum explanatum	7.26		Bile ducts	No	Goil (1957)
Schistosoma mansoni, ♀	0.9	3–5	Blood stream	Yes	Bueding and Koletsky (1950); Robinson (1956)
Schistosoma mansoni, ♂	2.8–3.8	14–29	Blood stream	Yes	Bueding and Koletsky (1950); Robinson (1956)
Cestodes					
Cysticercus fasciolaris	4.4–7.3	20–28	Liver	?	Salisbury and Anderson (1939); von Brand and Bowman (1961)
Diphyllobothrium latum	1.9	20	Intestine	No	Smorodincev and Bebesin (1936)
Echinococcus granulosus, scoleces	2.8	19	Liver	?	Agosin et al. (1957)
Hymenolepis citelli	9.8		Intestine	No	Read and Rothman (1957b)
Hymenolepis diminuta	9.8	26–48	Intestine	No	Fairbairn et al. (1961); Goodchild (1961); Goodchild and Vilar-Alvarez (1962)

Species			Location	Anaerobic	References
Ligula intestinalis		34	Body cavity	?	Markov (1939)
Moniezia expansa	2.7–3.2	24–32	Intestine	No	Weinland (1901a); von Brand (1933); Wardle (1937)
Raillietina cesticillus	6.5	32	Intestine	No	Reid (1942)
Schistocephalus solidus, plerocercoids	16	51	Body cavity	?	Hopkins (1950, 1952)
Taenia saginata	7.4	60	Intestine	No	Smorodincev and Bebesin (1936)
Taenia solium	2.2	25	Intestine	No	Smorodincev and Bebesin (1936)
Acanthocephala					
Macracanthorhynchus hirudinaceus	1.2–2.3	7–13	Intestine	No	von Brand (1938, 1940); Ward (1952)
Moniliformis dubius	0.7–7.1		Intestine	No	Read and Rothman (1958); Graff and Allen (1963)
Nematodes					
Ancylostoma caninum	1.6		Intestine	Yes	von Brand and Otto (1938)
Ascaridia galli	3.6–4.7		Intestine	No	Reid (1945a,b)
Ascaris lumbricoides	3.3–8.7	14–24	Intestine	No	Weinland (1901a); Flury (1912); Smorodincev and Bebesin (1936); von Brand (1937); Cavier and Savel (1951)
Dipetalonema gracilis	0.2		Abdominal cavity	Yes	von Brand (1950)
Dirofilaria immitis	1.9	10	Heart	Yes	von Brand (1950)
Dirofilaria uniformis	1.7		Subcutaneous	Yes	von Brand *et al.* (1963)

TABLE X (Continued)

Glycogen Content of Parasitic Worms and Arthropods[a]

Species	Glycogen in per cent of		Habitat	Availability of significant amounts of oxygen	References
	Fresh weight	Dry weight			
Eustrongylides ignotus, larvae	6.9	28	Various organs	Yes	von Brand (1938)
Heterakis gallinae	2.7	11.8	Intestine	No	Glocklin and Fairbairn (1952)
Litomosoides carinii	0.8	5	Pleural cavity	Yes	Bueding (1949)
Parascaris equorum	2.1–3.8	10–23	Intestine	No	Schimmelpfennig (1903); Toryu (1933)
Porrocaecum decipiens, larvae		55	Muscle	?	Fairbairn (1958a)
Strongylus vulgaris	3.5		Intestine	No	Toryu (1933)
Trichuris vulpis	2.3		Intestine	No	Bueding *et al.* (1960)
Arthropods					
Gastrophilus intestinalis, larvae	5.0–9.0	14–31	Stomach	Variable	von Kemnitz (1916); Dinulescu (1932)
Gastrophilus inermis, larvae	8.9		Rectum	No	Dinulescu (1932)
Gastrophilus nasalis, larvae	2.9–9.4		Stomach, duodenum	Variable	Dinulescu (1932)
Gastrophilus haemorrhoidalis, larvae	3.0–4.6		Stomach	Variable	Dinulescu (1932)

[a] Further quantitative data on glycogen in helminths will be found in the papers by von Brand (1934, 1957); von Brand *et al.* (1952); Vernberg and Hunter (1956); Odlaug (1955); Daugherty and Taylor (1956); Pandya (1961); Goil (1961); Dunagan (1964).

tissue helminths, on the other hand, is not readily influenced by host starvation. This has been shown for larval *Eustrongylides ignotus* which showed an entirely normal polysaccharide level after its hosts *(Fundulus)* had been starved for 65 days (von Brand, 1938). Furthermore, the glycogen content of *Clinostomum attenuatum* was not reduced by a 2-month starvation period of its hosts *(Rana pipiens),* as shown by Odlaug (1955).

It is not necessary to starve hosts completely to demonstrate an effect on sensitive parasites, including effects on their glycogen stores. Read and his co-workers have emphasized that there is a close connection between the amount and the nature of the carbohydrates in the host's diet and (1) the ability of several tapeworm species to establish themselves in the intestine, and (2) their rate of growth (Read, 1959; Read and Rothman, 1957a,c; Read *et al.,* 1958; Read and Simmons, 1963). Similarly, surgical alteration of the host's intestine can lead to suppression of the development of *Hymenolepis diminuta,* for instance, when the flow of bile is diverted from the small intestine to the caecum. Shortening of the intestine leads to altered chemical composition, including reduced glycogen stores, of tapeworms developing in such abnormal environment (Goodchild, 1961; Goodchild and Vilar-Alvarez, 1962).

Whether or to what extent internal secretions of the host have an influence on the magnitude of the polysaccharide stores of parasites is hardly known. Graff and Allen (1963) found that male *Moniliformis dubius* recovered from either male or female rats were not significantly different in this respect, but that female worms isolated from female hosts stored significantly more polysaccharide than those isolated from male rats. It might be worthwhile to extend such studies to other forms, since it is known that the sex of the host, or the functional state of its gonads sometimes can play a rather pronounced role in the establishment of parasites. This has been shown, to mention only two examples, for *Cysticercus fasciolaris* (Curtis *et al.,* 1933; Campbell and Melcher, 1940), or *Hymenolepis diminuta* (Addis and Chandler, 1944; Addis, 1946; Beck and Chandler, 1950).

Considerable changes in polysaccharide content evidently take place during the life cycle of helminths, but no generalizations are possible. In respect to trematodes it may be mentioned that the primary sporocysts of schistosomes contained no glycogen, whereas secondary sporocysts did store some polysaccharide. The free-living stages, miracidia and cercariae, contained relatively large polysaccharide reserves (Axmann, 1947). Similarly, Cheng and Snyder (1962) found no glycogen in daughter sporocysts of *Glypthelmins pennsylvaniensis.* It appeared first in cercariae developing within the sporocysts and increased with developing maturity. On the other hand, the wall of rediae of *Echino-*

paryphium sp. contained relatively large amounts of glycogen and other polysaccharides (Cheng, 1963), but the cercariae followed the pattern described for the *Glypthelmins* cercariae. Cercariae of several other species have also been found with appreciable glycogen stores. They are often located primarily within the tail, where the polysaccharide seems to serve as energy reserve for the more or less vigorous swimming movements (Ginecinskaja, 1960; Palm, 1962; Bogitsh, 1963). A relatively extensive literature exists dealing with the distribution of glycogen in the body of adult trematodes as revealed by histochemical techniques. The parenchymal cells, especially those located in the suckers, are important storage places, while the muscle cells proper contain usually but little glycogen. The intestinal tract is in most cases glycogen-poor or glycogen-free, as is the excretory system. Conditions in the reproductive tract vary from species to species. In some flukes, as *Fasciola* or *Fascioloides,* the vitellaria are rich in glycogen, explaining the large glycogen stores of their uterine eggs. The vitellaria of schistosomes, to mention the other extreme, are glycogen-free and consequently the uterine eggs contain but little polysaccharide. The male reproductive system is usually glycogen-poor, although the sperm cells not rarely give distinct polysaccharide reactions which in some cases, e.g., *Clonorchis sinensis* can be quite pronounced. For further information concerning the localization of glycogen in trematodes reference is made to the following papers: Ortner-Schoenbach (1913); Prenant (1922); Kajiro (1927); Wilmoth and Goldfisher (1945); Fernando (1945); Axmann (1947); Singh (1958); Yoshimura and Yokogawa (1958); Rao (1959); Bruskin (1959); von Brand and Mercado (1961); Takagi (1962), and Melekh (1963).

In cestodes, as in the above trematodes, the glycogen content is to some extent dependent on the stage in the life cycle. Especially instructive are the relevant observations of Archer and Hopkins (1958), who found a high and constant polysaccharide level in the plerocercoids of *Diphyllobothrium* sp. During the 18- to 54-hour period following establishment in the intestine of the final host, the glycogen stores declined by about half, only to increase again during the 96- to 160-hour post-invasion period during which the worms are still immature. In mature worms high polysaccharide stores were found, but they were somewhat variable, probably as a consequence of nutritional variations. Other relevant observations are due to Lewert and Lee (1955) and Heyneman and Voge (1957) who found an increase in morphologically demonstrable glycogen correlated to increase in age in *Cysticercus fasciolaris* and *Hymenolepis* spp., respectively. In the latter worms most of the glycogen was deposited in the scolex and tail, while on the contrary Waitz (1963) found a decrease in parenchymal glycogen toward the posterior end of *Cysticercus fasciolaris.*

Whether a glycogen gradient occurs along the adult cestode strobila is not certain. Read (1956) found less glycogen in the anterior and posterior quarters of *Hymenolepis diminuta* than in the second and third quarters. Daugherty and Taylor (1956) divided worms belonging to the same species into 10-cm lengths, finding a high glycogen content near the scolex and lower amounts in the next 10 cm. In the remaining segments the polysaccharide content increased again to form a short plateau and then decreased progressively. Finally, Fairbairn *et al.* (1961) found identical high carbohydrate values in immature, mature, pregravid, and gravid proglottids of *Hymenolepis diminuta,* but lower values in infective ones (i.e., the terminal 50 mm), and especially in infective eggs. While these observations indicate some discontinuity in glycogen distribution, Hedrick and Daugherty (1957) could not observe a similar phenomenon by means of histochemical techniques in adult *Hymenolepis diminuta* and *Raillietina cesticillus.*

The intimate distribution of glycogen in cestodes follows essentially the pattern described above for trematodes. The main storage organ is the medullary parenchyma with sometimes large amounts in uterine eggs and other organs of the reproductive tract. A special feature in cestodes is that some glycogen occurs in the calcareous corpuscles (Chowdhuri *et al.,* 1955, 1962; von Brand *et al.,* 1960). Further details concerning the distribution of glycogen within the tissues of larval and adult tapeworms can be found in the following papers: Brault and Loeper (1904a,b); Busch (1905); Ortner-Schoenbach (1913); Smyth (1949); Yamao (1952); Marzullo *et al.* (1957b); Turchini and Khau-Van-Kien (1958); Takahashi (1959); Ogren (1959); Rybicka (1960); Kilejian *et al.* (1961); Waitz (1963); Cheng and Dyckman (1964).

In Acanthocephala, the studies of Miller (1943) showed that the acanthor of *Macracanthorhynchus hirudinaceus* lost all its polysaccharide upon liberation from the egg shell. Glycogen reappeared in traces only after 22 days' development. It increased from then on progressively until the fully developed acanthella contained relatively large amounts. In adult Acanthocephala (von Brand, 1939, 1940; Bullock, 1949), one of the most important glycogen storage organs is the subcuticle where the glycogen is deposited not only along the subcuticular fibers but also within the lacunar system. The occurrence of large amounts of glycogen within the lacunar system seems to indicate that glycogen can be transported as such from one part of the body to the other. In most other organisms polysaccharides are first degraded to low molecular compounds before being shifted from location to location. A considerable amount of glycogen occurs also in the muscles of Acanthocephala, but the deposition is limited to the noncontractile parts of the muscle cells. In contrast to other classes of worms, distinct glycogen granules have been encountered within the nerve cells of Acanthocephala. Their floating ovaries and the young embryos are poor in glycogen, but the mature embryo contains large amounts of polysaccharide in the region of the "Embryonalkern," which, however, is probably not all glycogen. The testes and the cement glands contain but little glycogen. In Acanthocephala, in contrast to flatworms, chemical analyses of isolated organ systems are possible. As Table XI shows, by far the greatest part of the total glycogen is deposited in the body wall, that is, essentially, the subcuticle and the muscular layer.

The eggs of parasitic nematodes frequently contain large polysaccharide stores. Thus, in unembryonated, decoated eggs of *Ascaris lumbricoides* glycogen accounts for 7.8 % of the dry matter, while the corresponding value for embryonated eggs is 6.9%. In contrast to trehalose, the glycogen is confined to the embryo and does not occur in the perivitelline fluid (Fairbairn and Passey, 1957). When *Ascaris* eggs were embryonated at 28°C and kept subsequently for 1 to 2 years at room temperature, no diminution of the histochemically demonstrable glycogen in the larvae was visible (Münnich, 1962). *Ascaris* larvae and the larvae of many other species of nematodes migrate through the body of the host before settling down at their final destination, and during this migration they increase their glycogen stores (Stepanow-Grigoriew and Hoeppli, 1926; Giovannola, 1936; Münnich, 1958). The attempt to link the migration and polysaccharide accumulation to the need for glycogen for a subsequent life in anaerobic habitats (Pintner, 1922), however, does not appear well founded.

In contrast to the long persistence of glycogen in *Ascaris* larvae, when confined to the eggs, a rapid depletion of polysaccharide stores occurs in the larvae of *Enterobius vermicularis,* if the eggs are incubated *in vitro* (Engelbrecht, 1963). There are evidently great variations in the glycogen relationships of nematode larvae. Thus *Trichinella spiralis* larvae contain appreciable polysaccharide stores (Giovannola, 1936). In contrast, the free-living stages of hookworms and of *Nippostrongylus* contain, if any, at most traces of glycogen (Busch, 1905; Payne, 1923; Giovannola, 1936) and those of the blood-inhabiting microfilariae of *Acanthocheilonema perstans* are completely free of histochemically demonstrable glycogen (Brault and Loeper, 1904b).

In adult nematodes by far the greatest part of the stored glycogen is found in the tissues of the body wall (Table XI). Because of the higher

TABLE XI

GLYCOGEN OF SOME ORGAN SYSTEMS OF HELMINTHS EXPRESSED AS PER CENT OF THE TOTAL BODY GLYCOGEN

Species	Body wall	Intestine	Female reproductive system	Male reproductive system	Body fluid	References
Ascaris lumbricoides, ♂	91.5–96.4			3.6–9.5		Cavier and Savel (1951)
Ascaris lumbricoides, ♀	59.0–67.2		32.8–41.0			Cavier and Savel (1951)
Parascaris equorum, ♂	95.8–97.5	2.1–2.3		0.3–2.3		Toryu (1933)
Parascaris equorum, ♀	53.7–75.5	1.2–2.9	22–41			Toryu (1933)
Macracanthorhynchus hirudinaceus, ♀	80		12		8	von Brand (1939)

glycogen concentration in the elements of the female reproductive tract than in those of the male system, the body wall of the females contains a smaller percentage of the total body glycogen than that of the males. The body wall glycogen is located primarily in the muscles, where the carbohydrate concentration (glycogen plus trehalose) reaches the surprising figure of 70% of the dry matter (Fairbairn and Passey, 1957) or 15.9% (14.8% glycogen, 1.1% trehalose) of the fresh tissues (Harpur, 1963).

The intimate distribution of glycogen in nematode tissues has been studied often by histochemical methods; in recent years a beginning has been made to demonstrate the intracellular glycogen localization by means of electron microscopy. These studies have shown that the cuticle is generally glycogen-free, but that the lateral lines are often very rich in polysaccharide. The main storage areas, however, are microscopically, as well as chemically, the muscle layers. In muscle cells of the body wall the glycogen occurs not so much in the contractile parts, but in the characteristic plasmatic bulbs. The intestinal cells often contain glycogen, and it is frequently concentrated in the middle region of the cells. Conditions in the reproductive tracts are somewhat variable. As an example it may be mentioned that in *Thelastoma bulhoesi* the germinal zone of the ovary contains but little glycogen, while the epithelium of that zone is well supplied with polysaccharide. Oogonia and ova contain some glycogen, but not particularly large amounts. The epithelium of the testis is well supplied, but the germinal zone, the growth zone, and the sperm cells are without glycogen (Lee, 1960).

More or less detailed discussions concerning the histochemical glycogen distribution in nematode tissues will be found in the following papers: Busch (1905); von Kemnitz (1912); Fauré-Fremiet (1913); Quack (1913); Martini (1916); Toryu (1933); Giovannola (1935); Hirsch and Bretschneider (1937); Marzullo *et al.* (1957a); Kessel *et al.* (1961); Monné (1959a); Beckett and Boothroyd (1962); and Wright (1963a,b).

Hardly anything is known about the distribution of glycogen in the body of parasitic arthropods. It has been established (Levenbook, 1951) that the polysaccharide content of the tracheal organ of *Gastrophilus intestinalis* undergoes a cycle which approximates that occurring in entire larvae (von Kemnitz, 1912). The highest concentration was reached in the third instar, where the glycogen content of the tracheal organ rose from 22% of the dry substance in December to the very high value of slightly over 40% in March. After that date a gradual decline occurred up to the time of pupation. During the initial stages of pupation a further marked decline could be observed.

V. STRUCTURAL POLYSACCHARIDES

One of the best-known structural polysaccharides occurring in animals is chitin. It is a complex polysaccharide which yields glucosamine and acetic acid upon acid hydrolysis. It forms the exoskeleton of endoparasitic arthropods, fulfilling the same function as in free-living ones. Von Kemnitz (1916) determined the chitin content of *Gastrophilus intestinalis* larvae as 1.38 to 3.12% of the fresh or 5.13 to 8.98 % of the dry substance.

Whether chitin occurs in parasitic protozoa is questionable. It has been reported as forming the spore capsule of *Nosema apis* (Koehler, 1921) and, tentatively, as constituting the cuticle of the ciliates *Cycloposthium bipalmatum* and *Ophryoscolex* sp. (Schulze, 1924). The tests applied are not entirely convincing, especially in view of recent observations of Wilson and Fairbairn (1961). They found that the oocyst capsule of *Eimeria acervulina* contains a substance which can be isolated by methods used for chitin, but it does not contain *N*-acetyl glucosamine nor is it attacked by chitinase and hence cannot be chitin. Monné and Hönig (1954a) had previously, on histochemical grounds, reached the conclusion that the oocyst shells of several *Eimeria* spp. and of *Isospora felis* do not contain chitin.

It is, however, a well-established fact that the eggshell proper of many nematode species consists at least in part of chitin. A rather extensive literature on the subject exists: Krakow (1892); Jammes and Martin (1910); Fauré-Fremiet (1912, 1913); Schulze (1924); Wottge (1937); Chitwood (1938); Jacobs and Jones (1939); Kreuzer (1953); Monné and Hönig (1954b); Monné (1955, 1963); Guevara Pozo (1957); and Crites (1958). The evidence for chitin in eggshells of nematodes is convincing. It has thus been shown that acid hydrolysis results in formation of glucosamine and *N*-acetyl glucosamine and that upon superheating of the membranes with strong alkali chitosan is formed. Furthermore, Fairbairn and Passey (1955) have shown that the chitinous layer is dissolved by chitinolytic bacteria. The amount of chitin within the shells seems to vary in different species. It is the main constituent of the "chitinous shell" in such forms as *Ascaris* or *Contracoecum,* but not the only one. Monné and Hönig (1954b), basing themselves mainly on optical observations, reached the conclusion that in Heterakidae the chitinous shell is not a uniform structure but that it is formed of alternating chitin layers and protein lamellae. In other nematodes, especially the Strongyloidea and *Echinuria uncinata* the eggs seem to contain only traces of chitin (Monné and Hönig, 1954b; Monné, 1955).

The eggs of Acanthocephala also contain true chitin. It has been reported for the innermost membrane of the *Macracanthorhynchus* egg (von Brand, 1940), for *Acanthocephalus jacksoni* and *Echinorhynchus gadi* (West, 1963). The egg shells of *Polymorphus botulus* and *Polymorphus minutus* apparently contain only traces of the polysaccharide (Monné and Hönig, 1954c).

While there can be no doubt that the nematode and acanthocephalan eggs contain chitin, it should be emphasized that the mere finding of the compound does not imply complete identity of worm and arthropod chitin. Indeed both differ in optical properties (Schmidt, 1936) and by the greater elasticity of the worm chitin (von Brand, 1940; Pick, 1947). The occurrence of chitin in other parts of the worm's body has never been demonstrated conclusively. It has been claimed that the lining of the stoma and esophagus of *Strongylus edentatus* is chitinous (Immink, 1924), but the studies of Chitwood (1938) on the corresponding structures of *Strongylus equinus* cast considerable doubt on this observation.

Much more widely distributed than chitin are mucopolysaccharides which can be separated into acid and neutral compounds. Both are characterized by having hexosamine as one constituent, but the acid mucopolysaccharides, in contrast to the neutral ones, contain either uronic acid, sulfate groups, or both.

Insofar as parasitic protozoa are concerned, there is only histochemical evidence available which seems to indicate that mucopolysaccharides are rather common. Thus hyaluronic acid types of mucopolysaccharide have been found both in the nucleus and the cytoplasm of *Entamoeba histolytica* (Loran *et al.,* 1955) and in the nucleus and the oocyst membranes of *Eimeria tenella,* while its cytoplasm contained mucoid sulfate (Gill and Ray, 1954b). The uncertainties in distinguishing between the various mucopolysaccharides by means of histochemical reactions alone are emphasized by the fact that Hara *et al.* (1954), in contrast to Loran *et al.* (1955), could not find hyaluronic acid in *Entamoeba histolytica;* they identified the acid mucopolysaccharide occurring in nucleus and cytoplasm as chondroitin or mucoitin sulfate. Small amounts of mucopolysaccharides have also been found in trichomonads (Nomura, 1957a; Gerzeli, 1959), hemogregarines (Gerzeli, 1954a), and polycystic gregarines (Stein, 1963). Occasionally compounds are encountered that give polysaccharide reactions, but that are neither glycogen nor mucopolysaccharides. They may be glycoproteins or mucoproteins. Examples are the substance observed by Lavette (1960) in the parabasal apparatus of *Joenia annectens* or the so-called "plastic granules" of *Eimeria* spp. (Patillo and Becker, 1955).

Chemical data on mucopolysaccharides are available for one group of helminths, the cestodes. Small amounts of a polysaccharide have been found in the scoleces of *Echinococcus granulosus* which yields upon acid hydrolysis galactose and glucosamine, but no uronic acid (Agosin *et al.*, 1957). Compounds with the same constituents have then been isolated from the laminated membranes, the scoleces, and the cyst fluid of hydatid cysts by Kilejian *et al.* (1962), who also determined their infrared spectra. An apparently different alkali-stable polysaccharide was encountered by von Brand *et al.* (1964) in larval and adult *Taenia taeniaeformis*. It yielded upon acid hydrolysis glucosamine and *N*-acetyl glucosamine, but no trace of galactose. Since it was not separated from glycogen, no decision is possible as to whether it contained glucose. It is probable that all these substances can be classified as neutral mucopolysaccharides. Less chemical evidence exists in respect to acid mucopolysaccharides. It is, however, probable that they do occur. Lynch and Bogitsh (1962) found in hydrolyzates of *Posthodiplostomum minimum* and its cyst wall uronic acids, besides glucose, galactose, and ribose, while hexosamines were found only in the parasite's body.

In view of these chemical findings it is not surprising that substances identified by histochemical procedures as mucopolysaccharides have been described for cestodes and other helminths. Specifically, they have been found in the scolex and the first proglottids, but not the mature proglottids of *Taenia saginata* by Marzullo *et al.* (1957b), as well as in the basement membrane of the embryophore and in the embryo proper of the same tapeworm by Chowdhuri *et al.* (1956). The occurrence of an acid mucopolysaccharide in the main cuticular layer of several cestode and trematode species has been described by Monné (1959b), but no mucopolysaccharide has been found in the vitellarian cells or in the eggshells of *Paragonimus ohirai* (Yokogawa and Yoshimura, 1957). Mucopolysaccharides have, however, been found in the postacetabular glands of *Schistosoma mansoni* and the mucoid glands of virgulate xiphidiocercariae by Stirewalt (1959) and Ortigoza and Hall (1963), respectively. Muco- or glycoprotein-like substances have been described from the metacercarial wall of *Notocotylus urbanensis* (Singh and Lewert, 1959) and *Posthodiplostomum minimum* (Bogitsh, 1962). Finally, acid mucopolysaccharides have been found throughout the bodies of the nematodes *Ancylostoma duodenale* and *Enterobius vermicularis* (Marzullo *et al.*, 1957a) and the eggshells of *Dictyocaulus* spp. and *Metastrongylus elongatus* (Monné, 1959a).

VI. SEROLOGICALLY ACTIVE POLYSACCHARIDES

Antigenic polysaccharides, or polysaccharide-protein complexes, have been isolated repeatedly from parasitic protozoa. The older studies by Senekjie (1941) and Muniz and DeFreitas (1944) are not supported by detailed chemical analysis. However, Feinberg and Morgan (1953) isolated from *Trichomonas foetus* an immunologically active complex which was homogeneous in a Tiselius apparatus and by ultracentrifuge analysis. After acid hydrolysis the following sugars were found in the polysaccharide moiety: rhamnose, fucose, galactose, xylose, and hexosamine, while the presence of glucose was not established unequivocally. The protein moiety consisted of lysine, arginine, aspartic and glutamic acids, glycine, serine, alanine, threonine, valine, and leucine (isoleucine). It is very curious that the corresponding fractions isolated from various strains of *Trichomonas foetus* were serologically not completely identical (Robertson, 1960), but the chemical basis of this diversity has not yet been elucidated. A similar complex has been isolated by Gonçalves and Yamaha (1959) from the culture form of *Trypanosoma cruzi*. It contained glucose, glucosamine, xylose, mannose, and galactose in the proportion 1:2:4:5:9, and also 11 amino acids.

Antigenic polysaccharide fractions have been isolated repeatedly from various parasitic worms (Campbell, 1936, 1937, 1939; Melcher and Campbell, 1942; Melcher, 1943; Oliver-Gonzalez, 1944; Oliver-Gonzalez and Torregrosa, 1944). A considerable variety of immunological properties has been described for such fractions. Thus, Oliver-Gonzalez (1953) reported that *Trichinella* and *Ascaris* polysaccharides inhibit blood agglutinins, and Heidelberger *et al.* (1954) observed that *Ascaris* glycogen precipitates antipneumococcal sera of various types. Cmelik (1952) isolated from *Echinococcus* cysts various active polysaccharide-containing fractions. The purest fraction consisted of unidentified aldohexoses, deoxypentoses, and glucosamine; it contained but little phosphorus and produced allergic and toxic reactions. Kent (1963) has emphasized that many antigenic fractions isolated from nematodes and cestodes are heteroproteins, often complexed with carbohydrates (frequently glycogen). As an example for nematodes, the ethanol-soluble antigen isolated by Sleeman (1961) from *Trichinella* larvae may be mentioned. It contained 13–17% carbohydrate, which yielded only glucose upon hydrolysis. Trematodes seem to have been studied less in this respect. However, Maekawa *et al.* (1954) purified and even crystallized an antigenic substance from *Fasciola hepatica* which was apparently largely proteinaceous in nature, but also contained carbohydrate, as indicated by a positive Molisch test.

There is some question whether glycogen, the main polysaccharide of many parasites, has antigenic properties. The yield of antigenic material during isolation of polysaccharides from helminths is often so large that the assumption of the active polysaccharide consisting mainly of glycogen seems unavoidable (Baldwin and King, 1942). These authors, however, thought it improbable that glycogen as such would be antigenic. They consider it possible that the antigen may have been present as an impurity in the glycogen fraction, or else that some active prosthetic group was attached to the glycogen. It should be recalled in this connection that Feinberg and Morgan (1953) found the *Trichomonas foetus* glycogen serologically inactive, in contrast to the polysaccharide-protein complex mentioned above, and Lukaskenko (1958) found the polysaccharides isolated from *Trichinella* larvae to be incomplete antigens. On the other hand, Heidelberger *et al.* (1954) used carefully prepared and highly purified glycogen samples from various sources, among them *Ascaris,* and found these polysaccharides definitely antigenic. Further studies along these lines seem indicated and should prove rewarding.

VII. INCOMPLETELY CHARACTERIZED POLYSACCHARIDES

A polysaccharide consisting of galactose, but contaminated with nucleic acid fragments, was isolated from the culture form of *Trypanosoma cruzi* by von Brand *et al.* (1959). The question whether it was split off from the antigenic polysaccharide described by Gonçalves and Yamaha (1959) by the KOH used in its isolation requires further study. Another polysaccharide yielding glucose, galactose, and arabinose upon acid hydrolysis was found in the culture form of *Leishmania donovani* (Chatterjee and Ghosh, 1959).

In helminths, a polysaccharide of unknown constitution has been found to account for a large part of the total polysaccharides of *Litomosoides carinii* (Bueding, 1949). Small amounts of a polysaccharide withstanding diastase digestion and yielding upon hydrolysis a substance giving reactions similar to those of galactose have been isolated from *Macracanthorhynchus hirudinaceus* (von Brand and Saurwein, 1942).

Histochemical evidence, unfortunately so far unsupported by chemical analysis, also points to the possibility that in helminths a greater variety of polysaccharides exists than hitherto suspected. The most common relevant findings are that the substances in question react positively with polysaccharide stains (e.g., the periodic acid-Schiff reaction), that they resist diastase digestion, and that they do not give the common mucopolysaccharide reactions (e.g., metachromasia). Such material has been found in the cuticle of several trematode species (Singh, 1958; Yoshimura and Yokogawa, 1958; Monné, 1959b), in the intestine, the vitellaria, and the ovaries of *Paragonimus westermani* (Hamada, 1959), and in the polar plugs of the eggs of several *Trichuris* spp. (Monné and Hönig, 1954d).

REFERENCES

Abdel-Akher, M., and Smith, F. (1951). *J. Am. Chem. Soc.* **73**, 994–996.

Abou Akkada, A. R., and Howard, B. H. (1960). *Biochem. J.* **76**, 445–451.

Addis, C. J. (1946). *J. Parasitol.* **32**, 574–580.

Addis, C. J., and Chandler, A. C. (1944). *J. Parasitol.* **30**, 229–236.

Agosin, M., and Brand, T. von (1955). *Exptl. Parasitol.* **4**, 548–563.

Agosin, M., Brand, T. von, Rivera, F., and McMahon, P. (1957). *Exptl. Parasitol.* **6**, 37–51.

Archer, D. M., and Hopkins, C. A. (1958). *Exptl. Parasitol.* **7**, 542–554.

Armer, J. M. (1944). *J. Parasitol.* **30**, 131–142.

Axmann, M. C. (1947). *J. Morphol.* **80**, 321–343.

Baldwin, E., and King, H. K. (1942). *Biochem. J.* **36**, 37–42.

Beck, J. W., and Chandler, A. C. (1950). *J. Parasitol.* **36** Suppl., 44.

Beckett, E. B., and Boothroyd, B. (1962). *Ann. Trop. Med. Parasitol.* **56**, 264–273.

Bell, D. J. (1944). *J. Chem. Soc.* pp. 473–476.

Bell, D. J. (1948). *Biol. Rev. Cambridge Phil. Soc.* **23**, 256–266.

Bell, D. J., Gutfreund, H., Cecil, R., and Ogston, A. G. (1948). *Biochem. J.* **42**, 405–408.

Bernard, C. (1859). *Compt. Rend. Soc. Biol.* **1**, [not seen, quoted in Lesser, E. J. (1909). *Ergeb. Physiol.* **8**, 742–796].

Bogitsh, B. J. (1962). *J. Parasitol.* **48**, 55–60.

Bogitsh, B. J. (1963). *Exptl. Parasitol.* **14**, 193–202.

Boxer, G. E., and Devlin, T. M. (1961). *Science* **134**, 1495–1501.

Brand, T. von (1932). *Z. Parasitenk.* **4**, 753–775.

Brand, T. von (1933). *Z. Vergleich. Physiol.* **18**, 562–596.

Brand, T. von (1934). *Z. Vergleich. Physiol.* **21**, 220–235.

Brand, T. von (1937). *J. Parasitol.* **23**, 68–72.

Brand, T. von (1938). *J. Parasitol.* **24**, 445–451.

Brand, T. von (1939). *J. Parasitol.* **25**, 329–342.

Brand, T. von (1940). *J. Parasitol.* **26**, 301–307.

Brand, T. von (1950). *J. Parasitol.* **36**, 178–192.

Brand, T. von (1957). *Z. Tropenmed. Parasitol.* **8**, 21–23.

Brand, T. von (1963). *Ergeb. Mikrobiol. Immunitaetsforsch. Exptl. Therapie* **36**, 1–58.

Brand, T. von, and Bowman, I. B. R. (1961). *Exptl. Parasitol.* **11**, 276–29.7.

Brand, T. von, and Mercado, T. I. (1961). *J. Parasitol.* **47**, 459–463.

Brand, T. von, and Otto, G. F. (1938). *Am. J. Hyg.* **27**, 683–689.

Brand, T. von, and Saurwein, J. (1942). *J. Parasitol.* **28**, 315–318.

Brand, T. von, Weinstein, P. P., Mehlman, B., and Weinbach, E. C. (1952). *Exptl. Parasitol.* **1**, 245–255.

Brand, T. von, McMahon, P., Tobie, E. J., Thompson, M. J., and Mosettig, E. (1959). *Exptl. Parasitol.* **8**, 171–181.

Brand, T. von, Mercado, T. I., Nylen, M. U., and Scott, D. B. (1960). *Exptl. Parasitol.* **9**, 205–214.

Brand, T. von, Bowman, I. B. R., Weinstein, P. P., and Sawyer, T. K. (1963). *Exptl. Parasitol.* **13**, 128–133.

Brand, T. von, McMahon, P., Gibbs, E., and Higgins, H. (1964). *Exptl. Parasitol.* **15**, 410–429.

Brault, A., and Loeper, M. (1904a). *J. Physiol. Pathol. Gen.* **6**, 295–301.

Brault, A., and Loeper, M. (1904b). *J. Physiol. Pathol. Gen.* **6**, 503–512.

Bruskin, B. P. (1959). *Dokl. Akad. Nauk SSSR* **127**, 1315–1316.

Bueding, E. (1949). *J. Exptl. Med.* **89**, 107–130.

Bueding, E. (1962). *Federation Proc.* **21**, 1039–1046.

Bueding, E., and Koletsky, S. (1950). *Proc. Soc. Exptl. Biol. Med.* **73**, 594–596.
Bueding, E., and Orrell, S. A. (1961). *J. Biol. Chem.* **236**, 2854–2857.
Bueding, E., Kmetec, E., Swartzwelder, C., Abadie, S., and Saz, H. J. (1960). *Biochem. Pharmacol.* **5**, 311–322.
Buetschli, O. (1885). *Z. Biol.* **21**, 603–612.
Bullock, W. L. (1949). *J. Morphol.* **84**, 201–225.
Bunge, G. (1883). *Z. Physiol. Chem.* **8**, 48–59.
Bunge, G. (1889). *Z. Physiol. Chem.* **14**, 318–324.
Busch, P. W. C. M. (1905). Dissertation, University of Utrecht.
Campbell, D. H. (1936). *J. Infect. Diseases* **59**, 266–280.
Campbell, D. H. (1937). *J. Parasitol.* **23**, 348–353.
Campbell, D. H. (1939). *J. Infect. Diseases* **65**, 12–15.
Campbell, D. H., and Melcher, L. R. (1940). *J. Infect. Diseases* **66**, 184–188.
Canning, E. U. (1963). *In* "Progress in Protozoology" (J. Ludvik *et al.,* eds.), pp. 439–442. Czech. Acad. Sci., Prague.
Cavier, R., and Savel, J. (1951). *Bull. Soc. Chim. Biol.* **33**, 447–454.
Chatterjee, A. N., and Ghosh, J. J. (1959). *Ann Biochem. Exptl. Med.* (Calcutta) **19**, 37–50.
Cheng, T. C. (1963). *Malacologia* **1**, 291–303.
Cheng, T. C., and Dyckman, E. (1964). *Z. Parasitenk.* **24**, 27–48.
Cheng, T. C., and Snyder, R. W. (1962). *Trans. Am. Microscop. Soc.* **81**, 209–228.
Chitwood, B. G. (1938). *Proc. Helminthol. Soc. Wash., D.C.* **5**, 68–75.
Chowdhuri, A. B., Das Gupta, B., Ray, H. N., and Bhadhuri, V. N. (1955). *Bull. Calcutta Sch. Trop. Med.* **3**, 52 [not seen, quoted in Chowdhuri *et al.,* (1962)].
Chowdhuri, A. B., Das Gupta, B., Ray, H. N., and Bhadhuri, V. N. (1956). *J. Indian Med. Assoc.* **26**, 295–301.
Chowdhuri, A. B., Das Gupta, B., and Ray, H. N. (1962). *Parasitology* **52**, 153–157.
Christophers, S. R., and Fulton, J. D. (1938). *Ann. Trop. Med. Parasitol.* **32**, 43–75.
Cleveland, L. R. (1925). *Biol. Bull.* **48**, 309–326.
Cmelik, S. (1952). *Biochem. Z.* **322**, 456–462.
Codounis, A., and Polydorides, J. (1936). *Proc. 3rd Intern. Congr. Comp. Pathol., Athens, 1936* Vol. 2, pp. 195–202. Eleftheroudakis, Athens.
Coleman, R. M., and Brand, T. von (1957). *J. Parasitol.* **43**, 263–270.
Colucci, A. V., Orrell, S. A., Saz, H. J., and Bueding, E. (1964). *Federation Proc.* **23**, 320.
Colucci, A. V., Orrell, S. A., Bueding, E., and Saz, H. J. (1965). *Federation Proc.* **24**, 512.
Crites, J. L. (1958). *Ohio J. Sci.* **58**, 343–346.
Curtis, M. R., Dunning, W. F., and Bullock, F. D. (1933). *Am. J. Cancer* **17**, 894–923.
Das Gupta, B. (1960). *Parasitology* **50**, 509–514.
Das Gupta, B., and Kulasiri, C. (1959). *Parasitology* **49**, 594–600.
Daugherty, J. W., and Taylor, D. (1956). *Exptl. Parasitol.* **5**, 376–390.
Dawes, B., and Muller, R. (1957). *Nature* **180**, 1217.
Dinulescu, G. (1932). *Ann. Sci. Nat., (Paris), Zool.* **15**, 1–183.
Dobell, C. (1919). "The Amoebae Living in Man," Bale & Danielson, London.
Dobell, C., and O'Connor, F. W. (1921). "The Intestinal Protozoa of Man." Bale & Danielson, London.
Dubosq, O., and Grassé, P. (1933). *Arch. Zool. Exptl. Gen.* **73**, 381–621.
Dunagan, T. T. (1963). *J. Parasitol.* **49**, No. 5, Sect. 2, 18–19.
Dunagan, T. T. (1964). *Proc. Helminthal. Soc. Wash., D.C.* **31**, 166–172.
Dutta, G. P. (1958). *Quart. J. Microscop. Sci.* **99**, 517–521.
Dutta, G. P. (1959). *Res. Bull. (N.S.) Panjab Univ.* **10**, Part I, 13–19.
Eadie, J. M., and Oxford, A. E. (1955). *J. Gen. Microbiol.* **12**, 298–310.

Eadie, J. M., Manners, D. J., and Stark, J. R. (1963). *Biochem. J.* **89**, 91P.
Emery, A. G., and Benedict, F. G. (1911). *Am. J. Physiol.* **28**, 301–307.
Engelbrecht, H. (1963). *Z. Parasitenk.* **23**, 384–389.
Fairbairn, D. (1957). *Exptl. Parasitol.* **6**, 491–554.
Fairbairn, D. (1958a). *Nature* **181**, 1593–1594.
Fairbairn, D. (1958b). *Can. J. Zool.* **36**, 787–795.
Fairbairn, D. (1960). *In* "Nematology" (J. N. Sasser and W. R. Jenkins, eds.), pp. 267–296. Univ. of North Carolina Press, Chapel Hill, North Carolina.
Fairbairn, D., and Passey, B. I. (1955). *Can. J. Biochem. Physiol.* **33**, 130–134.
Fairbairn, D., and Passey, R. F. (1957). *Exptl. Parasitol.* **6**, 566–574.
Fairbairn, D., Wertheim, G., Harpur, R. P., and Schiller, E. L. (1961). *Exptl. Parasitol.* **11**, 248–263.
Fauré-Fremiet, E. (1912). *Bull. Soc. Zool. France* **37**, 83–84.
Fauré-Fremiet, E. (1913). *Arch. Anat. Microscop. (Paris)* **15**, 435–757.
Feinberg, J. G., and Morgan, T. J. (1953). *Brit. J. Exptl. Pathol.* **34**, 104–118.
Fernando, W. (1945). *J. Parasitol.* **31**, 185–190.
Flury, F. (1912). *Arch. Exptl. Pathol. Pharmakol.* **67**, 275–392.
Flury, F., and Leeb, F. (1926). *Klin. Wochschr.* **5**, 2054–2055.
Forsyth, G., and Hirst, E. L. (1953). *J. Chem. Soc.* pp. 2132–2135.
Forsyth, G., Hirst, E. L., and Oxford, A. E. (1953). *J. Chem. Soc.* pp. 2030–2033.
Foster, M. (1865). *Proc. Roy. Soc.* **14**, 543–546.
Fouquey, C., Polonsky, J., and Lederer, E. (1957). *Bull. Soc. Chim. Biol.* **39**, 101–132.
Fouquey, C., Polonsky, J., and Lederer, E. (1958a). *Bull. Soc. Chim. Biol.* **40**, 315–325.
Fouquey, C., Lederer, E., Lüderitz, O., Polonsky, J., Staub, A. M., Stirm, S., Tinelli, R., and Westphal, O. (1958b). *Compt. Rend.* **246**, 2417–2420.
Fouquey, C., Polonsky, J., and Lederer, E. (1959). *Bull. Soc. Chim. France* pp. 803–810.
Gerzeli, G. (1954a). *Riv. Istochim.* **1**, 91–94.
Gerzeli, G. (1954b). *Riv. Istochim.* **1**, 205–210.
Gerzeli, G. (1955). *Riv. Parassitol.* **16**, 209–215.
Gerzeli, G. (1959). *Acta Histochim.* **8**, 191–198.
Gill, B. S., and Ray, H. N. (1954a). *Indian J. Vet. Sci. Animal Husbandry* **24**, 223–228.
Gill, B. S., and Ray, H. N. (1954b). *Indian J. Vet. Sci. Animal Husbandry* **24**, 229–237.
Ginecinskaja, T. A. (1960). *Dokl. Akad. Nauk SSSR* **135**, 1012–1015.
Giovannola, A. (1934). *Arch. Protistenk.* **83**, 270–274.
Giovannola, A. (1935). *Arch. Ital. Sci. Med. Colon.* **16**, 430–436.
Giovannola, A. (1936). *J. Parasitol.* **22**, 207–218.
Glocklin, V. C., and Fairbairn, D. (1952). *J. Cell. Comp. Physiol.* **39**, 341–356.
Goil, M. M. (1957). *Z. Parasitenk.* **18**, 36–39.
Goil, M. M. (1961). *Parasitology* **51**, 335–337.
Gonçalves, J. M., and Yamaha, T. (1959). *Res. Trab. Congr. Intern. Doenca Chagas,* Rio de Janeiro, 1959. pp. 159–160. Oficina Grafica, Universidade do Brasil.
Goodchild, C. G. (1961). *J. Parasitol.* **47**, 401–405.
Goodchild, C. G., and Vilar-Alvarez, C. M. (1962). *J. Parasitol.* **48**, 379–383.
Guevara Pozo, D. (1957). *Rev. Iberica Parasitol.* **17**, 117–148.
Graff, D., and Allen, K. (1963). *J. Parasitol.* **49**, 204–208.
Grant, P. T., and Fulton, J. D. (1957). *Biochem. J.* **66**, 242–250.
Hallman, F. A., Michaelson, J. B., Blumenthal, H., and DeLamater, J. N. (1955). *Exptl. Parasitol.* **4**, 45–53.
Halsall, T. G., Hirst, E. L., and Jones, J. K. N. (1947). *J. Chem. Soc.* pp. 1399–1400.
Hamada, M. (1959). *Shikoku Acta Med.* **14**, 165–186.

Hara, K., Oka, S., Sawada, T., and Fuse, M. (1954). *Gunma J. Med. Sci.* **3**, 249–265.
Harpur, R. P. (1963). *Can. J. Biochem. Physiol.* **41**, 1673–1689.
Harvey, S. C. (1949). *J. Biol. Chem.* **179**, 435–453.
Hedrick, R. M., and Daugherty, J. W. (1957). *J. Parasitol.* **43**, 497–504.
Heidelberger, M., Aisenberg, A. C., and Hassid, W. Z. (1954). *J. Exptl. Med.* **99**, 343–353.
Hellerman, L. (1947). *Trans. Macy Conf. Biol. Antioxidants* **2**, 78–92.
Heyneman, D., and Voge, M. (1957). *J. Parasitol.* **43**, 527–531.
Hirsch, G. C., and Bretschneider, L. H. (1937). *Cytologia (Tokyo)* Fuji Jubilee Vol. 424–436.
Hopkins, C. A. (1950). *J. Parasitol.* **36**, 384–390.
Hopkins, C. A. (1952). *Exptl. Parasitol.* **1**, 196–213.
Hungate, R. E. (1943). *Biol. Bull.* **84**, 157–163.
Hungate, R. E. (1955). *In* "Biochemistry and Physiology of Protozoa" (S. H. Hutner and A. Lwoff, eds.), Academic Press, New York. Vol. 2. pp.159–199.
Immink, B. D. C. M. (1924). *Arch. Anat. Histol. Embryol. Strasbourg* **3**, 281–326.
Jacobs, L., and Jones, M. F. (1939). *Proc. Helminthol. Soc. Wash., D.C.* **6**, 57–60.
Jammes, L., and Martin, A. (1910). *Compt. Rend.* **151**, 250–251.
Kajiro, Y. (1927). *Trans. Japan. Pathol. Soc.* **17**, 213–214.
Kemnitz, G. von (1912). *Arch. Zellforsch.* **7**, 463–603.
Kemnitz, G. von (1916). *Z. Biol.* **67**, 129–244.
Kent, N. H. (1957a). *Exptl. Parasitol.* **6**, 351–357.
Kent, N. H. (1957b). *Exptl. Parasitol.* **6**, 486–490.
Kent, N. H. (1963). *Am. J. Hyg., Monogr. Ser.* **22**, 30–45.
Kent, N. H., and Macheboeuf, M. (1947). *Compt. Rend.* **225**, 602–604.
Kent, N. H., Macheboeuf, M., and Neiadas, B. (1948). *Experientia* **4**, 193–194.
Kessel, R. G., Prestage, J. J., Sekhon, S. S., Smalley, R. L., and Beams, H. W. (1961). *Trans. Am. Microscop. Soc.* **80**, 103–118.
Keysselitz, G. (1906). *Arch. Protistenk.* **7**, 1–174.
Kilejian, A., Schinazi, L. A., and Schwabe, C. W. (1961). *J. Parasitol.* **47**, 181–188.
Kilejian, A., Sauer, K., and Schwabe, C. W. (1962). *Exptl. Parasitol.* **12**, 377–392.
Kjölberg, O., Manners, D. J., and Wright, A. (1963). *Comp. Biochem. Physiol.* **8**, 353–365.
Koehler, A. (1921). *Zool. Anz.* **53**, 84–87.
Krakow, N. P. (1892). *Z. Biol.* **29**, 177–198.
Kreuzer, L. (1953). *Z. Vergleich. Physiol.* **35**, 13–26.
Krijgsman, B. J. (1936). *Z. Vergleich. Physiol.* **23**, 663–711.
Kruidenier, F. J. (1953a). *J. Morphol.* **92**, 531–543.
Kruidenier, F. J. (1953b). *Am. Midland Naturalist* **50**, 382–396.
Kuenen, W. A., and Swellengrebel, N. H. (1913). *Zentr. Bakteriol. Parasitenk., Abt. I: Orig.* **71**, 378–410.
Kuenen, W. A., and Swellengrebel, N. H. (1917). *Geneesk. Tijdschr. Ned. Indie* **57**, 496–506.
Latteur, B. (1958). *Cellule* **109**, 271–296.
Laurie, J. S. (1959). *Exptl. Parasitol.* **8**, 188–197.
Lavette, A. (1960). *Compt. Rend.* **250**, 4202–4204.
Lee, D. L. (1960). *Parasitology* **50**, 247–259.
Lemaire, G., and Ribère, R. (1935). *Compt. Rend. Soc. Biol.* **118**, 1578–1579.
Lesuk, A., and Anderson, R. J. (1941). *J. Biol. Chem.* **139**, 457–469.
Levenbook, L. (1950). *Biochem. J.* **47**, 336–346.
Levenbook, L. (1951). *J. Exptl. Biol.* **28**, 173–180.
Lewert, R. M., and Lee, C. L. (1954). *J. Infect. Diseases* **95**, 13–51.

Lewert, R. M., and Lee, C. L. (1955). *J. Infect. Diseases* **97**, 177–186.

Lillie, R. D. (1947). *J. Lab. Clin. Med.* **32**, 76–88.

Lom, J. (1955). *Cesk. Biol.* **4**, 397–409.

Lom, J. (1960). *Zool. Anz.* **164**, 111–114.

Loran, M. R., Kerner, M. W., and Anderson, H. H. (1955). *Exptl. Parasitol.* **4**, 542–547.

Loran, M. R., Kerner, M. W., and Anderson, H. H. (1956). *Exptl. Cell Res.* **10**, 241–245.

Ludvik, J. (1958). *Zentr. Bakteriol. Parasitenk., Abt. I: Orig.* **172**, 330–350.

Lukaskenko, N. P. (1958). *Med. Parasitol. USSR* **27**, 82–88 [not seen, *Helminthol. Abstr.* (1958), **27**, 36].

Lynch, D. L., and Bogitsh, J. (1962). *J. Parasitol.* **48**, 241–243.

McKee, R. W., Ormsbee, R. A., Anfinsen, C. B., Geiman, Q. M., and Ball, E. G. (1946). *J. Exptl. Med.* **84**, 569–582.

Maekawa, K., Kitazawa, K., and Kushiba, M. (1954). *Compt. Rend. Soc. Biol.* **148**, 763–765.

Manners, D. J., and Ryley, J. F. (1955). *Biochem. J.* **59**, 369–372.

Manners, D. J., and Wright, A. (1961). *J. Chem. Soc.* pp. 2681–2684.

Mansour, T. E. (1959). *Biochim. Biophys. Acta* **34**, 456–464.

Markov, G. S. (1939). *Compt. Rend. Acad. Sci.* URSS **25**, 93–96.

Marshall, P. B. (1948). *Brit. J. Pharmacol.* **3**, 8–14.

Martini, E. (1916). *Z. Wiss. Zool.* **116**, 142–543.

Marzullo, F., Squadrini, F., and Taparelli, F. (1957a). *Boll. Soc. Med. Chir. Modena* **57**, 84–88.

Marzullo, F., Squadrini, F., and Taparelli, F. (1957b). *Boll. Soc. Med. Chir. Modena* **57**, 327–331.

Masson, F. M., and Oxford, A. E. (1951). *J. Gen. Microbiol.* **5**, 664–672.

Mazzocco, P. (1923). *Compt. Rend. Soc. Biol.* **88**, 342–343.

Melcher, L. R. (1943). *J. Infect. Diseases* **73**, 31–39.

Melcher, L. R., and Campbell, D. H. (1942). *Science* **96** 431–432

Melekh, D. A. (1963). *Vestn. Leningrad Univ.* **18**, Ser. Biol. No. 2, 5–13 [not seen, *Chem. Abstr.* (1963), **59**, 9120].

Miller, M. A. (1943). *J. Morphol.* **73**, 19–41.

Monné, L. (1955). *Arkiv Zool.* [2] **9**, 93–113.

Monné, L. (1959a). *Arkiv Zool.* [2] **12**, 99–122.

Monné, L. (1959b). *Arkiv Zool.* [2] **12**, 343–358.

Monné, L. (1963). *Z. Parasitenk.* **22**, 475–483.

Monné, L., and Hönig, G. (1954a). *Arkiv Zool.* [2] **7**, 251–256.

Monné, L., and Hönig, G. (1954b). *Arkiv Zool.* [2] **7**, 261–272.

Monné, L., and Hönig, G. (1954c). *Arkiv Zool.* [2] **7**, 257–260.

Monné, L., and Hönig, G. (1954d). *Arkiv Zool.* [2] **6**, 559–562.

Monteoliva, H. M., and Guevara, P. D. (1958). *Rev. Iberica Parasitol.* **18**, 107–115.

Morita, Y. (1938). *J. Oriental Med.* **28**, No. 3, 38 (English summary).

Mould, D. L., and Thomas, G. J. (1958). *Biochem. J.* **69**, 327–337.

Münnich, H. (1958). *Naturwiss.* **45**, 551–552.

Münnich, H. (1962). *Naturwiss.* **49**, 66–67.

Muniz, J., and DeFreitas, G. (1944). *Rev. Brasil. Biol.* **4**, 421–438.

Nomura, H. (1957a). *Keio Igaku* **34**, 75–88.

Nomura, H. (1957b). *Keio Igaku* **34**, 131–140.

Nouvel, H. (1929). *Bull. Soc. Zool. France* **54**, 124–128.

Nouvel, H. (1931). *Arch. Zool. Exptl. Gen. (Notes et Rev.)* **71**, 53–61.

Odlaug, T. O. (1955). *J. Parasitol.* **41**, 258–262.

Oesterlin, M., and Brand, T. von (1934). *Z. Vergleich. Physiol.* **20**, 251–254.

Ogren, R. E. (1959). *J. Parasitol.* **45**, 575–579.
Oliver-Gonzalez, J. (1944). *J. Infect. Diseases* **74**, 81–84.
Oliver-Gonzalez, J. (1953). *Proc. Soc. Exptl. Biol. Med.* **82**, 559–561.
Oliver-Gonzalez, J., and Torregrosa, M. V. (1944). *J. Infect. Diseases* **74**, 173–177.
Orrell, S. A., and Bueding, E. (1958). *J. Am. Chem. Soc.* **80**, 3800.
Orrell, S. A., and Bueding, E. (1964). *J. Biol. Chem.* **239**, 4021–4026.
Ortigoza, R. O., and Hall, J. E. (1963). *Exptl. Parasitol.* **14**, 160–177.
Ortner-Schoenbach, P. (1913). *Arch. Zellforsch.* **11**, 413–449.
Oxford, A. E. (1951). *J. Gen. Microbiol.* **5**, 83–90.
Palm, V. (1962). *Z. Parasitenk.* **22**, 261–266.
Pandya, G. T. (1961). *Z. Parasitenk.* **20**, 466–469.
Panzer, T. (1913). *Z. Physiol. Chem.* **86**, 33–42.
Passey, R. F., and Fairbairn, D. (1957). *Can. J. Biochem. Physiol.* **35**, 511–525.
Patillo, W. H., and Becker, E. R. (1955). *J. Morphol.* **96**, 61–96.
Payne, F. K. (1923). *Am. J. Hyg.* **3**, 547–597.
Pick, F. (1947). *Compt. Rend. Soc. Biol.* **141**, 983–986.
Pintner, T. (1922). *Sitzber. Akad. Wiss. Wien., Math.-naturw. Kl., Abt. I* **131**, 129–138.
Prenant, M. (1922). *Arch. Morphol. Gen. Exptl.* **5**, 1–474.
Quack, M. (1913). *Arch. Zellforsch.* **11**, 1–50.
Rao, K. H. (1959). *J. Parasitol.* **45**, 347–351.
Read, C. P. (1949). *J. Parasitol.* **35**, Suppl., 96.
Read, C. P. (1956). *Exptl. Parasitol.* **5**, 325–344.
Read, C. P. (1959). *Exptl. Parasitol.* **8**, 365–382.
Read, C. P. (1961). *In* "Comparative Physiology of Carbohydrate Metabolism in Hetero-thermic Animals" (A. W. Martin, ed.), pp. 3–34. Univ. of Washington Press, Seattle, Washington.
Read, C. P., and Rothman, A. H. (1957a). *Exptl. Parasitol.* **6**, 1–7.
Read, C. P., and Rothman, A. H. (1957b). *Exptl. Parasitol.* **6**, 280–287.
Read, C. P., and Rothman, A. H. (1957c). *Exptl. Parasitol.* **6**, 294–305.
Read, C. P., and Rothman, A. H. (1958). *Exptl. Parasitol.* **7**, 191–197.
Read, C. P., and Simmons, J. E. (1963). *Physiol. Rev.* **43**, 263–305.
Read, C. P., Schiller, E. L., and Phifer, K. (1958). *Exptl. Parasitol.* **7**, 198–216.
Reid, W. M. (1942). *J. Parasitol.* **28**, 319–340.
Reid, W. M. (1944). *J. Parasitol.* **30**, Suppl., 12.
Reid, W. M. (1945a). *Am. J. Hyg.* **41**, 150–155.
Reid, W. M. (1945b). *J. Parasitol.* **31**, 406–410.
Ro, M. (1939). *Acta Japon. Med. Trop.* **1**, 29–36.
Robertson, M. (1960). *J. Hyg.* **58**, 207–213.
Robinson, D. L. H. (1956). *J. Helminthol.* **29**, 193–202.
Rogers, W. P. (1945). *Parasitology* **36**, 211–218.
Rybicka, K. (1960). *Exptl. Parasitol.* **10**, 268–273.
Ryley, J. F. (1955). *Biochem. J.* **59**, 353–361.
Ryley, J. F. (1956). *Biochem. J.* **62**, 215–222.
Salisbury, L. F., and Anderson, R. J. (1939). *J. Biol. Chem.* **129**, 505–517.
Schimmelpfennig, G. (1903). *Arch. Wiss. Prakt. Tierheilk.* **29**, 332–376.
Schindera, M. (1922). *Arch. Protistenk.* **45**, 200–240.
Schmidt, W. J. (1936). *Z. Zellforsch. Mikroskop. Anat.* **25**, 181–203.
Scholtyseck, E. (1964). *Z. Zellforsch.* **64**, 688–707.
Schopfer, W. H. (1932). *Rev. Suisse Zool.* **39**, 59–194.
Schulte, H. (1917). *Arch. Ges. Physiol.* **166**, 1–44.
Schulze, P. (1924). *Z. Morphol. Oekol. Tiere* **2**, 643–666.

Seaman, G. R. (1956). *Exptl. Parasitol.* **5**, 138–148.

Senekjie, H. A. (1941). *Am. J. Hyg.* **34**, Sect. C, 63–66.

Singh, K. S. (1958). *Indian J. Helminthol.* **8**, 122–126.

Singh, K. S., and Lewert, R. M. (1959). *J. Infect. Diseases* **104**, 138–141.

Sleeman, H. K. (1961). *Am. J. Trop. Med. Hyg.* **10**, 834–838.

Smorodincev, I., and Bebesin, K. (1936). *Compt. Rend. Acad. Sci. URSS* [N.S.] **2**, 189–191.

Smyth, J. D. (1949). *J. Exptl. Biol.* **26**, 1–14.

Stein, G. A. (1963). *In* "Progress in Protozoology" (J. Ludvik *et al.*, eds.), pp. 294–295. Czech. Acad. Sci., Prague.

Stepanow-Grigoriew, J., and Hoeppli, R. (1926). *Arch. Schiffs- u. Tropen- Hyg.* **30**, 577–585.

Stewart, H. M. (1938). *Am. J. Hyg.* **28**, 80–84.

Stirewalt, M. A. (1959). *Exptl. Parasitol.* **8**, 199–214.

Stirewalt, M. A., and Evans, A. S. (1960). *Exptl. Parasitol.* **10**, 75–80.

Sugden, B., and Oxford, A. E. (1952). *J. Gen. Microbiol.* **7**, 145–153.

Sukhanova, K. M. (1963). *In* "Progress in Protozoology" (J. Ludvik *et al.*, eds.). p. 296. Czech. Acad. Sci., Prague.

Takagi, K. (1962). *Tokushima J. Exptl. Med.* **9**, 60–66.

Takahashi, T. (1959). *Kiseichugaku Zasshi* **8**, 669–676.

Toryu, Y. (1933). *Sci. Rept. Tohoku Imp. Univ., Fourth Ser.* **8**, 65–74.

Trier, H. J. (1926). *Z. Vergleich. Physiol.* **4**, 305–330.

Tsunoda, K., and Ichikawa, O. (1955). *Govt. Expt. Sta. Animal Hyg., Expt. Rept.* **29**, 73–82.

Turchini, J., and Khau-Van-Kien, L. (1958). *Bull. Zool. France* **83**, 251.

Vernberg, W. B., and Hunter, W. S. (1956). *Exptl. Parasitol.* **5**, 441–448.

von Brand, T., *see* Brand, T. von.

von Kemnitz, G., *see* Kemnitz, G. von.

Waitz, J. A. (1963). *J. Parasitol.* **49**, 73–80.

Wantland, W. W., Wantland, E. M., and Weidman, T. A. (1962). *J. Parasitol.* **48**, 305.

Ward, H. L. (1952). *J. Parasitol.* **38**, 493–494.

Wardle, R. A. (1937). *Can. J. Res.* **D15**, 117:126.

Weineck, E. (1931). *Jena Z. Naturw.* **65**, 739–750.

Weinland, E. (1901a). *Z. Biol.* **41**, 69–74.

Weinland, E. (1901b). *Z. Biol.* **42**, 55–90.

Weinland, E., and Brand, T. von (1926). *Z. Vergleich. Physiol.* **4**, 212–285.

Wendel, W. B. (1946). *Federation Proc.* **5**, 406–407.

West, A. J. (1963). *J. Parasitol.* **49**, No. 5, Sect. 2, 42–43.

Westphal, A. (1934). *Z. Parasitenk.* **7**, 71–117.

Williamson, J., and Desowitz, R. S. (1961). *Exptl. Parasitol.* **11**, 161–175.

Wilmoth, J. H., and Goldfisher, R. (1945). *J. Parasitol.* **32**, Suppl., 22.

Wilson, P. A. G., and Fairbairn, D. (1961). *J. Protozool.* **8**, 410–416.

Wottge, K. (1937). *Protoplasma* **29**, 31–59.

Wright, K. A. (1963a). *J. Ultrastruct. Res.* **9**, 143–155.

Wright, K. A. (1963b). *J. Morphol.* **112**, 233–259.

Yamao, Y. (1952). *Zool. Mag. Tokyo* **61**, 317–322.

Yokogawa, M., and Yoshimura, H. (1957). *Kiseichugaku Zasshi* **6**, 546–554.

Yoshimura, H., and Yokogawa, M. (1958). *Kiseichugaku Zasshi* **7**, 363–369.

Chapter 3

CARBOHYDRATES II:
METABOLISM OF CARBOHYDRATES

I. ASSIMILATION AND LEAKAGE OF CARBOHYDRATES

Many protozoan and metazoan parasites are dependent on the availability of carbohydrates in their environments. Thus, the blood-stream form of African pathogenic trypanosomes die in a few minutes if kept *in vitro* in sugar-free surroundings (literature in von Brand, 1951); on the other hand, the culture form of *Trypanosoma cruzi* remains alive for hours in sugar-deficient media (von Brand and Agosin, 1955) and the culture forms of *Trypanosoma gambiense* develop equally well in sugar-poor and sugar-rich culture media (Reichenow, 1937). As to metazoan parasites, a definite carbohydrate requirement has been demonstrated for cestodes and Acanthocephala (literature in C. P. Read and Simmons, 1963). It finds its expression in a low percentage of establishment in the final host, and/or poor growth or egg production when the host's diet is either deficient in quantity or quality of carbohydrate.

An interesting question is whether the absorption of soluble sugars involves active transport mechanisms. Little work along such lines has been done with parasitic protozoa, but the analysis of the galactose and fructose uptake by the culture form of *Trypanosoma cruzi* (Warren and Kitzman, 1963; Warren and Patrzek, 1963) indicates the functioning of such mechanisms. However, in addition to them, a diffusion component becomes evident at high external substrate concentrations. The interaction of these two components results in two bisecting lines when galactose utilization is plotted as a function of substrate concentration (Lineweaver-Burke plot). There is good evidence that active mechanisms are involved in cestodes. Phifer (1960a,b,c) has shown that the glucose absorption of *Hymenolepis diminuta* is independent of the environmental potassium concentration and of the external glucose concentration above a certain level, and that it takes place against a concentration gradient. In this tapeworm sodium transport and glucose uptake seem not to be linked, nor does cholinesterase play a role. Lee *et al.* (1963) have shown that the inhibition of sodium transport by strophanthin G did not alter the rate of glucose absorption, nor did inhibition of cholinesterase activity through preincubation of the worms with eserine sulfate. It is quite evident, however, that these findings cannot be generalized. Thus, Schwabe (1959) and Schwabe *et al.* (1961) found that cholinesterase has an influence on the permeability of the *Echinococcus* cysts and that eserine affects the movement of glucose through its wall. A different type of evidence is available for the adults of *Taenia taeniaeformis*. Von Brand *et al.* (1964) have demonstrated for it (but not for the larval form) a very distinct glucose absorption against a concentration gradient, but in this case the glucose absorption has an absolute sodium requirement, apparently corresponding closely to the sodium pump of vertebrate tissues.

Some indications exist that the sites of entry may not be identical for all hexoses. Pointing in this direction is the observation that both in the culture form of *Trypanosoma cruzi* (Warren, 1961) and in *Taenia taeniaeformis* (von Brand *et al.* 1964) the glucose absorption is, within wide limits, independent of the external concentration, while the galactose absorption, on the contrary, is clearly dependent on environmental concentration. Furthermore, Phifer's (1960c) finding that sugars other than glucose and sugar derivatives, even when present in twice the concentration of glucose, do not interfere with the glucose absorption of *Hymenolepis diminuta* is suggestive. However, C. P. Read (1961b) found that galactose, allose, 1-deoxyglucose, 6-deoxygalactose, and some sugar derivatives inhibit glucose absorption competitively, while fructose, mannose, fucose, and some other carbohydrates are ineffective in this respect. Separate systems for the permeation of glucose and galactose into this tapeworm are also indicated by Rothman's (1959) observation that sodium taurocholate interferes only with anaerobic glycolysis when glucose is the substrate, but not when galactose is.

It is evident that the absorption of soluble carbohydrates takes place through the surface in cestodes and Acanthocephala. In nematodes the site of absorption is undoubtedly the intestinal canal. The cuticle of *Ascaris lumbricoides* is impermeable to soluble sugars (Cavier and Savel, 1952); in the case of *Ascaridia galli* a glucose uptake through the cuticle has been described (Weatherly *et al.* 1963), but it was quantitatively totally insignificant. The role of the intestinal canal in trematodes is rather obscure, since Mansour (1959a) found, surprisingly, that *Fasciola hepatica* removes practically identical amounts of glucose from the medium whether the intestine is prevented from absorbing by a ligature at the anterior end or whether it has an opportunity to function normally. The electron microscopic studies of Threadgold (1963) have shown that pinocytosis may be involved in cuticular absorption.

While soluble sugars can then be absorbed through the external surface or through some internal surface, such as the intestinal tract, these are not the only possibilities of acquiring carbohydrate. Incorporation of soluble carbohydrates by pinocytosis may occur also in parasitic protozoa, since the process has been demonstrated for the free-living amoeba *Chaos chaos* (Chapman-Andresen and Holter, 1955). Related to this latter type of food intake is the incorporation of formed carbohydrates by means of food vacuoles. It is well known that such protozoa as parasitic amoebas (Dobell and Laidlaw, 1926; newer data in D. L. Hopkins and Warner, 1946; Benham and Havens, 1958; and others) and rumen ciliates (Trier, 1926; Westphal, 1934; Sugden and Oxford, 1952) avidly engulf starch granules both *in vivo* and *in vitro*. However, the nature of the starch granules is of great importance, not all starches being equally well suited as food material. In some ciliates the decisive factor may be the size of the granules, the size range engulfed being determined by the size of the cytostome. On this basis Oxford (1955) explains the fact that *Isotricha intestinalis* ingests larger starch granules than *Isotricha prostoma*. Other unknown factors are, however, sometimes of even greater importance. For instance, *Isotricha* readily engulfs rice starch, but only trace amounts of the relatively small amylopectin granules deposited in its body, when the latter are offered in the medium (Eadie and Oxford, 1955). In view of the way in which parasitic amoebas incorporate formed food particles it does not seem probable that the size of the starch granules, of course within limits, determines their uptake. It has been shown, nevertheless, that the cultivation of *Entamoeba histolytica* is favored by the following sequence of starches: wheat > potato > yucca > white sweet potato > plantain > corn. Corn starch was utilized only in traces, if at all and did not allow maintenance of cultures over long periods (T. R. Read and Faust, 1958). Curiously enough, different strains of the amoeba did not respond in entirely identical fashion to the various starches tested (Faust and Read, 1959).

Of the methods used in determining whether a given carbohydrate can be utilized by parasites, by far the most satisfactory one is demonstration of substrate disappearance by enzymatic or chemical procedures. Nearly as convincing is the search for increased oxygen consumption or anaerobic carbon dioxide production induced by a sugar. Results gained by other indirect methods, such as demonstration of deposition of reserve carbohydrate, acid formation, prolongation of life or motility *in vitro,* or increased growth in cultures should be interpreted with caution. The possibility of secondary effects on metabolic sequences different from those of interest at the moment, or the masking of the measured criterion by concomitant metabolic reactions (e.g., neutralization of excreted acids by ammonia) can lead to misinterpretations. The availability of many carbohydrates and related compounds (such as alcohols, or glycosides) to many species of parasitic protozoa and worms has been tested by one or the other of these methods. It is impossible to show all the results of these investigations; a few examples are given in Tables XII and XIII.

As a result of these investigations the generalization that relatively few protozoa consume pentoses, sugar alcohols, or glycosides is permissible. Many use several hexoses and disaccharides freely. Fructose is in many cases consumed at a rate comparable to that of glucose, while galactose is commonly used at lower rate. A few points only require special mention.

A study of the literature reveals that in some cases an author reports a given sugar as utilized by a certain species of protozoa, while another finds it is not absorbed. Differences in technique may be responsible for some of the divergent results, but they do not explain all such cases. There is no question but that strain differences occur. A case in point is *Crithidia fasciculata;* as shown in Table XII one strain consumes xylose, another does not. Other similar instances have been described by Guttman (1963) for trypanosomids and by Teras (1963) for *Trichomonas vaginalis.* In this latter case the acid production from various sugars was apparently fairly similar from strain to strain, but remarkable differences in gas production were observed.

A curious situation exists in respect to mannose. It is rather freely utilized by many protozoa, indeed at a somewhat higher rate than glucose by the blood-stream form of *Trypanosoma lewisi* (Mercado, 1947) and *Plasmodium knowlesi* (Maier and Coggeshall, 1941). On the contrary, the sugar is toxic to the holotrich rumen protozoa (Sugden and Oxford, 1952), as are, incidentally, glucosamine and galactosamine. In fact, Oxford (1958) used overnight exposure of mixed material of holotrichs and of *Epidinium ecaudatum* to 0.5% mannose to eliminate the holotrich ciliates and thus to achieve purification of his *Epidinium* material.

The disaccharide trehalose is used by several trichomonads (C. P. Read, 1957a; Doran, 1957), but not by all species (Doran, 1958). Weinman (1957, 1960) and Geigy *et al.* (1959) reported that normally non-infectious cultures of *Trypanosoma gambiense* and *Trypanosoma rhodesiense* developed forms infective to vertebrates if grown in the presence of trehalose and provided that the cultures had been isolated fairly recently from a vertebrate host. However, no proof of causal connection between trehalose and developing infectivity was brought forward. Indeed, later studies (Bowman, *et al.*, 1960a) showed that neither the African trypanosomes nor *Trypanosoma cruzi* utilized trehalose when it is present in the culture medium, but that the usual culture media contain a trehalase which breaks down the disaccharide to glucose rather rapidly, which then, of course, is consumed by the flagellates. The nonavailability of trehalose seems to be a character common to most, if not all trypanosomids (cf. the data presented for various species by Cosgrove, 1959, and Zeledon, 1960a).

Of alcohols, only glycerol is utilized by many protozoan species. It is consumed by some trypanosomes (Harvey, 1949; Thurston, 1958) or plasmodia (Fulton, 1939; Maier and Coggeshall, 1941; Marshall, 1948a) at approximately the same, or occasionally even at higher rate, than glucose. Ryley (1962) has shown recently that the culture forms of *Trypanosoma rhodesiense* use glycerol in preference to glucose aerobically and anaerobically, when both substrates are offered simultaneously. The blood-stream forms, on the contrary, withdraw aerobically both glucose and glycerol from a mixture of both substrates, but only glucose in the absence of oxygen. Only occasionally is a species found that uses freely alcohols other than glycerol. An example is *Crithidia fasciculata,* whose endogenous oxygen consumption is raised by 200 to 300% when the following compounds are available as only substrates: ethyl, *n*-propyl, *n*-butyl, isobutyl, and *n*-amyl alcohol (Cosgrove, 1959).

The rates of glucose utilization of various species of protozoa are evidently different in many cases, but it is difficult to present precise and meaningful figures, since the sugar consumption is usually referred to a unit number of organisms rather than to unit weight, because of technical difficulties of obtaining reliable weight figures. Occasionally data are presented on a nitrogen or dry weight basis; some of the pertinent experiments are shown in Table XIV. The glucose consumption of the bloodstream forms of the African pathogenic trypanosomes is especially high. Older experiments (Christophers and Fulton, 1938) already had shown that it approximates 50 to 100% of their dry weight in 1 hour, a figure in fair agreement with the newer ones reported by Ryley (1956). Undoubtedly, differences in the rates of glucose consumption occur between the various stages in the life cycle of parasitic protozoa. It is thus quite certain that the culture forms of the African trypanosomes (corresponding to the stages occurring in the intestine of the tsetse fly) consume less sugar than the blood-stream forms (von Brand *et al.*, 1955; Ryley, 1962). Indeed it has been assumed that the presumptive scarcity of sugar in the

TABLE XII

UTILIZATION OF SOME CARBOHYDRATES BY SOME PARASITIC PROTOZOA[a,b]

Species	Ribose	Xylose	Glucose	Fructose	Mannose	Galactose	Maltose	Saccharose	Lactose	Raffinose	Glycerol	References
Trypanosomids												
Blastocrithidia culicis	x	–	x	x	x	x	–	–		–		Cosgrove (1963)
Crithidia acanthocephali	x	–	x	x	x	x	–	x		x		Cosgrove (1963)
Crithidia fasciculata C	x	x	x	x	x	x	x	x		x		Cosgrove (1963)
Crithidia fasciculata N	x	–	x	x	x	x	x	x		x		Cosgrove (1963)
Crithidia flexonema	x	–	x	x	x	x	–	x		x		Cosgrove (1963)
Endotrypanum schaudinni			x	x	x	x	x	x		(x)		Zeledon (1960a)
Leishmania enrietti	x		x	x	x	x	x	x		x		Zeledon (1960a)
Leptomonas collosoma		–	x	x	x	x	–	x		x		Cosgrove (1963)
Strigomonas oncopelti			x	x	x	x	x	x	x			Ryley (1955a)
Trypanosoma cruzi			x	x	x	x	x	–		–	x	Zeledon (1960a)
Trypanosoma lewisi, blood-stream form		–	x	x	x	–	–		–		x	Ryley (1951)
Trypanosoma rhodesiense			x	x	x	–					x	Ryley (1962)
Trichomonads												
Trichomonas gallinae			x	x	x	x	x	x		–	–	C. P. Read (1957a); Lindblom (1961)
Trichomonas foetus			x	x	x	x	x	x	x	–		Ryley (1955b); Doran (1957); Lindblom (1961); Bellelli and Bonacci (1961)

Trichomonas vaginalis	—	x	x	x	x	—	—	—	Tsukahara (1957, 1961)
Sporozoa									
Plasmodium knowlesi	—	x	x	x	—	x	—	—	x	Fulton (1939); Maier and Coggeshall (1941)
Ciliates									
Dasytricha ruminantium	—	x	—	x	x	x	—	x	Oxford (1951); Heald and Oxford (1953); Howard (1959a)
Isotricha intestinalis + *Isotricha prostoma*	—	x	x	—	x	—	x	Gutierrez (1955); Howard (1959a)

[a] Data on the usability of other carbohydrates and related compounds, as well as on additional species will be found in several of the papers quoted in this table. Further relevant material will be found in the following papers: For trypanosomids: Kudicke and Evers (1924); Colas-Belcour and Lwoff (1925); Noguchi (1926); Kligler (1926); Ivanov and Jakovlev (1943); Plunkett (1946); Mercado (1947); Chang (1948); Fulton and Joyner (1949); Chatterjee and Ghosh (1959); Cosgrove (1959); Guttman (1963); for trichomonads: Cailleau (1937); Trussell and Johnson (1941); Plastridge (1943); Cole (1950); Ninomiya and Suzuoki (1952); Suzuoki and Suzuoki (1951a); Baba *et al.* (1957); Doran (1958); for ciliates: Sugden and Oxford (1952); Williams *et al.* (1961); G. S. Coleman (1962).

[b] Key: x indicates that a compound is utilized; (x) indicates utilization in traces only; — indicates that a compound is not used.

TABLE XIII
Utilization of Some Carbohydrates by Helminths[a,b]

Species	Glucose	Fructose	Mannose	Galactose	Maltose	Saccharose	Lactose	Trehalose	References
Trematodes									
Entobdella bumpusi	—								Laurie (1961)
Himasthla quissetensis	x	—	x						Vernberg and Hunter (1963)
Macraspis cristata	x			—	—	—			Laurie (1961)
Schistosoma mansoni	x	x	x	—	—	—	—	—	Bueding (cited in von Brand, 1952)
Cestodes									
Calliobothrium verticillatum	x	(x)	(x)	x					C. P. Read (1957b); Laurie (1961)
Cittotaenia sp.	x	—	—	x	x	x	—	—	C. P. Read and Rothman (1958a)
Hymenolepis citelli	x	—	—	x	—	—	—	—	C. P. Read and Rothman (1958a)
Hymenolepis diminuta	x	—	(x)	x	—	—	—	—	Laurie (1957)
Hymenolepis nana	x	—	—	x	—	—	—	—	C. P. Read and Rothman (1958a)
Lacistorhynchus tenuis	x	—	—	x	—	—		—	C. P. Read (1957b)
Multiceps serialis, adult	x	x		—		—			Esch (1964)
Multiceps serialis, larva	x	—		—					Esch (1964)
Taenia taeniaeformis, adult	x	—	(x)	x					von Brand et al. (1964)
Taenia taeniaeformis, larva	x	(x)	(x)	x					von Brand et al. (1964)

Acanthocephala								
Moniliformis dubius	x	x	x	x	—	—		Laurie (1957, 1959)
Neoechinorhynchus pseudemydis	x	x	x	x	—	x		Dunagan (1962)
Nematodes								
Ascaris lumbricoides	x	x	—	x	x	—		Cavier and Savel (1952)
Ascaris lumbricoides, eggs	x	x	x	x	x			Hoshino and Suzuki (1956)
Litomosoides carinii	x	x	x	—				Bueding (1949a)

[a] Data on the availability of other carbohydrates and related compounds, as well as on additional species will be found in this table. Further relevant material will be found in the following papers: Weinland and Ritter (1902); Stephenson (1947a); von Brand and Simpson (1944).

[b] KEY: x indicates that a compound is utilized; (x) indicates utilization in traces only or questionable utilization; — indicates that a compound is not utilized.

tsetse's intestine is responsible for the rapid transition from the un-economic pyruvic acid fermentation shown by the blood-stream forms to the more complete degradation of sugar characterizing the metabolism of the culture forms (von Brand et al., 1953). Similarly, it is well known that the blood stages of malarial parasites consume large amounts of glucose (see literature in Table XIV), and it can be assumed, although no

TABLE XIV

AEROBIC AND ANAEROBIC GLUCOSE CONSUMPTION OF SOME TRYPANOSOMATIDAE[a,b]

Species	Temperature °C	Aerobic (μmole glucose in 1 mg dry tissue in 1 hour)	Anaerobic (μmole glucose in 1 mg dry tissue in 1 hour)
Trypanosoma cruzi, blood-stream form	37	0.63	1.05
Trypanosoma cruzi, culture form	30	0.24	0.33
Trypanosoma lewisi, blood-stream form	37	0.91	0.81
Strigomonas oncopelti, culture form	30	2.76	3.35
Trypanosoma congolense, blood-stream form	37	1.58	1.77
Trypanosoma vivax, blood-stream form	37	1.37	0.98
Trypanosoma rhodesiense, blood-stream form	37	1.50	1.67
Trypanosoma gambiense, blood-stream form	37	0.80	1.35
Trypanosoma brucei, blood-stream form	37	3.74	1.38
Trypanosoma evansi, blood-stream form	37	4.00	3.10
Trypanosoma equinum, blood-stream form	37	3.22	2.82
Trypanosoma equiperdum, blood-stream form	37	1.71	2.05

[a] Calculated from Ryley's 1956 data.
[b] Further data on glucose consumption of parasitic protozoa will be found in the papers of the following authors: For Trypanosomatidae: Regendanz (1930); Geiger et al. (1930); Yorke et al. (1929); von Issekutz (1933); von Brand (1933b); Chen and Geiling (1945); Moulder (1947, 1948b); von Brand and Tobie (1948, 1959); Agosin and von Brand (1954); von Brand et al. (1955); Ryley (1962); for Trichomonadidae: Andrews and von Brand (1938); Cole (1950); for Sporozoa: Christophers and Fulton (1938); Fulton (1939); Wendel (1943); McKee et al. (1946); Marshall (1948a); Ball et al. (1948); Manwell and Feigelson (1949); Warren and Manwell (1954); Khabir and Manwell (1955); Manwell and Loeffler (1964).

precise data are yet available, that the parasites have not access to similar quantities once they have reached the intermediate host (von Brand, 1963).

In view of the fact that nearly all parasitic protozoa studied so far utilize, or even seem to require, soluble carbohydrates, it is not surprising that the latter are usually a component of the media used for cultivation. It is evident that a utilization of these carbohydrates by the protozoa can only be deduced if the cultures are axenic. In the presence of other microorganisms indirect effects cannot be ruled out. It has thus been claimed that *Entamoeba histolytica* cannot utilize glucose directly, but, at least in the Shaffer-Frye medium, only degradation products of glucose liberated by the penicillin-inhibited *Streptobacillus* present in the cultures (Hallman *et al.*, 1954; Loran *et al.*, 1956). Other authors, however, have found that the amoeba can utilize glucose directly (Kun and Bradin, 1953; Nakamura *et al.*, 1953; Becker and Geiman, 1955; Entner and Hall, 1955); strain differences may lie at the root of these divergent results.

The soluble carbohydrate added to routine cultures of parasitic protozoa is usually glucose. To give a few examples: Glucose has been employed in the defined media used to cultivate *Leishmania tarentolae* (Trager, 1957), *Strigomonas oncopelti* (Newton, 1957), or *Crithidia fasciculata* (Kidder and Dutta, 1958), or the complicated and chemically undefined media used in the cultivation of *Trypanosoma cruzi* and the African pathogenic trypanosomes (von Brand *et al.*, 1949; Tobie *et al.*, 1950; Citri, 1954). Other types of carbohydrates, though employed frequently in cultures for experimental purposes, are only rarely added to routine cultures serving maintenance of strains. An example is maltose which is used by Kupferberg (1955) in his defined medium allowing maintenance of *Trichomonas vaginalis*. Quinn *et al.* (1962) have developed a synthetic medium allowing short-time cultures of axenic rumen ciliates; it contains a variety of carbohydrates (cellobiose, fructose, glucose, maltose, sucrose, and xylose).

While the spectrum of utilizable carbohydrates is broad in the majority of parasitic protozoa studied so far, it is quite restricted in many cestodes (see Table XIII), consisting essentially of glucose and galactose. A few exceptions to this rule have been reported, however. Thus, *Cittotaenia* sp. (C. P. Read and Rothman, 1958a) and *Phyllobothrium foliatum* (Laurie, 1961) utilize maltose at an even faster rate than glucose. Of interest also is the case of *Multiceps serialis;* the adult, in contrast to the larval form, is able to utilize fructose (Esch, 1964), a sugar appearing to be a regular constituent of the diet of the adult worm's host (coyote). It is rather curious that, in contrast to all other cestodes studied to date, neither larval nor adult *Multiceps* seem able to consume appreciable amounts of galactose. However, caution in accepting this finding as final may be indicated. Esch's conclusion is based on the observation that environmental galactose does not raise the oxygen consumption above the endogenous rate. However, a replacement of endogenous metabolism by degradation of absorbed galactose cannot be ruled out. A case in point is *Fasciola hepatica,* where the presence of glucose in the medium does not alter materially the rate of oxygen consumption, even though it can be shown by chemical methods that the worms absorb large amounts of the sugar (Mansour, 1959a).

The few Acanthocephala studied have a broader range of utilizable carbohydrates than cestodes, as have nematodes. In the case of trematodes too few sugars have been tried to allow any deductions. Some details concerning these groups are shown in Table XIII.

Great variations in the rates of glucose consumption are found in different species of helminths (Table XV). In such forms as *Schistosoma mansoni* (Bueding *et al.,* 1947), *Litomosoides carinii* (Bueding, 1949a), *Dracunculus insignis* (Bueding and Oliver-Gonzalez, 1950), or *Dirofilaria uniformis* (von Brand *et al.,* 1963) they are very high, the amounts of glucose taken from the medium corresponding in 24 hours to 50 to 80% of the worm's fresh body weight. The other extreme is represented by the larval *Eustrongylides ignotus* (von Brand and Simpson, 1944) which consumes in 24 hours glucose corresponding to less than 1% of its body weight.

Just as in the previously discussed cultures of protozoa, carbohydrates are often used as constituents of media employed to culture or simply to maintain helminths *in vitro.* Only a few examples for such uses can be given here. Senft and Senft (1962) added 100 mg% of glucose to the medium employed by them for culturing *Schistosoma mansoni,* the same amount used by Taylor (1963) during corresponding experiments with *Taenia crassiceps.* Berntzen (1962), on the other hand, employs in one of his media used in culturing *Hymenolepis nana* glycogen, glucose, and maltose, and in a second one sucrose, fructose, and glucose. While it can be assumed that in these cases the presence of carbohydrate is beneficial, or even essential to the worms, Friedl (1961) found only a questionable degree of beneficial influence of glucose and galactose in his attempts to keep rediae of *Fascioloides magna* alive *in vitro.* Finally, in cultivating the free-living stages of *Nippostrongylus muris* and *Necator americanus,* Weinstein (1953) added 100 mg% of glucose to the media, a concentration also useful for cultivating the infective stages of *Nippostrongylus* (Weinstein and Jones, 1959), while Earl's (1959) media for the *in vitro* maintenance of *Dirofilaria immitis* contained 250 mg% glucose.

TABLE XV
AEROBIC AND ANAEROBIC GLUCOSE CONSUMPTION OF SOME HELMINTHS[a]

Species	Temperature (°C)	Aerobic (μmole glucose in 1 mg dry tissue in 1 hour)	Anaerobic (μmole glucose in 1 mg dry tissue in 1 hour)	References
Trematodes				
Fasciola hepatica	37.5	0.15	0.19	Mansour (1959a)
Schistosoma mansoni	37.5	1.10		Bueding et al. (1947)
Cestodes				
Anthobothrium variable	20	0.11		Laurie (1961)
Calliobothrium verticillatum	20	0.11		Laurie (1961)
Disculiceps pileatum	20	0.017		Laurie (1961)
Hymenolepis diminuta	38	0.43		Fairbairn et al. (1961)
Inermiphyllidium pulvinatum	20	0.16		Laurie (1961)
Lacistorhynchus tenuis	20	0.18		Laurie (1961)
Onchobothrium pseudo-uncinatum	20	0.040		Laurie (1961)
Orygmatobothrium dohrnii	20	0.038		Laurie (1961)
Phyllobothrium foliatum	20	0.009		Laurie (1961)
Taenia taeniaeformis	37	0.07	0.10	von Brand et al. (1964)
Nematodes				
Eustrongylides ignotus	37	0.0007		von Brand and Simpson (1944)
Litomosoides carinii	37.5	0.68		Bueding (1949a)

[a] Data on other species in Bueding and Oliver-Gonzalez (1950); Warren and Guevara (1962); von Brand et al. (1963).

It is a curious fact that several species of tapeworms leak carbo-hydrate when kept outside the host. This phenomenon has been de-scribed by Daugherty and Taylor (1956) for *Hymenolepis diminuta,* by Schwabe *et al.* (1961) for the hydatid cyst, and by Esch (1964) for *Multiceps. Calliobothrium* and *Lacistorhynchus* leak carbohydrate only when exposed to phloridzin (Laurie, 1961). The most detailed information is available for larval and adult *Taenia taeniaeformis.* Von Brand and Bowman (1961) established that the larval worms excreted much larger amounts than the adult ones and they identified by specific enzymatic assay the largest fraction of eliminated carbohydrate as glucose. How-ever, two other unidentified carbohydrates were eliminated in smaller amounts. Von Brand *et al.* (1964) reported later that in glucose-containing media the transition from leakage to absorption took place at external glu-cose concentrations of 100 to 200 mg% in the case of the larva, but at 12.5 mg% in that of the adults. Presence of relatively high concentrations of sugars other than glucose, such as galactose, fructose, or mannose, did not prevent glucose leakage, a fact also observed by Esch (1964) for *Multiceps.* Indeed, the adult *Taenia* excreted in the presence of galac-tose more glucose than in a completely sugar-free medium. The glucose leakage reached very high levels when adult worms were kept in a sodium-free Tyrode solution. The significance of carbohydrate leakage in cestodes is obscure. At the present stage of our knowledge it is most likely that it is a pathological process in response to unphysiological *in vitro* conditions.

II. POLYSACCHARIDE SYNTHESIS

The polysaccharides stored by endoparasites seem to be derived in most, but not all cases, from exogenous carbohydrate. It has thus been shown that *Entamoeba histolytica* specimens taken from starch-contain-ing cultures are very rich in glycogen (Morita, 1938) and that a parallel-ism exists between the starch content of the medium, the degree of starch uptake, and the polysaccharide deposition in rumen ciliates (Usuelli, 1930; Trier, 1926; Westphal, 1934). The polysaccharide synthesis pro-ceeds in these latter protozoa at a very rapid rate. Previously starved *Diplodinium maggii* show the beginning of intracellular polysaccharide deposition 2 hours after having been fed cellulose (Hungate, 1943b) and similar observations have been reported for sugar-fed holotrich rumen ciliates (Oxford, 1951; Gutierrez, 1955). It is rather remarkable that *Isotricha* can accumulate so much amylopectin that it finally bursts open, indicating that it does not possess regulatory mechanisms limiting the deposition of polysaccharide (Sugden and Oxford, 1952). The observa-tions reviewed so far are derived from experiments carried out *in vitro.*

There can be little doubt that analogous relationships also hold *in vivo.* It has thus been shown that the polysaccharide content of *Nyctotherus ovalis* is greatly increased in specimens taken from roaches kept on a high carbohydrate diet as compared to those isolated from starving insects or hosts kept on high protein or high fat diet (Armer, 1944).

A rapid rate of glycogen synthesis from exogenous carbohydrates has been described for several helminths. The older relevant experiments of Weinland and Ritter (1902) with *Ascaris,* and those of Wardle (1937) and Markov (1939) with cestodes are not entirely convincing because the worms were not kept in an axenic condition. In more recent years experiments with either aseptically isolated worms, or with worms sterilized by antibiotics have definitely proved the utilization of exogenous carbohydrates for polysaccharide synthesis. For trematodes, Mansour (1959a) has shown that worms starved for 24 hours *in vitro* and then fed glucose for 24 hours resynthesize practically all the glycogen lost and histochemical evidence (von Brand and Mercado, 1961) indicates that the resynthesized polysaccharide is deposited in the same organs from where it was lost, especially the suckers and the parenchyma. Bueding and Orrell (1961) have shown that during starvation high molecular weight glycogen disappears to a greater extent than the fraction with lower molecular weight. However, after refeeding the balance between the two fractions is reestablished. In the case of *Hymenolepis diminuta* more UC^{14}-glucose is incorporated into the low than the high molecular weight fraction during resynthesis of glycogen after previous severe glycogen depletion (Colucci *et al.,* 1964). However, when glycogen synthesis is studied in worms which had undergone previously moderate or no glycogen depletion, higher specific activity appeared in the high than the low molecular weight fraction, apparently indicating that the relationships between the two fractions are complex (Colucci *et al.,* 1964). It is probable that glycogen synthesis from glucose is involved in maintaining the glycogen levels of *Schistosoma mansoni* (Robinson, 1956) or *Haplometra cylindracea* (Dawes and Muller, 1957) normal even after several weeks' survival *in vitro.*

Not all cestode species respond identically to exogenous glucose. Rapid glycogen synthesis *in vivo* and *in vitro* has been demonstrated repeatedly for *Hymenolepis diminuta* (C. P. Read, 1956; Daugherty, 1956; C. P. Read and Rothman, 1957; Fairbairn *et al.,* 1961). Of special interest is that the *in vitro* glycogen synthesis of this worm is nearly completely dependent on the presence of carbon dioxide in the environment (Fairbairn *et al.,* 1961; Kilejan, 1963). Appreciable glycogen synthesis in the presence of glucose has also been found in *Lacistorhynchus tenuis, Onchobothrium pseudo-uncinatum,* and *Inermiphyllidium pul-*

vinatum (Laurie, 1961). *Hymenolepis citelli* (Read and Rothman, 1957), *Calliobothrium verticillatum, Phyllobothrium foliatum* (Laurie, 1961), and *Taenia taeniaeformis* (von Brand *et al.*, 1964) cannot be induced to increase their glycogen stores *in vitro,* indicating that the requirements for glycogenesis are not uniform in this group.

Of Acanthocephala only one species seems to have been studied so far in this respect. *Moniliformis dubius* rapidly synthesizes glycogen, when the host is fed starch (C. P. Read and Rothman, 1958b), or when maintained *in vitro* in the presence of glucose, fructose, mannose, or maltose (Laurie, 1959). In contrast to *Hymenolepis* glycogenesis is not dependent on the presence of environmental carbon dioxide (Kilejan, 1963). Male *Moniliformis,* when isolated from starved hosts (in contrast to those taken from fed rats) incorporated more C^{14}-glucose into glycogen than females (Graff, 1964).

As to nematodes, Bueding (1949a) observed rapid glycogen synthesis of *Litomosoides carinii* upon incubation in glucose-containing media. Fernando and Wong (1964) observed glycogen synthesis by *Ancylostoma caninum* from glucose essentially only when the incubation medium contained serum. Cavier and Savel (1952) showed that *Ascaris lumbricoides* synthesizes glycogen *in vitro* from glucose, fructose, sorbose, maltose, and saccharose, but not from mannose, galactose, lactose, glycerol, and various sugar alcohols. Entner and Gonzalez (1959) finally found that upon feeding radioactive glucose to *Ascaris* the highest activity appears after 24 hours in glycogen, while proteins, lipids, nucleic acids, the acid-soluble fraction, and carbon dioxide are labeled to a lesser degree.

The first step in the chain of biochemical mechanisms leading to the synthesis of polysaccharides in animals is phosphorylation of glucose to glucose-6-phosphate by means of hexokinase. Glucomutase then transforms this compound into glucose-1-phosphate. The Cori ester in turn reacts enzymatically with uridine triphosphate to form uridine diphosphate glucose which serves for the synthesis of a linear polysaccharide of the amylose type. The final step, transformation of amylose into a branched compound of the amylopectin or glycogen type is due to the so-called branching enzyme which severs some of the α-1,4 bonds of amylose and forms α-1,6 bonds, their sites representing the branching sites. Synthesis of a linear polysaccharide from glucose-1-phosphate by reversal of phosphorolysis has often been mentioned in the older literature. There is no doubt that this mechanism can be realized in *in vitro* systems, such as those described in the experiments of Rogers and Lazarus (1949) with *Ascaridia galli* or those of Cavier and Savel (1953) with *Ascaris lumbricoides.* It is, however, unlikely that these experiments have much relevancy to the synthetic processes occurring *in vivo.* Within living cells phosphorylase seems to be important for the degradation rather than the synthesis of polysaccharides, probably because *in vivo* the glucose-1-phosphate concentration necessary to drive the reaction toward synthesis is not reached.

There is little concrete evidence concerning the mechanisms actually realized in parasites leading to polysaccharide synthesis. As mentioned previously, the amylopectin of rumen ciliates does not contain amylose. It must hence be postulated that they contain a very potent branching system. However, the actual demonstration of the branching enzyme has been very difficult and could be achieved only indirectly because of interference by amylase present in the same fraction (Mould and Thomas, 1958). The possibility that uridine diphosphate synthetase is involved in the glycogen synthesis of *Echinococcus granulosus* has been mentioned, but has not yet been proved (Agosin and Repetto, 1963). In this organism a pathway for carbohydrate synthesis from $C^{14}O_2$ and C^{14}-acetate appears to exist, but the details remain to be elucidated. *In vitro* synthesis of the disaccharide trehalose by homogenates of *Macracanthorhynchus* and *Moniliformis* is markedly enhanced by the addition of adenosine triphosphate, uridine triphosphate, and uridine diphosphoglucose, indicating similarity of the synthetic processes to those described for yeast and insects (Fisher, 1964).

Relatively little is known about the nature of nonsugar glycogenic compounds. Besides acetate, mentioned above, it has been reported that pyruvate is a suitable substrate for glycogen formation in the case of *Hymenolepis diminuta* (Daugherty, 1956), as is glutamic acid (J. Schwade, unpublished observations quoted in C. P. Read and Simmons, 1963). Of considerable interest are the observations of Passey and Fairbairn (1957) who found that in the developing *Ascaris* egg glycogen and trehalose are resynthesized, following an initial decrease in both substances. Careful analysis ruled out protein, nonprotein nitrogen-containing substances, and several other potentially glycogenic substances as source of the newly formed carbohydrate. Passey and Fairbairn (1957) reached the conclusion that the latter originated from fatty acids of triglycerides. The direct evidence for this process is as follows: The increase in lipid-free dry weight corresponded closely to the increase in carbohydrates. The amount of lipid carbon disappearing equalled the sum of carbon dioxide and carbohydrates produced, while the oxygen consumption was too low to allow assumption of total oxidation of lipids. Passey and Fairbairn (1957) assume that the carbon of partially oxidized fragments of fatty acids, possibly acetyl CoA was incorporated into glycogen and trehalose. The great significance of this finding rests on the fact that the interconversion of fat to carbohydrate was for many years an unproved and controversial matter. It may occur in other parasites besides *Ascaris*. Wilson and Fairbairn (1961) found indications for the process in the oocysts of *Eimeria acervulina*.

III. DIGESTION OF CARBOHYDRATES

Carbohydrases of various kinds are widely distributed among parasitic protozoa. Their presence has been inferred in some cases because starch granules disintegrate more or less rapidly after having been ingested by such forms as *Entamoeba histolytica* (D. L. Hopkins and Warner, 1946) or rumen ciliates (Trier, 1926; Westphal, 1934). Amylases, however, which have not been fully characterized, have been described from *Entamoeba histolytica, Entamoeba gingivalis,* and *Dientamoeba fragilis* (Hallman and DeLamater, 1953; Baernstein *et al.,* 1954; Kaneko, 1956; Hilker *et al.,* 1957), trichomonads (Adler, 1953; Nomura, 1957), and *Balantidium coli* (Glaessner, 1908). More is known about a sucrase occurring in *Leishmania donovani* (Chatterjee and Ghosh, 1958). The enzyme is of a purely hydrolytic type with an optimal pH of 7.1 to 8.0, a K_m of $5 \times 10^{-3} M$, and a Q_{10} of approximately 2. It is fully active up to a temperature of 44°C. By far the most detailed information, however, is available for rumen ciliates.

Mould and Thomas (1958) found in extracts of holotrich species an amylase which, upon acting on potato starch, led to the formation of glucose, maltose, and maltotriose, and hence shows the characteristics of an α-amylase. The enzyme has a pH optimum of 5.5 and an optimal temperature of 50°C. In contrast to salivary amylase it is not activated by $CaCl_2$, NaCl, or $MgSO_4$. Electrophoretic purification showed that actually two enzymes were present which could be ascribed to two protozoan species represented in the material. One was characteristic for *Isotricha;* it transformed amylose essentially only into maltose and maltotriose, while the second enzyme, ascribed to *Dasytricha,* also showed considerable activity against maltose and maltotriose.

Similar amylases were also found in the oligotrich ciliates *Epidinium* and *Entodinium* by Bailey (1958) and by Abou Akkada and Howard (1960). The amylases isolated from both species were contaminated with maltase, but the latter could be eliminated essentially from the *Entodinium* material by suitable purification procedures. The purified enzyme produced almost exclusively maltose from amylose, but small amounts of maltotriose and traces of glucose were also found. One rather curious observation was made with the *Epidinium* amylase. Although amylases usually are not able to attack intact starch grains and although the *Epidinium* enzyme conforms to this pattern in respect to potato starch grains, it does readily attack starch grains from clover. It may be signifi-

cant in this connection that *Epidinium* develops especially large popula-
tions in the rumen when the host's diet consists of starch-containing
clover (Oxford, 1958).

The maltases of *Dasytricha ruminantium, Epidinium ecaudatum,* and
Entodinium caudatum were studied in detail by Bailey and Howard
(1963a). The enzymes are true maltases and not general α-glucosidases.
Slight differences in pH optima were observed between the enzymes isolated from the three species and greater ones in respect to temperature
optima. The latter was 38°C for the *Epidinium* and *Entodinium* enzymes,
the activity of both declining sharply above 40°C. The *Dasytricha*
enzyme, on the contrary, showed maximal activity at 50°C and was still
moderately active at 60°C. Another difference between the enzymes of
the two oligotrichs and *Dasytricha* was that the former are activated by
citrate ions, while the latter, in common with all other known maltases,
is not. The three maltases also showed transferase activity when incubated with high maltose concentrations. *Epidinium* and *Entodinium*
enzymes transferred glucose to C_4 of maltose, forming maltotriose, while
the *Dasytricha* enzyme transferred it to both C_4 and C_6 of maltose, in the
latter case producing panose. Since the two oligotrich species swallow
and digest starch granules, the biological role of maltase seems clear. It is
not so clear in the case of *Dasytricha* which does not ingest starch. Although it utilizes the amylopectin granules deposited in its own body, an
intervention of maltase is questionable, since *Isotricha* which has the
same capability does not have a maltase.

In addition to maltase, *Epidinium ecaudatum* also contains an iso-
maltase with a pH optimum of 6.0 and transferase activity leading to
isomaltotriose (Bailey and Howard, 1963b).

Holotrich rumen ciliates contain an invertase (Mould and Thomas,
1958) the properties of which were studied in detail by Howard (1959b).
The enzyme was more active in *Isotricha* than in *Dasytricha* extracts and
showed characteristics of a general β-fructosidase, attacking insulin and a
bacterial levan in addition to saccharose. In contrast to the invertase of
Leishmania mentioned previously the ciliate enzyme shows also trans-
fructosylase activity, a fact of special interest since the synthetic properties of animal invertases are so far unknown. Howard (1959b) recognized
three trisaccharides as end products of the synthetic processes: 6^F-
β-fructosylsucrose (kestose), 1^F-β-fructosylsucrose, and 6^G-β-fructo-
sylsucrose. Tetra- and higher oligosaccharides were produced only in
traces. Transfer of the fructosyl group to raffinose did not lead to sucrose,
but to a disaccharide of unidentified constitution.

Despite an early controversy concerning the question as to whether
rumen ciliates digest cellulose (Braune, 1914; Dogiel, 1925; Schulze,

1924; Margolin, 1930; Westphal, 1934; Weineck, 1934), it is now well known that some species, such as the *Diplodinium* species, are capable of utilizing cellulose, while others (e.g., *Entodinium, Isotricha, Dasytricha, Buetschlia*) are not (Hungate, 1942). Hungate (1942) was the first to demonstrate a cellulase and cellobiase in *Eudiplodinium neglectum* and he also found a cellulase in *Diplodinium maggii* (Hungate, 1943b). Oxford (1955), however, pointed out that Hungate did not give a strict proof for the occurrence of a true cellulase, since he used as substrate cellulose which might have been chemically somewhat altered. The enzymes might therefore have been unspecific β-glucosidases; an enzyme of this latter type has actually been found in *Dasytricha* (Howard, 1959b). However, Sugden (1953) showed that *Diplodinium medium* can utilize genuine cellulose and it is therefore probable that the organisms do contain true cellulase (Oxford, 1955). The various steps involved in cellulose digestion by rumen ciliates are essentially unknown. It is possible that cellobiose is an intermediate product, since a cellobiase has been found in several species (Hungate, 1942; Mould and Thomas, 1958) and a cellodextrinase in *Eudiplodinium neglectum* (Bailey and Clarke, 1963). It must be recognized, however, that the mere finding of cellobiase does not prove the above assumption, since it has been found that *Dasytricha* can ferment cellobiose without being able to utilize cellulose (Gutierrez, 1955; Howard, 1959a).

Cellulose digestion is not limited to rumen protozoa; it has been known for a long time that the symbiotic flagellates of the termite intestine have this ability. Indeed, some species, such as *Trichomonas termopsidis* (Trager, 1934) or the large flagellates of *Kalotermes* (Visintin, 1941) appear to be limited to cellulose as food. This is not true for the *Zootermopsis* flagellates which can utilize, besides cellulose, glucose and various other simple sugars, but not starch (Cook, 1943). Curious, and unexplained in its mechanism, is the observation by Gutierrez (1956) that *Trichonympha* isolated from starved termites can utilize cellulose only when the diet is supplemented with yeast extract, while the latter is not required when organisms isolated from fed hosts are studied. The cellulose-digesting enzymes of termite flagellates have been investigated by Trager (1932). He showed that the intestinal fauna of the roach *Cryptocercus punctulatus* and the termites *Reticulitermes flaviceps* and *Termopsis angusticollis* contain both a cellulase and a cellobiase. The enzymes were partially purified and glucose was identified as an end product of the digestive processes. Trager (1934) also found a cellulase in *Trichomonas termopsidis*. Quantitative data on cellulose utilization by termite protozoa were presented by Hungate (1943a), indicating fairly high rates.

Pectic substances are common constituents of ruminant food; it is therefore not too surprising that at least some rumen ciliates possess the two enzymes required for degradation of pectins: pectinesterase, which liberates polygalacturonic acid, and polygalacturonase. Wright (1960), working with mixed material of holotrich and oligotrich ciliates, found both enzymes. More uniform material was subsequently employed by Abou Akkada and Howard (1961). *Entodinium* did not contain the above two enzymes; their activity was low in *Dasytricha* and quite pronounced in *Isotricha*. The pectinesterase of this latter species and its polygalacturonase had surprisingly high pH optima; 8.6 to 8.8 and 8.7 to 9.0, respectively. While Wright (1960) had found galacturonic acid as the main end product of the digestive process, Abou Akkada and Howard (1961) found only little of this acid produced; the main end products in their experiments were oligouronides. Curious is the fact that *Isotricha* appears incapable of utilizing degradation products of pectic provenience (methanol, polypectate, galacturonic acid) in its fermentative metabolism.

Another class of compounds frequently occurring in the diet of ruminants is hemicelluloses. *Epidinium ecaudatum* is so far the only rumen ciliate with the demonstrated ability of digesting plant hemicelluloses (Bailey *et al.,* 1962). During the degradation process arabinose was liberated initially, followed by xylobiose, and finally xylose, glucose, galactose, and uronic acid. It is probable that the hydrolysis of complex hemicelluloses (such as wheat flower xylan or clover stem hemicellulose) involves several enzymes for which the collective term hemicellulases can be used. It is probable, however, that the enzyme attacking xylobiose is a separate entity. However, whether in the case of *Epidinium* a specific xylobiase or a less specific β-1,4-glycosidase is involved remains to be elucidated. A xylanase has more recently also been reported for *Eudiplodinium neglectum* (Bailey and Clarke, 1963).

Epidinium ecaudatum possesses an exceptionally wide spectrum of digestive enzymes; besides those mentioned in the foregoing paragraphs, it also contains an α-galactosidase (Bailey and Howard, 1963b) which readily hydrolyzes galactosylgalactosylglycerol and at a somewhat slower rate melibiose and other compounds containing α-(1$\longrightarrow$6)-linked galactose. The enzyme also liberates galactose from intact clover galactosyl lipids, but does not appear to have true lipase activity. Finally, it can act as a transferase. Thus, after incubation with high concentrations of melibiose, manninotriose was produced, and upon incubation with suitable concentrations of galactosylgalactosylglycerol a compound appeared which chromatographically moved like galactosylgalactosylgalactosylglycerol.

Related to the digestive enzymes discussed above, but of less obvious biological significance, are enzymes occurring in *Trichomonas foetus,* but not in *Trichomonas vaginalis* or *Strigomonas oncopelti,* which attack water-soluble blood-group substances (Watkins, 1953). The serological activity of these substances is destroyed by the enzymatic activity and usually reducing sugars are liberated during digestion. Ikeda (1955) identified fucose as the sugar set free; his preparations had a pH optimum of 6.6 and a temperature optimum of 45°C. Watkins (1962) purified cell-free extracts of *Trichomonas foetus* by zone electrophoresis on starch columns in phosphate buffer at pH 6.2 or 7.0 and obtained in this way three preparations. One was active against the human blood-group substances A, B, and Le^a, the second one only against H, and the last one against B and Le^a. About 20% reducing sugars are liberated from these substances and they were identified as fucose, galactose, and *N*-acetylhexosamine (Watkins, 1959).

Watkins and Morgan (1955) considered the possibility that the enzyme active against the B substance could be a specific galactosidase, a view finding apparent support by Watkins' (1956) isolation of a purified enzyme which set free almost exclusively galactose. However, Watkins (1959) reported later on, that *Trichomonas foetus* can cleave an entire series of α- and β-galactosides, but the enzymes involved could not be identified with the one attacking the B substance. The flagellates are able to decompose, besides galactosides, α- and β-glucosides, *N*-acetyl-α- or β-glucosaminides, *N*-acetyl-α- or β-galactosaminides, α-L-fucoside, and α-L-rhamnoside. To what extent the enzymes involved in the degradation of these compounds correspond to those attacking the blood-group substances is at present problematical. It is probable that the latter are fairly specific and it can be assumed that the enzymes degrading the H and Le^a substances have specific α-fucosidase activity (Watkins and Morgan, 1955).

In contrast to the large body of information available for parasitic protozoa, relatively little is known about carbohydrases of helminths. It has been established (Myuge, 1957, 1960; Zinovev, 1957; Goffart and Heiling, 1962; Krusberg, 1960) that many species of plant-parasitic nematodes, such as *Ditylenchus* spp. or *Heterodera* spp., secrete an amylase and an invertase from their salivary glands into the surroundings. A chitinase and cellulase have been reported for *Ditylenchus* spp. (Tracey, 1958), as well as a pectinesterase (Krusberg, 1960; Goffart and Heiling, 1962), the latter enzyme also being found in *Heterodera.* However, no polygalacturonase activity could be detected in *Ditylenchus,* that is, the full enzyme complement necessary for complete cellulose digestion has not been demonstrated. Later experiments by

Dropkin (1963) demonstrated the presence of a cellulase, or possibly various cellulases, in some species of plant-parasitic nematodes. The general properties of the enzyme corresponded to those described for cellulases isolated from other sources. Similar experiments by Morgan and McAllen (1962) proved the occurrence of pectinase and cellulase in *Pratylenchus* and *Heterodera*. As Fairbairn (1960) has pointed out it is at present not possible to distinguish between those secretions of plant-parasitic nematodes that assist in penetration of the host tissues and those directly concerned with digestion of food material. It is of course questionable whether a strict distinction is possible. Fairbairn (1960) emphasized that soluble sugars originating from the dissolution of a cellulose cell wall during penetration may well be used as nutrients by the worms. Similarly, end products of chitin digestion could be used as alimentation. However, the main function of a chitinase found by Rogers (1958) in the hatching fluid of *Ascaris* eggs is undoubtedly facilitation of hatching by destroying the chitinous layer of the eggshell.

In the case of helminths parasitizing animals some older and newer experiments were done with tissue extracts or homogenates of entire worms, partly because the small size of some worms or their organization makes the isolation of the intestine difficult if not impossible. It is clear that in such instances no distinction can be drawn between tissue enzymes acting on some reserve substance and enzymes involved in preparing food material for absorption. For example, amylolytic enzymes derived from such experiments have been described by Kobert (1903) from a dog ascarid or by Guevara and Monteoliva (1959) for *Ascaridia galli*. In this latter case the end products of digestion were identified as glucose, maltose, and high oligosaccharides. The enzyme clearly had the characteristics of an α-amylase.

Carbohydrases found in the body fluid of nematodes evidently cannot act on food present in the gut lumen; they definitely fall into the class of tissue enzymes. Thus a starch-degrading enzyme has been found in the perivisceral fluid of *Parascaris equorum* (Schimmelpfennig, 1903) and an amylase as well as a saccharase and maltase in that of *Ascaris lumbricoides* (Cavier, 1951; Monteoliva, 1961). It is of interest to note that during maintenance of *Ascaris in vitro* in non-nutrient solution a decrease in the amylase activity of the perivisceral fluid was observed, the level reached after 5 days being 2/3 of that found in freshly isolated worms (Ichii *et al.*, 1959).

The presence of true digestive enzymes can be considered as proved when they are demonstrated in gut extracts. Flury (1912) was apparently the first to show that extracts of the *Ascaris* intestine are able to split glycogen and starch. Very suggestive is also the observation by Enigk (1938) that *Graphidium strigosum,* although not able to digest raw starch, can digest starch heated previous to feeding for 30 minutes at 60°C.

A more detailed study of the amylolytic enzymes of nematodes is credited to Rogers (1940). He extracted the intestines of *Strongylus edentatus* and *Ascaris lumbricoides* and studied with the extracts both the amyloclastic action, that is, the progressive loss of the blue color of starch due to iodine, and the saccharogenic action, the gradual appearance of reducing sugar. He observed distinct differences between the enzymes of both species (Fig. 3). Lee (1958), using a similar isolation technique, found in the intestine of *Leidynema appendiculata* an amylase with a pH optimum of 4.5 and a maltase with an optimum of pH 5.0 to 6.0. Considerable differences between the enzymes of various species exist in respect to their response to inorganic salts. While the *Strongylus* and *Ascaris* enzymes were essentially unaffected by NaCl, but stimulated by Na_2HPO_4, sodium chloride stimulated the *Leidynema* enzyme by 29%. Potassium iodide activated the *Strongylus* amylase, but was ineffective in the case of the *Ascaris* enzyme. However, exactly the reverse held true when the activating influence of sodium bicarbonate was tested.

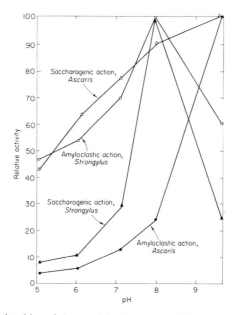

Fig. 3.   pH relationships of the amylolytic enzymes of *Ascaris* and *Strongylus*. (After Rogers, 1940.)

Very few data on carbohydrases of endoparasitic arthropods have been reported so far. Roy (1937) did not find an amylase in the salivary glands of *Gastrophilus intestinalis* larvae, but more recently Tatchell (1958) demonstrated in their secretion an amylase with a pH optimum of 6, as well as an invertase and maltase. Both authors agree that the midgut contains an amylase and Tatchell (1958) observed that the enzyme is somewhat stimulated by NaCl. He found in addition to amylase also maltase and invertase activity in the mid-gut. All investigators have found a powerful amylase in the body fluid of the larvae (von Kemnitz, 1914, 1916; Roy, 1937; Tatchell, 1958). It is assumed that it serves to convert the glycogen derived from the tracheal cells to glucose. The salivary gland and mid-gut carbohydrases can hardly be understood on the basis of purely blood-feeding habits of the larvae. Roy (1937) thinks that they derive their main food from the fluid content of the horse's stomach which surrounds them. The larvae of *Cordylobia anthropophaga* have no amylase in their body fluid. Their salivary glands do contain an amylase and an invertase, and amylase, maltase, and invertase were found in their mid-gut (Blacklock *et al.*, 1930).

IV. UTILIZATION OF ENDOGENOUS CARBOHYDRATE RESERVES

Endogenous carbohydrate, essentially glycogen, is most frequently an energy reserve; it may be utilized by purely fermentative processes, by oxidations, or during aerobic fermentation. These aspects will be treated in the following sections. It should be realized, however, that the production of energy is not always the sole purpose of a polysaccharide accumulation.

Glycogen will unquestionably be utilized by endoparasitic arthropods, just as by free-living ones, for the synthesis of the chitin of the exoskeleton. It is entirely possible that in parasites like *Peltogaster* which store but little polysaccharide this function is in the foreground. It would be interesting to study whether in this and similar instances cyclic variations in glycogen content occur depending on the molting cycle, as they do, for example, in free-living crustacea.

Similarly, glycogen, though certainly only a small part of the total metabolized, is used for chitin synthesis in those previously mentioned nematodes and Acanthocephala that produce chitinous egg membranes. It has been found that in ascarids about half the glycogen deposited in the oocytes is utilized to form the glucosamine built into the chitin of the egg membrane (Fauré-Fremiet, 1913; Szwejkowska, 1929).

It is also possible that in special cases the polysaccharide reserves are used for other, as yet unidentified, purposes. For example, the rapid appearance and equally rapid disappearance of a large glycogen vacuole in young *Entamoeba* cysts is a puzzling phenomenon.

No quantitative data on the utilization of endogenous polysaccharides are available for parasitic protozoa. The qualitative observations by Westphal (1934), Hungate (1943b), Abou Akkada and Howard (1960), and Oxford (1951) suggest a high rate of amylopectin utilization in starving rumen ciliates. The glycogen vacuole of *Iodamoeba buetschlii,* on the other hand, disappears only gradually and very slowly (von Brand, 1932) and in gregarines starving within the mealworm intestine no significant decrease in polysaccharide could be demonstrated histochemically (von Brand, 1950). Apparently, therefore, considerable differences between species exist in this respect.

The rate of endogenous glycogen consumption of helminths is determined generally by keeping the worms in inorganic solutions under either aerobic or anaerobic conditions, that is, conditions fairly far removed from those prevailing in the intestine of a starving host. On the whole it seems, nevertheless, that the values obtained reflect rather closely the rates prevailing *in vivo.* This is indicated by the fact that dog ascarids (Weinland, 1901), *Ascaridia galli* (W. M. Reid, 1945), and *Hymenolepis diminuta* (C. P. Read, 1956) showed reasonably close rates of polysaccharide utilization when kept starving *in vitro* and *in vivo.* Furthermore, one of the worms studied, the larva of *Eustrongylides,* survives for very long periods *in vitro* and it can be assumed that the relatively short periods of starvation used for the determination of the polysaccharide consumption (von Brand and Simpson, 1945) did not seriously interfere with its vitality.

Some older and newer data on the utilization of endogenous glycogen reserves are shown in Table XVI. It is evident that both in respect to aerobic and anaerobic consumption considerable species differences have been found. As C. P. Read (1961b) has pointed out, such rates are determined by various factors and no simple explanation can be given. One point to keep in mind is that the amount of carbohydrate consumed per unit weight and unit time decreases frequently with increasing length of incubation *in vitro,* as shown in Table XVII for *Ascaris.* However, the values assembled in Table XVI refer to experiments of greatly varying length (e.g., 3 hours for *Setaria cervi,* but 43 hours for *Macracanthorhynchus hirudinaceus*), making them not exactly comparable even though the values have been calculated for unit time. Of importance in determining the rates of glycogen consumption may be the size of the worms, smaller organisms usually metabolizing at a higher rate than large ones (von Brand, 1952), or their nutritional state, starvation commonly depressing the rate (Glocklin and Fairbairn, 1952; C. P. Read,

1956; Mansour, 1959a). The environment will undoubtedly be significant, at least in some cases. It has thus been shown that *Heterakis gallinae* uses twice as much glycogen when kept in CO_2-free environment than if the atmosphere contains 5% CO_2 (Glocklin and Fairbairn, 1952). It is known that this worm fixes CO_2 (Fairbairn, 1954). However, although *Ascaris lumbricoides* also does so (Saz and Vidrine, 1959), its glycogen consumption is apparently not subject to a similar CO_2 effect (Table XVII). Motility may be significant. Mansour (1959b) found serotonin-induced increase in motility of *Fasciola hepatica* accompanied by a distinct increase in carbohydrate turnover.

Of greater importance, possibly, may be the type of metabolism prevailing in various species of helminths, since it must be expected that different types of aerobic and anaerobic fermentations will release different amounts of energy. Unfortunately, direct evidence along this line is only available for *Ascaris,* and this evidence is not entirely satisfactory. Krummacher (1919) determined the heat produced by this worm, but his data are difficult to interpret since his experiments were conducted under conditions that were neither clearly aerobic or anaerobic. Meier (1931), working with the same parasite, found an anaerobic heat production of 0.300 gm cal/gm worm/hour and he estimates the energy yield of the fermentation as 22%. This value is unquestionably much too high (von Brand and Jahn, 1942), since he used Weinland's (1901) figures on glycogen consumption for his calculations which are derived from experiments lasting much longer periods than his own. This must have caused a rather considerable error since, as mentioned above, the glycogen consumption of *Ascaris* decreases as the experimental periods increase in length.

The data of Table XVI also illustrate the point that in most helminths studied so far there is but little difference in the rates of carbohydrate consumption whether a given species is kept aerobically or anaerobically. In most free-living invertebrates (data on a variety of species in von Brand, 1946) the anaerobic glycogen consumption is from several to many times greater than the aerobic rate because they oxidize carbohydrate completely in the presence of sufficient oxygen. In other words, they utilize a process releasing the maximum of energy from a given amount of carbohydrate. In the absence of oxygen they must mobilize a greater amount of carbohydrate in order to gain even the minimum of energy required for the sustenance of life from uneconomical fermentative processes. The metabolism of parasites, both protozoan and metazoan, is characterized, on the other hand, by the prevalence of aerobic fermentations. This fermentative use of carbohydrate even in the presence of ample oxygen drives the aerobic consumption of carbohydrate

TABLE XVI

CONSUMPTION OF ENDOGENOUS POLYSACCHARIDES
BY PARASITIC HELMINTHS AND ARTHROPODS[a,b]

Species	Carbohydrate consumption		References
	Anaerobic	Aerobic	
Trematodes			
Fasciola gigantica		4.56	Goil (1961)
Fasciola hepatica	6.16		Mansour (1959a)
Paramphistomum explanatum		6.33	Goil (1957)
Gastrothylax crumenifer		6.55	Goil (1957)
Cestodes			
Echinococcus granulosus,			
scoleces	1.98	1.60	Agosin (1957)
Hymenolepis diminuta		4.88	C. P. Read (1956)
Taenia taeniaeformis,			
larval	6.96	7.80	von Brand and Bowman (1961)
Taenia taeniaeformis,			
adult	9.36	6.48	von Brand and Bowman (1961)
Acanthocephala			
Macracanthorhynchus			
hirudinaceus	0.78	0.62	Ward (1952)
Moniliformis dubius		6.48	Laurie (1959)
Nematodes			
Ascaridia galli	3.60	2.80	Reid (1945); Monteoliva and Guevara (1958)
Ascaris lumbricoides	1.39	1.18	von Brand (1934)
Eustrongylides ignotus,			
larva	0.73	0.24	von Brand and Simpson (1945)
Heterakis gallinae	3.74	3.30	Glocklin and Fairbairn (1952)
Setaria cervi		♀18.7; ♂8.8	Pandya (1961)
Trichuris vulpis	4.37	3.96	Bueding *et al.* (1961)
Arthropods			
Gastrophilus intestinalis,			
larva	0.7	1.3	von Kemnitz (1916)

[a] Further relevant data will be found in the following papers: For trematodes: Weinland and von Brand (1926); Vernberg and Hunter (1956); for cestodes: von Brand (1933a); Reid (1942); C. A. Hopkins (1950, 1952); Fairbairn *et al.* (1961); for Acanthocephala: Weinland (1910); von Brand (1940); for nematodes: Toryu (1936); von Brand *et al.* (1952).

[b] In gm/100 gm wet weight/24 hours at $36°-41°C$.

TABLE XVII
UTILIZATION OF ENDOGENOUS GLYCOGEN RESERVES
BY FEMALE *Ascaris lumbricoides* STARVING *in Vitro*

	After von Brand (1937)		After Harpur (1963)	
Medium	Na 156 mM, Cl 156 mM		Na 135 mM, K 24 mM, Ca 1 mM, Mg 5 mM, Cl 150 mM, SO$_4$ 5 mM, PO$_4$ 0.5 mM, HCO$_3$ 10 mM	
Temperature, °C	37		39	
Gas atmosphere	100% H$_2$		90% N$_2$, 5% O$_2$, 5% CO$_2$	
	In vitro period	gm glycogen/ 100 gm wet weight	*In vitro* period	gm glycogen/ 100 gm wet weight
	0–24 hours	1.32	0–18 hours	1.20
	24–48 hours	1.06	18–42 hours	1.11
	48–72 hours	0.67	42–66 hours	0.63

up to a level nearly equal to that of the anaerobic rate. Whether there is a fundamental difference between parasites and free-living invertebrates in this respect is a debatable point. On the one hand, free-living species, e.g., some snails, have been found which consume aerobically almost as much carbohydrate as anaerobically (von Brand *et al.,* 1950). On the other hand, the relatively low aerobic rate as compared to the anaerobic rate found in *Eustrongylides* points to the possibility that parasites may exist that behave like the majority of free-living organisms in this respect. It might be of interest to search for such instances among parasites with very free access to oxygen, such as monogenetic trematodes or the nematodes parasitizing the swim bladder of fish or the trachea of birds.

V. END PRODUCTS OF AEROBIC AND ANAEROBIC FERMENTATIONS

The end products of parasitic aerobic and anaerobic fermentations are more varied than those occurring in vertebrate tissues where lactic acid is formed almost exclusively. They are less varied, however, than those characterizing yeasts and bacteria where an almost unending array of substances is encountered.

Hydrogen, a gas produced by many bacteria, is formed by some groups of parasitic protozoa, but has not yet been found among the excreta of metazoan parasites. It has been reported from termite flagellates (Cook, 1932, 1943; Cook and Smith, 1942; Hungate, 1939, 1943a), the symbiotic

protozoa of *Cryptocercus punctulatus* (Gilmour, 1940), various holotrich (Heald and Oxford, 1953; Gutierrez, 1955; Howard, 1959a) and
oligotrich rumen ciliates (Abou Akkada and Howard, 1960; Williams
et al., 1961), and several *Trichomonas* species (Andrews and von Brand,
1938; Suzuoki and Suzuoki, 1951a; Ryley, 1955a; Doran, 1957, 1958;
C. P. Read, 1957a; Lindblom, 1961). A curious situation exists in respect to *Trichomonas vaginalis,* some strains producing appreciable
amounts of hydrogen, while others appear to be completely devoid of
this faculty (Kupferberg *et al.*, 1953; C. P. Read and Rothman, 1955;
Wellerson *et al.*, 1959). The significance of this variable behavior is
obscure.

Little is known about the production of combustible gases other than
hydrogen. Methane has been reported in small quantities as an admix-
ture to the hydrogen produced by *Trichomonas foetus* (Suzuoki and Suzuoki, 1951a), and an unidentified gas giving CO_2 upon combustion
accompanied the hydrogen given off by *Cryptocercus*-parasitizing
protozoa (Gilmour, 1940).

Entamoeba histolytica, when having access to both sugar and cysteine,
according to Kun and Bradin (1953), forms both CO_2 and H_2S. It is
assumed that the amoeba has a triosephosphate oxidase which transmits
hydrogen to the sulfur of cysteine (Kun *et al.*, 1956).

Carbon dioxide, on the other hand, is an almost universal end product
of both aerobic and anaerobic fermentations. However, its sources and
significance are probably not always identical. Carbon dioxide can be
of "inorganic" origin, that is, it can be liberated from bicarbonates
present either in the parasite's body or in the medium by acids stronger
than carbonic acid, when the former are produced during the fermentative processes. Or else carbon dioxide can be true respiratory CO_2,
that is, the carbon atom is derived from an organic compound, such as
glucose.

Pure lactic acid or pyruvic acid fermentations do not lead to any true
respiratory CO_2, as the following over-all formulations indicate:

$$C_6H_{12}O_6 \longrightarrow 2CH_3 \cdot CHOH \cdot COOH \text{ and}$$
$$C_6H_{12}O_6 + O_2 \longrightarrow 2CH_3 \cdot CO \cdot COOH + 2H_2O$$

Characteristically, the respiratory quotient of the blood-stream forms of
African pathogenic trypanosomes, which transform glucose almost quantitatively into pyruvic acid, is extremely low, namely, less than 0.1 (e.g.,
von Brand *et al.*, 1955; Ryley, 1956). On the other hand, true respiratory
CO_2 is formed during many parasitic fermentations, especially the fatty
acid fermentations. An example is the dismutation of pyruvic acid to

acetic and lactic acids by *Litomosoides* (Bueding, 1949a) which can be formulated as follows:

$$2 CH_3 \cdot CO \cdot COOH + H_2O \longrightarrow CH_3COOH + CO_2 + CH_3 \cdot COH \cdot COOH$$

In the earlier literature dealing with the metabolism of helminths (nematodes: Weinland, 1901; Schulte, 1917; von Brand, 1934; trematodes: Weinland and von Brand, 1926; Harnisch, 1932; cestodes: von Brand, 1933a) and arthropods (von Kemnitz, 1916) no distinction between CO_2 of inorganic and metabolic origin was made; it is therefore dangerous to introduce these figures into quantitative carbon balances (Bueding, 1949b). However, the proportion between CO_2 evolved and organic acids formed makes it very probable that at least some of the CO_2 found was of true metabolic origin (von Brand, 1950). Because of evident technical difficulties the origin of excreted CO_2 has not yet been established definitely for large nematodes such as *Ascaris,* or for tapeworms which possess in their calcareous corpuscles an immense carbonate reserve, but it was possible to prove the occurrence of true metabolic CO_2 in the case of small helminths (e.g., the larvae of *Trichinella spiralis* according to Stannard *et al.,* 1938). The reverse of carbon dioxide elimination, carbon dioxide fixation has been found in several parasites, especially under anaerobic conditions and in species that produce larger amounts of succinic acid; this process will be dealt with in greater detail later.

The relatively great variety of partially oxidized metabolic end products produced during aerobic and anaerobic fermentations by parasitic protozoa and helminths is shown in Tables XVIII and XIX. Before discussing them it should be realized that essentially all studies dealing with parasite metabolism by necessity have been conducted under conditions far removed from what they are *in vivo*. It is therefore possible that at least in some instances biochemical potentialities of a given organism have been studied rather than realities as they occur *in vivo*. Definite indications exist that changes in environmental conditions can shift certain metabolic pathways. These changes may be reflected simply in alterations of the relative abundance of the various metabolites produced, but can, in some instances, perhaps even constitute qualitative changes. To give just a few examples: In the blood-stream form of *Trypanosoma congolense* the question whether or not larger amounts of succinic acid are produced depends on whether the organisms are kept in a CO_2-containing or CO_2-free environment, as the apparent contradictory results of Ryley (1956) and Agosin and von Brand (1954) indicate. Another example refers to the same organism. Agosin and von Brand (1954), keeping the flagellates in whole blood or rabbit serum, found an oxygen/glucose ratio of 2.40, while Ryley (1956), using a Ringer/ bicarbonate medium, found the low value of 0.50 and, when he employed plasma as medium, the high one of 2.11. He assumes that in the inorganic medium the aerobic processes "decay" faster than the anaerobic ones. As to helminths, Weinland and von Brand (1926), as well as Stephenson (1947b), reported higher fatty acids as a main end product of the carbohydrate metabolism of *Fasciola hepatica,* while Mansour (1959a) found them only in small amounts. In his experience acetic and propionic acids were the metabolites accounting for most of the carbon of the decomposed carbohydrate. C. P. Read (1956) and Laurie (1957) considered lactic acid as predominating among the excreta of *Hymenolepis diminuta,* while Fairbairn *et al.* (1961) found only small amounts of that acid, but very large amounts of succinic acid. No valid reasons exist to suspect analytical inadequacies to explain these contradictions, but as yet they cannot be ascribed to any definite cause. The only fair statement possible at present is the assumption that under the influence of unknown stimuli originating in the medium some organisms can readily change metabolic pathways. It is important in this connection to realize that biochemical lesions, and some of the above examples may well fall into this category, can rather readily be induced. Typical examples of such lesions can be found when comparing the metabolites formed by intact nematodes and by homogenates of the worms. Intact *Ascaris* adults (von Brand, 1934) or *Trichinella* larvae (von Brand *et al.,* 1952) produce only very small amounts of lactic acid, while this acid definitely predominates when the metabolism of homogenates or minces is studied (*Ascaris:* Bueding and Yale, 1951; Rathbone and Rees, 1954; *Trichinella:* Goldberg, 1958; Agosin and Aravena, 1959a).

In evaluating the data of Tables XVIII and XIX, it should be kept in mind therefore that experiments conducted under completely biological conditions could change somewhat the nature or relative importance of various metabolites excreted. At the present state of our knowledge it can be stated that most parasitic protozoa excrete some lactic acid, accounting for nearly 100% of the excreted acids in *Plasmodium gallinaceum* (Silverman *et al.,* 1944). At the other extreme of the scale are the blood-stream forms of the African pathogenic trypanosomes which excrete, contrary to the early views of von Fenyvessy and Reiner (1924, 1928) and Geiger *et al.* (1930), only traces, if indeed any lactic acid (e.g., Ryley, 1956). Similar differences exist in the case of helminths. Thus, lactate accounts for practically all the carbon of the metabolized glucose in the case of *Dirofilaria uniformis* (von Brand *et al.,* 1963) and for nearly all of it in *Litomosoides carinii, Dracunculus insignis,* and *Schistosoma mansoni* (Bueding, 1949a, 1950; Bueding and Oliver-

Gonzalez, 1950), while at most traces of lactate have been reported for *Heterakis gallinae* (Glocklin and Fairbairn, 1952) and *Moniliformis dubius* (Laurie, 1959).

Pyruvic acid is the most important aerobic metabolic end product of the blood-stream forms of pathogenic African trypanosomes and various control experiments have demonstrated conclusively that this applies also to *in vivo* conditions (Grant and Fulton, 1957; R. M. Coleman and von Brand, 1957). Anaerobically, the excretion of pyruvate is reduced and part of the glucose carbon is accounted for by glycerol. In worms, pyruvate is eliminated only occasionally, mainly under aerobic conditions.

Lower fatty acids predominate among the excreta of several parasitic worms, especially nematodes. It is of historic interest to note that the assumption of a causal connection between volatile fatty acids and helminth metabolism, first described by Weinland (1901), has several times been severely criticized and doubted (e.g., Fischer, 1924; Slater, 1925, 1928), mainly because of the unwillingness to concede that in invertebrate tissues metabolic pathways may exist that are different from those prevailing in vertebrates. This controversy was first unequivocally decided by Epps *et al.* (1950), who succeeded in sterilizing specimens of *Ascaris lumbricoides* by means of antibiotics and found that these worms did produce large amounts of volatile fatty acids.

The complexity of the fatty acid mixture excreted by some nematodes is considerable and even greater than indicated by the data of Table XIX because several isomers of C_5 acids can be formed. While the larvae of *Trichinella spiralis* (von Brand *et al.*, 1952) and the adults of *Trichuris vulpis* (Bueding *et al.*, 1961) excrete only *n*-valeric acid, *Ascaris lumbricoides* specimens eliminate *n*-valeric, α-methylbutyric, and *cis*-α-methylcrotonic (tiglic) acid (Bueding and Yale, 1951; Bueding, 1953). The situation is still more complicated by the fact that the volatile fatty acids excreted by *Ascaris* are not completely identical with those occurring in abundance in the perienteric fluid, indicating perhaps selective excretion. Data concerning the fatty acids of the body fluid have been presented by Moyle and Baldwin (1952) and Ueno (1960).

The only C_6 acid regularly excreted by *Ascaris* is α-methylvaleric acid (Saz and Gerzon, 1962; Whitlock and Strong, 1963) while the tentative identification of isocaproic acid (Ellison *et al.*, 1960) proved to be erroneous. Quantitatively, α-methylvaleric acid is more significant than *n*-valeric, tiglic, propionic, or butyric acids. Traces of other C_6 acids, probably *n*-hexanoic acid, appear occasionally (H. J. Saz, personal communication, 1965).

Of dibasic acids, succinic acid is most commonly excreted. It is a major end product of both aerobic and anaerobic fermentations of protozoa and

TABLE XVIII
Organic End Products of Aerobic and Anaerobic Fermentations of Parasitic Protozoa[a,b]

Species	Anaerobic										Aerobic									References
	Lactic acid	Pyruvic acid	Acetic acid	Propionic acid	Butyric acid	Succinic acid	Glycerol	Ethyl alcohol	Carbon dioxide	Hydrogen	Lactic acid	Pyruvic acid	Acetic acid	Propionic acid	Butyric acid	Succinic acid	Glycerol	Ethyl alcohol	Carbon dioxide	
Flagellates																				
Crithidia fasciculata C	x	x	(x)			x		x	x	x		x	x			x		x	x	Schwartz (1961); Cosgrove (1959)
Leishmania donovani C	x	x	x			x		x	x		x	x	x			x		x	x	Chang (1948); Fulton and Joyner (1949); Crowther *et al.* (1954); Chatterjee and Ghosh (1959)
Strigomonas oncopelti C	(x)	x	(x)			x		x	x		(x)	x	(x)			x	x	x	(x)	Ryley (1955a); Clausen (1955); Bauchop (1962)
Termite flagellates			x						x	x										Hungate (1939, 1943a)
Trichomonas batracharum	x								x	x	x									Doran (1958)
Trichomonas foetus	x	(x)	x			x			–	x	x		x			x			x	Suzuoki and Suzuoki (1951a); Ryley (1955b); Doran (1957); Lindblom (1961)
Trichomonas vaginalis	x								x	x[c]										Kupferberg *et al.* (1953); C. P. Read and Rothman (1955); Wellerson *et al.* (1959)
Trypanosoma brucei B	(x)	x					x		(x)			x				x			(x)	Glowazky (1937); Ryley (1956)
Trypanosoma lewisi B	x	x					(x)		–		x	(x)				x[a]		(x)	x	Reiner *et al.* (1936); Ryley (1956)
Trypanosoma congolense B	(x)	x					x		–		(x)					x			(x)	Agosin and von Brand (1954); Ryley (1956)

												References
Trypanosoma congolense C	x	x		x	(x)		(x)	x	x	x	(x)	x	von Brand and Tobie (1959)
Trypanosoma cruzi B	x	(x)	x	x			x	(x)	x	x	(x)	x	Ryley (1956)
Trypanosoma cruzi C			x	x			(x)	(x)	x	x		x	Chang (1948); Ryley (1956)
Trypanosoma equinum B	(x)	x	x		x	(x)			x	x		(x)	Ryley (1956)
Trypanosoma equiperdum B	(x)	x	(x)	(x)	x	(x)	(x)	x	(x)	x	x	(x)	Reiner *et al.* (1936); Ryley (1956)
Trypanosoma evansi B	(x)	x	(x)	x	x		(x)	x	(x)	x	x	(x)	Marshall (1948b); Ryley (1956)
Trypanosoma gambiense B	(x)	x		x				x	(x)			(x)	von Brand *et al.* (1955); Ryley (1956)
Trypanosoma gambiense C							(x)	x	x	x			von Brand *et al.* (1955)
Trypanosoma hippicum B		x			x				x				Harvey (1949)
Trypanosoma rhodesiense B	(x)	x		(x)	x	(x)	(x)	x	(x)	x	(x)	(x)	Fulton and Stevens (1945); Ryley (1956); Grant and Fulton (1957)
Trypanosoma rhodesiense C		x		x					(x)	(x)		x	Ryley (1962)
Trypanosoma vivax B	x	x	(x)		x	(x)	x	x	x	x	x	x	Ryley (1956)
Rhizopods													
Entamoeba histolytica	x			x	x	x	x	x	x				Entner and Anderson (1954); Bragg and Reeves (1962)

TABLE XVIII (Continued)

Organic End Products of Aerobic and Anaerobic Fermentations of Parasitic Protozoa[a,b]

Species	Anaerobic										Aerobic									References
	Lactic acid	Pyruvic acid	Acetic acid	Propionic acid	Butyric acid	Succinic acid	Glycerol	Ethyl alcohol	Carbon dioxide	Hydrogen	Lactic acid	Pyruvic acid	Acetic acid	Propionic acid	Butyric acid	Succinic acid	Glycerol	Ethyl alcohol	Carbon dioxide	
Sporozoa																				
Plasmodium berghei											x	(x)	(x)			(x)			(x)	Fulton and Spooner (1956); Bowman et al. (1960b)
Plasmodium gallinaceum	x										x	(x)	(x)			(x)				Silverman et al. (1944); Speck et al. (1946)
Plasmodium knowlesi											x	(x)								Wendel (1943); McKee et al. (1946)
Toxoplasma gondii	x	(x)	x	(x)	(x)															Fulton and Spooner (1960)
Ciliates																				
Entodinium caudatum	x	(x)	x						x	x										Abou Akkada and Howard (1960)
Epidinium ecaudatum	(x)	(x)	x						x	x										Gutierrez and Davis (1962)
Isotricha + Dasytricha spp.	x	(x)	x						x	x										Heald and Oxford (1953); Gutierrez (1955); Howard (1959a)
Ophryoscolex caudatum	(x)		x						x	x										Williams et al. (1961)

[a] Essentially after von Brand (1963).

[b] Key: C = culture forms; x = end product produced in large to moderately large amounts; (x) = end product produced in small amounts only; − indicated CO_2 fixation; B = blood-stream form.

[c] Some strains of *Trichomonas vaginalis* do not produce hydrogen.

[d] The blood-stream form of *Trypanosoma congolense* produces larger amounts of succinic acid only when CO_2 tension is high.

helminths. Its formation frequently involves CO_2 fixation and it is characteristic that the succinate production is often much more pronounced under anaerobic conditions than in the presence of oxygen (e.g., in trypanosomes, as shown by Ryley, 1951, 1956, 1962, and Bowman *et al.*, 1963, and in some tapeworms, as found by Agosin, 1957, and von Brand and Bowman, 1961).

Little information is available concerning the excretion of other dicarboxylic acids or of tricarboxylic acids. A little fumaric and more malic acid has been found in media in which *Taenia taeniaeformis* had been kept (von Brand and Bowman, 1961). While relatively large amounts of succinic acid occur in the perienteric fluid of *Ascaris* (Bueding and Farrow, 1956), little oxaloacetic acid and no fumaric, malic, aconitic, or citric acids could be isolated (Ueno *et al.*, 1960).

Little is also known about the production of nonacidic organic metabolic end products referable to carbohydrate catabolism. One of the best documented cases is the anaerobic glycerol production by the bloodstream forms of African trypanosomes, the glycerol accounting for almost exactly 50% of the carbon of the metabolized glucose (e.g., Harvey, 1949; Ryley, 1956). Metazoan parasites seem in general not to eliminate glycerol. Only in *Taenia taeniaeformis* has a little glycerol been identified among the end products of aerobic and anaerobic fermentation (von Brand and Bowman, 1961). Appreciable amounts of acetoin (acetylmethyl-carbinol) have been found in incubates of *Litomosoides, Ascaris,* and *Setaria* (Bueding, 1951; Yonesawa, 1953; Saz *et al.*, 1958).

There can be little doubt that future research will reveal still more different nonacidic and acidic metabolic end products formed by parasites. Pointing in this direction is, for example, the fact that paperchromatographic analysis of the acids excreted by *Trichomonas vaginalis* (Wellerson *et al.*, 1959), *Toxoplasma gondii* (Fulton and Spooner, 1960), and *Taenia taeniaeformis* (von Brand and Bowman, 1961) revealed a slow moving spot that could not be identified with any of the reference acids tested.

VI.   GLYCOLYSIS

Typical glycolysis, as realized in vertebrate tissues, leads from carbohydrate to lactic acid, the individual steps of the sequence being catalyzed by specific enzymes. Glycolysis is independent of oxygen and can therefore serve as main energy-producing sequence under anaerobic conditions. In vertebrate tissues the same intermediate glycolytic steps are encountered in the absence and the presence of oxygen until the level of pyruvic acid is reached; from there on the pathways of anaerobic and aerobic degradation separate. The first steps of the glycolytic sequence

TABLE XIX

Organic Metabolites Excreted by Parasitic Helminths and Arthropods[a]

Species	Anaerobic												Aerobic												References
	Lactic acid	Pyruvic acid	Formic acid	Acetic acid	Propionic acid	Butyric acid	C_5 acids	C_6 acids	Higher fatty acids	Succinic acid	Acetoin	Ethyl alcohol	Lactic acid	Pyruvic acid	Formic acid	Acetic acid	Propionic acid	Butyric acid	C_5 acids	C_6 acids	Higher fatty acids	Succinic acid	Acetoin	Ethyl alcohol	
Trematodes																									
Fasciola gigantica																									Goil (1961)
Fasciola hepatica	(x)			x	x				x				(x)			x	x							x	Flury and Leeb (1926); Weinland and von Brand (1926); Stephenson (1947b); Mansour (1959a,b)
Schistosoma mansoni	x												x												Bueding *et al.* (1947)
Cestodes																									
Echinococcus granulosus, larva	x			x						x						x						x		x	Agosin (1957)
Hymenolepis diminuta	x			x						x		x	x	x											C. P. Read (1956); Laurie (1957); Fairbairn *et al.* (1961)
Moniezia expansa	x								x	x			x								x	x			Alt and Tischer (1931); von Brand (1933a)
Oochoristica symmetrica	x																								Read (1956)
Phyllobothrium foliatum													x												Laurie (1961)
Taenia taeniaeformis, larva	x	x		x								x	x	x		x						x		x	von Brand and Bowman (1961)
Taenia taeniaeformis, adult	x	(x)		x								x	x	x		x						x		(x)	von Brand and Bowman (1961)

Organism												References
Acanthocephala												
Moniliformis dubius	x	x	(x)								(x)	Laurie (1959)
Nematodes												
Ancylostoma caninum								x	x	x	x	Crowley and Warren (1963); Warren and Guevara (1962)
Ascaris lumbricoides	x	(x)	x x x				(x)	x x x x x x x			x x	Weinland (1904); Flury (1912); von Brand (1934); Waechter (1934); Krueger (1936); Oesterlin (1937); Epps *et al.* (1950); Bueding and Yale (1951); Saz *et al.* (1958); Bueding *et al.* (1959); Ellison *et al.* (1960); Harpur and Waters (1960); Saz and Gerzon (1962); Whitlock and Strong (1963)
Heterakis gallinae		x x (x)		x		(x) (x)	x x (x)				x	Glocklin and Fairbairn (1952); Fairbairn (1954)
Litomosoides carinii	x	x			x	x	x				x	Bueding (1949a; personal communication, 1952)
Dracunculus insignis	x					x						Bueding (1949c); Bueding and Oliver-Gonzalez (1950)
Parascaris equorum	x	x	x			x	x x					Fischer (1924); Toryu (1936)
Trichinella spiralis, larvae	(x)	x x	x x			(x)						von Brand *et al.* (1952); Goldberg (1958); Agosin and Aravena (1959a)
Trichuris vulpis	(x)	x x (x) x x				(x)	x x x x x				Bueding *et al.* (1961); Bueding (personal communication, 1965)
Dirofilaria uniformis		x				x						von Brand *et al.* (1963)
Arthropods												
Gastrophilus intestinalis, larvae	x		x									von Kemnitz (1916); Blanchard and Dinulescu (1932)

[a] KEY: x = compound excreted in significant amounts; (x) = compound excreted in very small amounts only.

117

differ when glucose or glycogen serve as substrate. In the former case the first reaction is phosphorylation of glucose to glucose-6-phosphate by means of hexokinase, while in the latter case this compound is formed only over glucose-1-phosphate as intermediate, requiring the intervention of two enzymes (phosphorylase and phosphoglucomutase).

Phosphorylative glycolysis is apparently widely distributed among parasites. Relevant evidence has been arrived at by different routes. One line of investigation has been the search for glycolytic enzymes within the tissues of parasites. As the data of Tables XX and XXI indicate, such enzymes do occur both in parasitic protozoa and worms. It is also obvious, however, that the evidence for the existence of a complete glycolytic sequence is in many cases incomplete, only one or a few of the required enzymes having been demonstrated. This is due, in part, to the fact that some investigators were interested just in one particular enzyme. In other cases, however, a negative search for some key enzymes of the glycolytic chain have been reported. Thus, to mention only one example, Hilker and White (1959) were unable to find a phosphotriose dehydrogenase in *Entamoeba histolytica*. However, in this and some similar cases an inactivation of the missing enzymes during processing of the material cannot be ruled out. Furthermore, it should be kept in mind that in most investigations intended as survey of the enzymatic equipment of a given parasite (be the survey restricted to the glycolytic sequence or dealing with the enzymes of the pentose-phosphate shunt, or those of the tricarboxylic acid cycle), systems were employed patterned after those found adequate for the corresponding mammalian enzymes. In one or the other case they may well have been inadequate for the parasite enzymes. Some of the differences in requirements of glycolytic enzymes isolated from various parasites will be mentioned later.

In some instances, however, there is evidence for a modified glycolysis because of the lack, or perhaps only the very low activity, of a certain enzyme. In normal glycolysis, for instance, reduction of pyruvic acid to lactic acid serves to reoxidize the reduced form of diphospho-pyridine nucleotide (DPNH) formed during triose oxidation and this process, however it is achieved, prevents glycolysis from coming to a complete standstill. The blood-stream forms of the trypanosomes of the *brucei* group do not produce appreciable amounts (if indeed any) of lactic acid. It is probable that glyceraldehyde phosphate serves as hydrogen acceptor for the reoxidation of DPNH, a process leading to phospho-glycerol. Glycerol, one of the main end products of the anaerobic metabolism of these organisms, would then be liberated by a phosphatase. The required enzymes have been demonstrated in trypanosomes: glycerophosphate dehydrogenase (Harvey, 1949; Grant and Sargent, 1960) and phosphatases (Harvey, 1949; Gerzeli, 1955). The previously mentioned multitude of anaerobic metabolic end products (Tables XVIII and XIX) is indicative of the fact that classical glycolysis (that is, the carbohydrate-lactic acid sequence) occurs only in few parasites as the only sequence of anaerobic carbohydrate degradation. While the intermediate steps, those leading to pyruvic acid, appear fairly uniform, the terminal steps are quite variable.

In addition to the demonstration of typical glycolytic enzymes, two other lines of study have been employed to demonstrate the occurrence of glycolytic types of carbohydrate degradation. One such line is the search for phosphorylated intermediates of glycolysis. As Table XXII indicates, typical intermediates have been found in several parasites and it can be surmised that they are widely distributed. Radiocarbon from C^{14}-glucose has been found in hexose-, mono- and diphosphates in the cases of *Leishmania tropica, Endotrypanum schaudinni, Trypanosoma cruzi*, and *Trypanosoma rhodesiense* (Shaw *et al.*, 1964).

Finally, glucose labeled in various positions has been offered parasites and subsequent elucidation of radioactivity in metabolic end products served to assess the relative importance of various metabolic pathways, among them glycolysis. To mention first some experiments with protozoa, Grant and Fulton (1957) found that pyruvic acid and glycerol formed by *Trypanosoma rhodesiense* from uniformly labeled glucose under both aerobic and anaerobic conditions were labeled to the same degree. This was true only for aerobiosis when glucose-1-C^{14} served as substrate, while under anaerobic conditions most of the label appeared in glycerol. In similar experiments with *Plasmodium berghei*, Bowman *et al.* (1961) found the greatest amount of activity in lactic acid and only a very small amount in respiratory CO_2, the latter of course not originating from true glycolysis. Fundamentally, these experiments uphold the view that a glycolytic pattern of metabolism characterizes many parasitic protozoa.

As to helminths, no relevant experiments seem as yet to have been done with species presumably having a more or less purely glycolytic type of metabolism, such as *Dirofilaria uniformis*. However, data are available for some species characterized by fatty acid fermentations; in other words, species where glycolytic reactions in the narrow sense of the word are only part of the sequence. Thus, Entner and Gonzalez (1959) offered glucose labeled in various positions to *Ascaris lumbricoides*. They found an appreciable amount of labeling regularly in the C_2 to C_6 acids produced, while carbon dioxide was especially highly labeled when derived from uniformly labeled glucose, indicating probably

TABLE XX
Glycolytic Enzymes in Parasitic Protozoa[a,b]

Species	Phosphorylase	Phosphoglucomutase	Hexokinase	Phosphohexose isomerase	Phosphohexokinase	Aldolase	Phosphotriose isomerase	Phosphotriose dehydrogenase[c]	Phosphoglyceromutase	Enolase	Pyruvic kinase	Lactic dehydrogenase	References
Flagellates													
Crithidia fasciculata			X										Schwartz (1961)
Leishmania donovani			X										Chatterjee et al. (1958)
Strigomonas oncopelti	X	X	X	X									Ryley (1955a)
Trichomonas foetus		X	X	X	X	X		X	X				Ryley (1955b); Lindblom (1961)
Trichomonas gallinarum			X	X	X	X				X			Lindblom (1961)
Trichomonas suis			X	X		X				X			Lindblom (1961)
Trichomonas vaginalis	X	X	X	X		X	X		X	X	X	X	Wirtschafter (1954); Wirtschafter and Jahn (1956); Baernstein (1959); Wellerson and Kupferberg (1962)
Trypanosoma cruziC				X	X	X	X	X			X	X	Baernstein and Rees (1952); Baernstein (1953a); Raw (1959); Warren and Guevara (1964)
Trypanosoma equiperdum B						X		X					Chen and Geiling (1946)
Trypanosoma hippicum B					X			X					Harvey (1949)
Trypanosoma lewisi B			X									X	Ryley (1951)

120

					References
Trypanosoma rhodesiense **B**	x		x	x	Grant and Sargent (1960); Ryley (1962)
Trypanosoma rhodesiense C	x			x	Ryley (1962)
Rhizopods					
Entamoeba histolytica	x	x	x	x	Hilker and White (1959); Kun *et al.* (1956); Bragg and Reeves (1962)
Sporozoa					
Plasmodium berghei	x	x			Fraser and Kermack (1957); Bowman *et al.* (1961)
Plasmodium gallinaceum	x		x	x	Speck and Evans (1945)
Plasmodium knowlesi					McKee *et al.* (1946)
Plasmodium lophurae					Sherman (1961)
Toxoplasma gondii	x				Fulton and Spooner (1960); Capella and Kaufman (1964)

[a] In part after von Brand (1963).
[b] KEY: C = culture forms; B = blood-stream forms; x = enzyme in significant amounts.
[c] In some cases the dehydrogenase was not demonstrated specifically, but a triosephosphate-oxidizing system is then mentioned.

TABLE XXI

Glycolytic Enzymes in Parasitic Worms[a,b]

Species	Phosphorylase	Phosphoglucomutase	Hexokinase	Phosphohexose isomerase	Phosphohexokinase	Phosphotriose isomerase	Aldolase	Phosphotriose dehydrogenase	Enolase	Lactic dehydrogenase	References
Trematodes											
Fasciola hepatica					x						Mansour (1962)
Schistosoma mansoni	x	x	x	x	x	x		x		x	Bueding (1949b); Bueding and Yale (1951); Mansour and Bueding (1953, 1954); Bueding and Mackinnon (1955); Bueding and Mansour (1957); Bueding (personal communication, 1965)
Cestodes											
Echinococcus granulosus	x	x	x	x		x	x	x		x	Agosin and Aravena (1959b, 1960)
Hymenolepis diminuta		x	x	x		x	x	x		x	C. P. Read (1951)
Taenia crassiceps						x					Phifer (1958)
Taenia taeniaeformis	x	x	x	x		x		x		x	Waitz (1963)
Nematodes											
Ascaris lumbricoides	x	x	x	x		x			x	x	Cavier and Savel (1953); Rathbone and Rees (1954); Saz and Hubbard (1957)
Ditylenchus dipsaci		x	x							x	Krusberg (1960)
Trichinella spiralis, larva			x	x		x		x	x	x	Goldberg (1958); Agosin and Aravena (1959a); Mancilla and Agosin (1960)
Acanthocephala											
Moniliformis dubius				x				x		x	C. P. Read (1961b)
Neoechinorhynchus emydis				x						x	Dunagan (1964)

[a] In part after Read (1961).

[b] KEY: x = enzyme in significant amounts.

TABLE XXII

PHOSPHORYLATED GLYCOLYTIC INTERMEDIATES IN SOME PARASITES[a,b]

Species	Glucose-1-phosphate	Glucose-6-phosphate	Fructose-6-phosphate	Fructose-1,6-phosphate	Triose-phosphate	Phosphoglyceric acid	Phosphopyruvic acid	References
Flagellates								
Trichomonas vaginalis	x	x	x	x		x		Wirtschafter and Jahn (1956)
Trypanosoma equiperdum B			x	x				Chen and Geiling (1946)
Trypanosoma evansi B		x	x	x	x	x	x	
Trypanosoma hippicum B	x			x	x			Marshall (1948b) Harvey (1949)
Sporozoa								
Plasmodium berghei		x	x					Bowman *et al.* (1961)
Plasmodium gallinaceum		x	x	x	x	x	x	Marshall (1948a)
Trematodes								
Fasciola hepatica			(Sugar phosphates x)				x	Bryant and Williams (1962)
Schistosoma mansoni		x	x	x				Bueding and Mansour (1957)
Cestodes								
Hymenolepis diminuta		x	x	x	x	x		C. P. Read (1951)
Nematodes								
Strongyloides ratti, filariform larvae	x	x	x	x	x	x		Jones *et al.* (1955)

[a] Some further data in Shaw *et al.* (1964).

[b] KEY: B = blood-stream form; x = intermediate in significant amounts.

that it was derived largely from the 3 and 4 carbons of the sugar. The methyl group of the acetate, on the other hand, was especially radioactive when derived from glucose-1-C^{14}. These experiments of Entner and Gonzalez (1959) can be interpreted as indicating a prevalence of glycolysis in *Ascaris* when the word is used in a broad sense, but they also indicate that the pentose phosphate pathway or some other mechanism plays a role, though probably only a minor one. In this connection it should be mentioned that Saz and Vidrine (1959) compared the incorporation of glucose-1-C^{14}, glucose-2-C^{14}, and glucose-6-C^{14} into succinate. They found no significant difference between the 1 and the 6 carbons of glucose, thus proving that the pentose shunt cannot be a significant factor in the oxidative pathway of the *Ascaris* muscle. Similar experiments done by Scheibel and Saz (personal communication) with *Hymenolepis diminuta* led to the same conclusion, since it was observed again that the 1 and 6 carbons of glucose were equivalent in labeling of succinate. In similar experiments with the miracidia and adults of *Fasciola hepatica,* Bryant and Williams (1962) found relatively high percentages of the labeled carbon in glycolytic intermediates, such as sugar phosphates, or end products, such as lactic acid. Furthermore, labeled alanine was found which presumably originated from pyruvic acid by transamination and therefore reinforces the impression that the glycolytic sequence down to pyruvate is realized in both stages. This will be true in many parasites, both protozoa and metazoa, as the three lines of evidence reviewed above indicate.

Labeled carbohydrate as substrate has, in addition to the above studies, served to elucidate the pathways of formation of many metabolic end products. Before mentioning these cases, some details concerning the glycolytic enzymes will be reviewed.

An interesting variety of properties has been reported for hexokinases. In the case of *Leishmania donovani* apparently a single enzyme phosphorylates glucose, fructose, mannose, galactose, and glucosamine; it seems not to depend on functional sulfhydryl groups for activity (Chatterjee *et al.,* 1958). On the contrary, several distinct hexokinases have been found in parasitic worms. *Schistosoma mansoni* has at least four different hexokinases, one solely active respectively with glucose, fructose, mannose, and glucosamine (Bueding *et al.,* 1954; Bueding and Mackinnon, 1955). They could be separated from each other by fractionation with alumina gel. To give an example of their properties, it may be mentioned that the glucokinase was inhibited by SH-inhibitors, glucose-6-phosphate, sorbose-1-phosphate, and adenosine diphosphate (ADP), resembling in these respects brain hexokinase, but differing from the mammalian enzyme in affinity for glucose, adenosine triphosphate (ATP), and Mg^{++}. Four corresponding hexokinases have also been found in the scoleces of *Echinococcus granulosus* by Agosin and Aravena (1959b). While they proved on the whole similar to the schistosome enzymes, they differed in detail from the latter. Thus, the tapeworm is unable to phosphorylate 2-deoxyglucose, while the fluke can. The fructokinase of *Schistosoma* is competitively inhibited by ADP, that of *Echinococcus* noncompetitively; the former enzyme is not inhibited by glucose-6-phosphate, the latter is, and so forth.

The various sugars mentioned above are used by many parasites (Tables XII and XIII). It can be assumed that phosphorylations are involved. This has been shown specifically for the larvae of *Trichinella spiralis* (Agosin and Aravena, 1959a), but it is not known whether one or more kinases are involved. Curiously, little attention seems to have been devoted to the question whether galactose is phosphorylated by a special enzyme. Some indication for transformation of galactose to glucose-6-phosphate via galactokinase, galactose uridyl transferase, and phosphoglucomutase have been reported by Waitz (1963) for *Taenia taeniaeformis*. The kinase involved seems to require ATP and Mg^{++} for activity.

Even less is known about the enzymes allowing mannose utilization. A phosphomannose isomerase has been found in the scoleces of *Echinococcus granulosus* (Agosin and Aravena, 1959b).

Phosphoglucose isomerase has been purified partially; in the case of *Schistosoma mansoni* 20- to 30-fold by ammonium sulfate precipitation followed by treatment with calcium phosphate gel (Bueding and Mackinnon, 1955), while an essentially similar procedure led to 48-fold purification in the case of *Trichinella spiralis* larvae (Mancilla and Agosin, 1960). The optimum pH of the schistosome enzyme was 8.2 to 8.6, that of the *Trichinella* enzyme 8.0. In both instances the ratio of glucose-6-phosphate/fructose-6-phosphate at equilibrium was 65/35, but both enzymes differed from one another by the fact that the K_m for fructose-6-phosphate was 1×10^{-4} and 4.25×10^{-3}, respectively, for the fluke and roundworm enzyme. The latter did not require metals for activation, but Co^{++} and Mg^{++} were inhibitory; the enzyme does not depend on sulfhydryl groups for activity.

The phosphofructokinase of *Schistosoma mansoni* is inhibited by trivalent organic arsenicals, such as stibophen or antimony potassium tartrate (Mansour and Bueding, 1954). The consequent induced lower-than-normal concentration of fructose-1, 6-diphosphate results in a decrease in aldolase activity with the end result that glycolysis of the homogenates is definitely inhibited (Bueding and Mansour, 1957). It is remarkable that the phosphofructokinase of *Fasciola hepatica* is stimulated by serotonin both *in vivo* and *in vitro* (Mansour, 1962).

The aldolases of several parasites have been studied in greater or lesser detail and some interesting differences between species have become known. The enzyme of the culture form of *Trypanosoma cruzi* appears not to be metal-activated since it is not inhibited by dipyridyl (Baernstein and Rees, 1952). This may be a common characteristic of the trypanosome aldolases, since Ryley (1953), working with the intact blood-stream form of *Trypanosoma lewisi* rather than homogenates as employed by Baernstein and Rees (1952) arrived at essentially similar conclusions. The aldolase of a tapeworm, the larva of *Taenia crassiceps* is also not influenced by metal-binding agents, nor by ferric, cobaltous, magnesium, stannous, or nickel salts (Phifer, 1958). The tapeworm enzyme has a somewhat higher pH optimum (8.4 to 9.0 versus 7.3 to 7.6) than the trypanosome enzyme, and a somewhat higher Michaelis-Menten constant (6.1×10^{-3} M versus 1.2×10^{-3} M hexosediphosphate).

The aldolase of *Trichomonas vaginalis*, on the other hand, differs sharply from the above aldolases by its metal relationships. It is strongly inhibited by dipyridyl and ethylene diamine tetraacetate, but can be reactivated by ferrous and cobaltous salts. Cu^{++} and Zn^{++} are inhibitory, while Mg^{++} and Mn^{++} have little effect. The pH optimum is 7.0 and K_m 10^{-3} M (Baernstein, 1954). A dipyridyl sensitivity has also been demonstrated for the aldolase of *Trichomonas foetus* (Ryley, 1955b) and may therefore be a common characteristic for the trichomonad enzymes.

The lactic dehydrogenase of *Trichomonas vaginalis* has been partially purified by Baernstein (1959). It is mainly DPN-linked, giving with TPN only 16% of the DPN activity. The enzyme attacks only L(+) lactate; the D(−) isomer is completely inactive. The K_m for DPNH is 1.7×10^{-5} M, that for pyruvate 2×10^{-4} M. The enzyme requires functional SH-groups; they are, however, not very reactive, being inhibited by *p*-chloromercuribenzoate, but not by iodoacetic acid or arsenite. The lactic dehydrogenase of *Plasmodium lophurae* during electrophoresis on a starch block has a single cathodal peak, which differs from that of the host cell enzyme. Both enzymes have identical pH optima (7.5) and K_m for pyruvate (1.8×10^{-5} M at pH 7.6), but their kinetic constants differ. The parasite's dehydrogenase is more efficient at low pH and high pyruvate concentration than the erythrocyte isozyme, while the reverse holds true for high pH and low pyruvate concentration (Sherman, 1961).

VII. TERMINAL ANAEROBIC PROCESSES

As mentioned in a preceding section, glycolysis proceeds in parasites quite generally in a typical fashion until pyruvate is formed. From this level on a greater variety of pathways leading to the final products of anaerobic sugar degradation is found than in vertebrate tissues. The classical final step of glycolysis, formation of lactic acid from pyruvic acid, has already been mentioned as occurring in pure form in only few parasites and will not be reviewed further. In this section, the pathways leading to various other metabolic end products will be discussed.

Little is known about the formation of ethanol. The classical alcoholic fermentation, as realized, for example, in yeast, consists in decarboxylation of pyruvic acid to acetaldehyde which is reduced by means of an alcohol dehydrogenase to ethyl alcohol during which process DPNH is oxidized. It is probable that this pathway prevails in those trypanosomids that produce ethanol. A pyruvate decarboxylase and an alcohol dehydrogenase have been observed in *Strigomonas oncopelti* and *Crithidia fasciculata* (Ryley, 1955a; Schwartz, 1961; Bauchop, 1962). The process has been studied in greatest detail by Bauchop (1962), who found cell-free extracts of *Strigomonas oncopelti* to metabolize pyruvate to acetaldehyde and CO_2. The formation of both these metabolites was inhibited by thiol-binding agents and it was found that the system is dependent on thiamine pyrophosphate.

Even less definite information is available concerning the mechanism of hydrogen formation. Umbreit (1952) assumed, on the basis of observations by Suzuoki and Suzuoki (1951b) that in the case of *Trichomonas foetus* a lyase splits off hydrogen from formic acid. Lindblom (1961) did find in some trichomonad species a formic acid dehydrogenase which sometimes is considered part of the lyase system, but he was unable to find definite indications for the presence of a true hydrogenlyase or hydrogenase. Ryley (1955a) considered it possible that a phosphoroclastic reaction is involved by which H_2, CO_2, and acetyl phosphate are formed from pyruvate without involvement of formic acid. Lindblom (1961) tried without success to demonstrate such a system in the trichomonad species studied by him, although they could develop hydrogen from pyruvate. He considers his negative evidence as inconclusive, since the system in question is very labile and could have been inactivated during processing of the organisms.

More has become known in recent years concerning the pathways leading to lower fatty acids. It has already been mentioned above that acetic acid arises in *Litomosoides carinii* from dismutation of pyruvic acid into CO_2, lactic, and acetic acids (Bueding, 1949a). Another system has been found in *Crithidia fasciculata* and the culture form of *Trypanosoma cruzi* (Seaman, 1956). It leads from succinic acid to acetic acid according to the following scheme:

$$\text{Succinic acid} + \text{DPNH} + 2\text{ATP} + 2\text{CoA} + 2\text{H}^+$$
$$\longrightarrow 2 \text{ acetyl CoA} + \text{DPN}^+ + 2\text{ADP} + 2\text{P}_i$$

Since the system leads to a reoxidation of the DPNH formed during glycolysis it is conceivable that it has some importance during anaerobic metabolism, but it seems hardly likely that all the acetic acid produced by these flagellates originates in this way. In *Ascaris lumbricoides* acetic acid is produced by decarboxylation of pyruvate, as indicated by the fact that C atoms of metabolized lactate-2-C^{14} appear in the methyl carbon of acetate, suggesting conversion of lactate to pyruvate, followed by de-carboxylation (Saz and Weil, 1960).

On the other hand, propionic acid seems not to originate directly from lactate in *Ascaris* muscle. Although propionic acid is labeled when muscle is incubated with lactate-1-C^{14}, malonate inhibits incorporation of lactate-2-C^{14} into propionate. This would not happen if this acid were produced by direct reduction of lactate, but agrees with the assumption that it is produced by decarboxylation of succinic acid (Saz and Vidrine, 1959).

Important metabolic end products of the *Ascaris* fermentation are two branched acids. Their origin has only recently been elucidated, a success made possible through the use of labeled compounds. The carbon chain of α-methylbutyric is produced (Fig. 4) by a condensation of the carboxyl carbon of acetate with the α-carbon of propionate (Saz and Weil, 1960; Bueding, 1962), while that of α-methyl valeric acid is formed by con-densation of the carboxyl atom of one propionic acid molecule (or strictly the acid's CoA ester) with the carbon of a second one (Saz and Weil, 1962).

Saz *et al.* (1958) found that homogenates of *Ascaris* muscle produce α-acetolactic acid. They assume that pyruvic acid is decarboxylated to form "active" acetaldehyde. The latter may then condense with pyruvic acid to form α-acetolactic acid, or with free dissociated acetaldehyde to form acetyl methyl carbinol. The acetyl methyl carbinol-forming system requires as cofactor diphosphothiamine and also Mn^{++}.

Succinic acid, one of the important intermediates of the tricarboxylic acid cycle, cannot originate under anaerobic conditions by the reactions of that cycle as they proceed under aerobiosis. Various pathways leading to anaerobic succinate production have been discussed. Although the succinate-splitting reaction (Seaman, 1956) mentioned above is reversi-ble, it is questionable whether it actually leads to succinate production under natural conditions since the equilibrium of the reaction favors splitting (Seaman, 1957). Another system that could lead to the anaerobic production of succinic acid with the anaerobic formation of high-energy phosphate bonds has been visualized by Seidman and Entner (1961) for the sarcosomes of *Ascaris* as follows:

$$2 \text{ Malate} + \text{ADP} + P_i \longrightarrow \text{pyruvate} + CO_2 + \text{succinate} + \text{ATP}$$
fumarate

The malate required for the reaction could be formed by CO_2 fixation on pyruvate and thus the entire system could function in the absence of oxygen. Most evidence, however, is available for anaerobic succinate

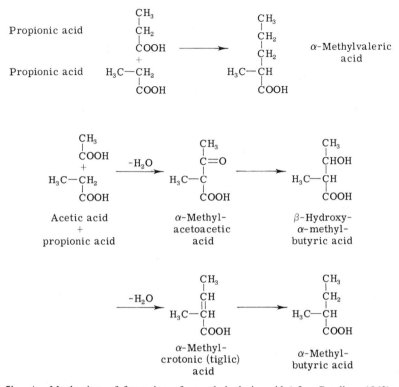

Fig. 4. Mechanism of formation of α-methylvaleric acid (after Bueding, 1962) and α-methylbutyric acid. (After Saz and Weil, 1960.)

production by reversal of some reactions of the Krebs cycle, coupled to an auxiliary reaction, such as formation of oxaloacetic acid by transamination or CO_2 fixation. Various CO_2-fixing mechanisms are known, the most important ones being carboxylation of pyruvic acid or phosphoenolpyruvic acid by pyruvate carboxylase and phosphoenolpyruvate carboxylase, respectively, resulting in the formation of oxaloacetic acid, or formation of malate from pyruvate by intervention of the "malic enzyme." The oxaloacetic acid, or malic acid originating in these ways can then be transformed into succinic acid by the successive intervention of malic dehydrogenase (in the case of oxaloacetic acid), fumarase, and succinic dehydrogenase.

The quantitative importance of transamination as source for oxaloacetic acid cannot be assessed properly at present; it can be stated that for some organisms oxaloacetic acid originating in this way will not be the main substrate for CO_2 fixation. *Trypanosoma cruzi*, for instance, fixes CO_2 and produces succinic acid in media containing glucose as the only organic substance; it is very unlikely that it stores sufficient aspartic acid in its body to explain succinate production via transamination. The occurrence of CO_2 fixation is well documented for trypanosomes. First evidence was adduced by Searle and Reiner (1940, 1941) and their findings were substantiated by the manometric experiments of Ryley (1956, 1962). Grant and Fulton (1957) proved CO_2 fixation in the case of the blood-stream form of *Trypanosoma rhodesiense* by the use of radioactive bicarbonate, recovering labeled carbon only from the carboxyl groups of succinic acid. Similar experiments by Bowman *et al.* (1963) with the culture form of *Trypanosoma cruzi,* involving utilization of variously labeled glucose and bicarbonate, led to the conclusion that both aerobic and anaerobic succinate production involved CO_2 fixation to pyruvate. However, no definite conclusion was reached as to whether a "malic enzyme" or oxaloacetic decarboxylase catalyzed the reaction. It can, however, be pointed out that Raw (1959) demonstrated in this organism a "malic enzyme." A similar mode of succinate production had already been described for *Ascaris* by Saz and Vidrine (1959), again with a "malic enzyme" probably involved in CO_2 fixation (Saz and Hubbard, 1957). It is of considerable interest that succinate production has been observed upon incubation of a purified particulate system from *Ascaris* muscle with fumarate and DPNH. This definitely implicates reversal of the succinoxidase system in succinate production (Kmetec and Bueding, 1961). Furthermore, it appears that the *Ascaris* system is more efficient in reducing fumarate than in oxidizing succinate, a feature possibly representing an adaptation to the worm's predominantly anaerobic life (Bueding, 1962). Incorporation of radioactive CO_2 into succinic acid has also been proven for the scoleces of *Echinococcus granulosus* (Agosin and Repetto, 1963). In this instance CO_2 appears to be fixed to pyruvic acid by more than one mechanism, namely, phosphoenolpyruvic acid carboxykinase and "malic enzyme," the latter enzyme probably being more important in this respect than the former (Agosin and Repetto, personal communication, 1964).

CO_2 fixation into succinic acid has also been made probable in the case of *Heterakis gallinae* (Fairbairn, 1954), but in this worm most of the label appeared in the carboxyl group of propionic acid. The monogenetic trematode *Entobdella bumpusi* initially incorporates C^{14} from labeled bicarbonate into malic acid, but also rapidly into other acids, among them fumaric and succinic acids (Hammen and Lum, 1962). Relatively high CO_2 tension in the environment favors many parasites and may be indicative for fixation processes. This has, for example, been shown for the worms *Hymenolepis diminuta* (Fairbairn *et al.*, 1961) and *Trichuris vulpis* (Bueding *et al.*, 1961), as well as for the protozoa *Epidinium ecaudatum* (Oxford, 1958), *Dasytricha ruminantium, Isotricha prostoma,* and *Isotricha intestinalis* (Gutierrez, 1955). It cannot be concluded, however, without further evidence that in these cases CO_2 fixation leads to succinic acid, since other possibilities exist. A case in point is *Trichomonas vaginalis.* Kupferberg *et al.* (1953) first recognized that this flagellate fixes CO_2. The label, however, appears not in succinic acid, but exclusively in the carboxyl group of lactic acid (Wellerson *et al.,* 1959, 1960). The organism seems not to be able to carboxylate pyruvic acid, and Wellerson *et al.* (1960) visualize a carboxylation of pentosediphosphate leading to 3-phosphoglyceric acid. This last compound would then be metabolized via the glycolytic pathway and eventually lead to carboxyl-labeled lactate. A somewhat different reaction series has recently been postulated for *Trichomonas foetus* by Magliocca (1963). He found only 50% of the fixed radioactivity in lactic acid; the other 50% was distributed between pyruvate, α-ketoglutarate, glycine, glutamate, and aspartate. He suggests the following route of synthesis: bicarbonate-α-ketoglutarate-lactate-pyruvate-amino acids.

VIII. THE PENTOSE PHOSPHATE AND ENTNER-DOUDOROFF PATHWAYS

The pentose phosphate pathway consists of a complicated series of reactions involving formation and degradation of phosphates of heptoses, hexoses, tetroses, and trioses, a sugar lactone, and gluconic acid. The end result is complete oxidation of glucose to CO_2 and water with the formation of 3 moles ATP per mole glucose utilized. The process is generally less important for the production of energy than it is as a basis for synthetic processes. It therefore would not be surprising if the sequence were widely distributed among parasites.

However, relatively little definite information is at present available insofar as parasitic protozoa are concerned. Only a few key enzymes of the sequence have been demonstrated (Table XXIII) and this is insufficient evidence to prove the presence of a functional cycle. Thus, *Entamoeba histolytica,* or at least one strain, has a glucose-6-phosphate dehydrogenase. Nevertheless, Hilker and White (1959) deny the presence of the pentose phosphate cycle because they could not find a 6-phosphogluconate dehydrogenase and because, according to Nakamura and Baker (1956) ribose-5-phosphate has to be added to culture media to ensure optimal growth. Hilker and White (1959) are of the opinion that in this case the so-called Entner-Doudoroff pathway is realized by which 6-phosphogluconate is split into pyruvic acid and glyceraldehyde-3-phosphate. This view is supported by Entner's (1958) finding that after providing the amoebas with glucose-1-C^{14} the greatest amount of radioactivity appears in the carboxyl group of lactic acid. The respiratory CO_2 remained unlabeled, in contrast to what would have happened if the pentose-phosphate cycle were functioning. The methyl group of lactic acid was labeled also, indicating that true glycolysis also was functioning. There is some question whether the above findings apply to all strains of *Entamoeba histolytica,* since Bragg and Reeves (1962) could not find one of the key enzymes of the Entner-Doudoroff scheme, glucose-6-phosphate dehydrogenase, in the so-called Laredo strain.

Comparable uncertainties exist in the case of the culture form of *Trypanosoma cruzi.* Raw (1959) denies the existence of the pentose phosphate pathway because the organisms are unable to split ribose-5-phosphate, although they attack 6-phosphogluconate. He considers it as possible that the flagellates produce pyruvate via the Wood and Schwerdt enzyme, which splits 6-phosphogluconate into pyruvate and glyceraldehyde-3 phosphate. In essence then a parallel to *Entamoeba* would exist. However, Ryley (1962) could not confirm the utilization of phosphogluconic acid by the culture form of *Trypanosoma cruzi,* nor did he observe such a faculty when using the culture form of *Trypanosoma rhodesiense.*

More evidence for a functional pentose phosphate cycle is available for helminths than for protozoa. While it is true that only two key enzymes have been sought for in the majority of worms studied, a much more complete set of data has been presented in two instances.

Agosin and Aravena (1960) identified, in addition to the enzymes shown in Table XXIII in *Echinococcus granulosus,* glucose, fructose, ribulose, ribose, sedoheptulose, and glyceraldehyde, all compounds derived from endogenous polysaccharide utilization. In the case of *Ascaris lumbricoides,* the formation of ribulose and sedoheptulose has been demonstrated (De Ley and Vercruysse, 1955; Entner, 1957). Some of the *Ascaris* enzymes have been partially purified, for instance, ribose-5-phosphate isomerase and transketolase, the two enzymes used by Entner (1957) to demonstrate ribulose formation. This investigator also showed the glucose-6-phosphate dehydrogenase and 6-phosphogluconate dehydrogenase to be strictly TPN specific.

On the whole then it seems likely that the above two worms have a functional pentose-phosphate pathway, although the failure to demonstrate a transaldolase reaction in *Ascaris* (Entner, 1957) casts some doubt on this conclusion.

IX. THE TRICARBOXYLIC ACID CYCLE

The tricarboxylic or Krebs cycle is of great importance to many aerobic organisms because the energy yield of the sequence is much greater than

TABLE XXIII

ENZYMES OF THE PENTOSE PHOSPHATE PATHWAY IN PARASITES[a,b]

Species	Glucose-6-dehydrogenase	6-Phosphogluconate dehydrogenase	Transketolase	Transaldolase	Phosphopentose isomerase	Ribokinase	3-Phosphoglyceraldehyde dehydrogenase	Triosephosphate isomerase	References
Ascaris lumbricoides	x	x	x		x				Entner (1957); DeLey and Vercruysse (1955)
Echinococcus granulosus	x	x	x	x	x	x	x	x	Agosin and Aravena (1960)

[a] KEY: x = enzyme in significant amounts.

[b] Glucose-6-dehydrogenase alone has been demonstrated in the following parasites: *Crithidia fasciculata* (Schwartz, 1961); *Trichomonas*, 4 spp. (Lindblom, 1961); *Trypanosoma rhodesiense*, bloodstream and culture forms (Ryley, 1962), and *Entamoeba histolytica* (Hilker and White, 1959); *Toxoplasma gondii* (Capella and Kaufman, 1964). Glucose-6-dehydrogenase and 6-phosphogluconate dehydrogenase have been found in the following parasites: *Trypanosoma cruzi*, culture form (Raw, 1959); *Fasciola hepatica, Dicrocoelium dendriticum; Anoplocephala perfoliata, Moniezia benedeni, Taenia saginata, Taenia pisiformis, Dipylidium caninum, Parascaris equorum, Toxocara canis, Ascaridia galli, Ascaridia columbae, Heterakis gallinae, Strongylus edentatus* (De Ley and Vercruysse, 1955); *Ditylenchus triformis*, and *Ditylenchus dipsaci* (Krusberg, 1960).

that resulting from glycolysis, because its intermediates can serve as substrates for various synthetic processes, and finally because it is linked not only to carbohydrate breakdown, but also to lipid metabolism (e.g., via fatty acids ⟶ acetoacetate ⟶ acetate ⟶ pyruvate), and protein metabolism (e.g., via alanine ⟶ pyruvic acid, or glutamate ⟶ α-ketoglutarate). The essence of the Krebs cycle is complete oxidation of pyruvic acid to carbon dioxide and water by a cyclic series of reactions. These involve condensation of a two-carbon derivative of pyruvic acid (acetyl CoA) with oxaloacetic acid to form tricarboxylic, then dicarboxylic acids, and completing the cycle with regeneration of oxaloacetic acid. The sequence can therefore proceed as long as pyruvic acid, regardless of its origin, is fed into the sequence. A complication arising in the case of practically all parasites is that they are, as mentioned in a preceding section, aerobic fermenters. That is, they excrete large amounts of organic acids, among them often acids, such as succinic acid, which originate from Krebs cycle reactions. It is evident that in these latter cases the cycle would soon come to a standstill if no oxaloacetic acid were resynthesized and refed into the cycle, since this acid can be considered as the "motor" of the sequence (Karlson, 1961). The necessity of synthesizing oxaloacetic acid may be the reason why CO_2 fixation takes place aerobically in such forms as *Trypanosoma cruzi* (Bowman *et al.*, 1963).

A typical Krebs cycle cannot function under anaerobic conditions. However, some of the reactions of the cycle may still be of importance either during enforced anaerobiosis, or normally for organisms leading *in vivo* a predominantly anaerobic life. It has thus been mentioned in the preceding section that anaerobic succinate production can often be explained by assuming a reversal of some of the Krebs cycle reactions.

Acetyl CoA, the starting compound of the Krebs cycle, is formed quite generally, if derived ultimately from carbohydrate catabolism, by oxidative decarboxylation of pyruvic acid, a process involving participation of thioctic acid, CoA, and DPN and mediated by a complicated enzyme complex, the pyruvic oxidase system. This initial step has been studied little in parasites, but a pyruvate oxidase has been reported from *Crithidia fasciculata* (F. R. Hunter, 1960) and the culture form of *Trypanosoma rhodesiense* (Ryley, 1962), while it was not found in the bloodstream form of this species.

More information is available in respect to other Krebs cycle enzymes (Tables XXIV and XXV) as a result of biochemical and histochemical investigations. Other relevant lines of investigation have been studies concerned with the detection of Krebs cycle intermediates in the bodies of parasites (Table XXVI) and investigations concerned with the question whether intermediates of the cycle can be utilized (Tables XXVII and XXVIII). In these latter studies various criteria have been applied: substrate utilization, influence on the rate of oxygen consumption, or in the case of some protozoa, influence on growth and multiplication. Adjuncts to these investigations have been studies dealing with the influence of fairly specific inhibitors of the tricarboxylic acid cycle, such as fluoroacetate and malonate.

A survey of the available evidence indicates that no generalizations are possible in respect to the question whether a typical tricarboxylic acid cycle is realized in parasites; one is furthermore impressed by the necessity of great caution in interpreting the data. Evidently if only one or a few enzymes have been found, or if only one or two intermediates are utilized, it would be premature to assume the presence of a complete cycle. But it would be equally premature to assume the absence of the cycle when several enzymes have not been found or intermediates have not been utilized. Differences in techniques often decide whether an enzyme is found or not. Typical in this respect is *Trypanosoma cruzi*. Baernstein and Tobie (1951) and Baernstein and Rees (1952) did not

TABLE XXIV

KREBS CYCLE ENZYMES IN PARASITIC PROTOZOA[a,b]

Species	Aconitase	Isocitric dehydrogenase	Succinic dehydrogenase	Fumarase	Malic dehydrogenase	References
Flagellates						
Crithidia fasciculata	x	x	x	x	x	F. R. Hunter (1960)
Strigomonas oncopelti			x	x	x	Ryley (1955a)
Trichomonas gallinarum					x	Lindblom (1961)
Trichomonas suis					x	Lindblom (1961)
Trichomonas vaginalis		(x)	(x)		x	Seaman (1953b); Wirtschafter et al. (1956); Asami (1956)
Trypanosoma cruzi C	x	x	x	x	x	Seaman (1953a,b); Baernstein (1953a,b); Agosin and von Brand (1955); Agosin and Weinbach (1956); Raw (1959); Chakravarty et al. (1962)
Trypanosoma lewisi B			x			Ryley (1951)
Trypanosoma rhodesiense B	x	x		x		Ryley (1962)
Trypanosoma rhodesiense C	x	x	x	x		Ryley (1962)
Rhizopods						
Entamoeba histolytica		x	x			Seaman (1953b); Takuma et al. (1958a,b)
Sporozoa						
Plasmodium gallinaceum			x			Speck et al. (1946)
Plasmodium lophurae			x			Seaman (1953b)
Toxoplasma gondii			x			Capella and Kaufman (1964)
Ciliates						
Opalina carolinensis	x	x	x		x	N. W. Hunter (1955)

[a] Essentially after von Brand (1963).
[b] KEY: C = culture form; B = blood-stream form; x = enzyme in significant amounts; (x) = indicates only indirect evidence for presence of enzyme.

find a succinic dehydrogenase, Seaman (1953c) found only a weak one, but Agosin and von Brand (1955) found a very strong one, the different results obtained by these investigators being readily explained by the different homogenization techniques employed. As to the utilization of intermediates, the question of penetration through cell membranes has

TABLE XXV

KREBS CYCLE ENZYMES IN PARASITIC WORMS[a]

Species	Condensing enzyme	Aconitase	Isocitric dehydrogenase	α-Ketoglutaric dehydrogenase	Succinic dehydrogenase	Fumarase	Malic dehydrogenase	References
Trematodes								
Fasciola hepatica					x		x	Pennoit-DeCooman and van Grembergen (1942)
Schistosoma japonicum					x			Huang and Chu (1962)
Cestodes								
Cysticercus pisiformis					x	(x)		Pennoit-DeCooman (1940)
Echinococcus granulosus, scoleces	x	x	x	x	x	x	x	Agosin and Repetto (1963)
Hymenolepis diminuta					x	x	x	C. P. Read (1952, 1953); Waitz and Schardein (1964)
Hymenolepis nana					x			Goldberg and Nolf (1954); Waitz and Schardein (1964)
Moniezia benedeni					x		x	Pennoit-DeCooman and van Grembergen (1942); van Grembergen (1944)
Nematodes								
Ancylostoma caninum					x			Warren (1963)
Ascaris lumbricoides					x	x		Bueding et al. (1955); Farber and Bueding (1956); Saz and Hubbard (1957); Rhodes et al. (1964)
Ascaris lumbricoides, eggs	x	x	x	x	x		x	Costello and Brown (1962); Smith et al. (1963); Oya et al. (1963)
Ditylenchus triformis	x		x		x	x	x	Krusberg (1960)
Necator americanus					x			Fernando (1963)
Strongyloides papillosus, larvae		x	x	(x)	x		x	Costello and Grollman (1959)
Trichinella spiralis, larvae	x	x		x	x	x	x	Goldberg (1957)
Trichuris vulpis					x			Bueding et al. (1961)

[a] KEY: (x) indicates that only indirect evidence is available for the presence of a given enzyme; x = enzyme in significant amounts.

TABLE XXVI

KREBS CYCLE INTERMEDIATES IN HELMINTHS[a]

Species	Citric acid	Aconitic acid	α-Ketoglutaric acid	Succinic acid	Fumaric acid	Malic acid	Oxaloacetic acid	References
Fasciola hepatica	x	x	x	x	x	x	x	Bryant and Williams (1962); Bryant and Smith (1963); Thorsell (1963)
Fasciola hepatica, miracidia	—		—	—	—			Bryant and Williams (1962)
Echinococcus granulosus, scoleces	x		x	x		x	x	Agosin and Repetto (1963)
Ascaris lumbricoides, body fluid	—	—	—	x	—	—	x	Bueding and Farrow (1956); Ueno et al. (1960)
Ascaris lumbricoides, muscle	—	—	x	x	—	—	—	Ueno et al. (1960)

[a] KEY: x = compound was demonstrated; — = compound was not found.

to be considered carefully. It is generally recognized that Krebs cycle acids are much more readily absorbed from acid than from neutral or alkaline surroundings. The studies by von Brand and Agosin (1955) and Zeledon (1960b) on trypanosomids clearly illustrate the point. It should furthermore be realized that enzymes usually ascribed to a functional Krebs cycle can actually be used for the synthesis of amino acids or other processes having no connection with the terminal respiration. The mere demonstration of the enzymes in an organism does therefore not necessarily prove the presence of a functional cycle, unless it is demonstrated that the reactions occur as an orderly sequence in accordance with the reactions of the cycle.

Finally, there are contradictions in the literature which are difficult to explain at present. Especially puzzling is the case of *Trichomonas vaginalis*. Wirtschafter *et al.*, (1956), in accord with Ninomiya and Suzuoki (1952) and C. P. Read (1957a), concluded that the organism does not have a Krebs cycle. They could not demonstrate the utilization of intermediates by suitably fortified homogenates, nor was the oxidation

TABLE XXVII

UTILIZATION OF KREBS CYCLE INTERMEDIATES BY PARASITIC PROTOZOA[a,b]

Species	Pyruvic acid	Oxaloacetic acid	Isocitric acid	Citric acid	cis-Aconitic acid	α-Ketoglutaric acid	Succinic acid	Fumaric acid	Malic acid	References
Flagellates										
Crithidia fasciculata	x			x	x	x	x	x	x	F. R. Hunter (1960)
Endotrypanum schaudinni C	x	x	—	(x)	—	x	x	x	x	Zeledon (1960b)
Leishmania brasiliensis C	x	x		x		x	x	x	x	Medina *et al.* (1955)
Leishmania enrietti C	x		x	—	(x)	x	x	x	x	Zeledon (1960b)
Leishmania tropica C	x			x	x	x	x	x	x	von Brand and Agosin (1955)
Trichomonas batrachorum	—		—	—		—	—	—	—	Doran (1958)
Trichomonas foetus	(x)	(x)	—	—		—	—	(x)	(x)	Suzuoki and Suzuoki (1951a); Doran (1957)
Trichomonas gallinae			x	x		x	x	x	x	C. P. Read (1957a)
Trichomonas vaginalis	x	(x)	—	—	(x)	(x)	(x)	(x)	(x)	Wirtschafter *et al.* (1956); Read (1957a); Baba *et al.* (1957); Tsukahara (1961)

Species									Reference
Trypanosoma cruzi C	x	(x)	x	x	(x)	x	x	x	x	von Brand and Agosin (1955); Zeledon (1960b)
Trypanosoma evansi B	(x)	–	–			(x)	–	–	(x)	Marshall (1948b)
Trypanosoma hippicum B	–	–	–			–	–	–		Harvey (1949)
Trypanosoma lewisi B	(x)	–	–	(x)		(x)	(x)	(x)	–	Moulder (1948a); Ryley (1951)
Trypanosoma rhodesiense C	x	x	x	x		x	x	x	x	Ryley (1962)
Trypanosoma vespertilionis C	x	–	(x)	x	–	x	x	x	x	Zeledon (1960b)
Sporozoa										
Plasmodium gallinaceum	x	(x)	x	x		x	x	x	x	Speck et al. (1946)
Plasmodium lophurae	x		x	x		x	x	–	x	Bovarnick et al. (1946)
Toxoplasma gondii	(x)		–	(x)		(x)	–	–	–	Fulton and Spooner (1960)

[a] Essentially after von Brand (1963).

[b] KEY: C = culture form; B = blood-stream form; x = compound is used at significant rate; – = compound is not utilized; (x) = compound is used at insignificant rate, or the available data are contradictory.

TABLE XXVIII

UTILIZATION OF KREBS CYCLE INTERMEDIATES BY HELMINTHS[a]

Species	Pyruvic acid	Oxaloacetic acid	Citric acid	α-Ketoglutaric acid	Succinic acid	Fumaric acid	Malic acid	References
Trematodes								
Fasciola hepatica					x		x	van Grembergen (1949)
Gynaecotyla adunca	−			−	x			Vernberg· and Hunter (1960)
Himasthla quissetensis	−			−	x			Vernberg and Hunter (1963)
Himasthla quissetensis, rediae	−			−	x			Vernberg and Hunter (1963)
Himasthla quissetensis, cercariae					−			Vernberg and Hunter (1963)
Cestodes								
Echinococcus granulosus scoleces	x	x	x	x	x	x	x	Agosin and Repetto (1963)
Hymenolepis diminuta	−		−	−	x		x	C. P. Read (1956)
Moniezia benedeni					x		x	van Grembergen (1944)
Nematodes								
Ascaridia galli	x	x		x	x	x	x	Massey and Rogers (1949, 1950)
Ascaris lumbricoides	−	−	−	x	x	x	x	Rathbone (1955)
Nematodirus spp.	x	x		x	x	x	x	Massey and Rogers (1949, 1950)
Neoaplectana glaseri	x	x		x	x	x	x	Massey and Rogers (1949, 1950)
Nippostrongylus muris, larvae	x				x	x		Schwabe (1957)

[a] KEY: x = compound is utilized; − = compound is not utilized.

of pyruvic acid inhibited by fluoroacetate or malonate. Finally, they could not find intermediates of the cycle in the bodies of the flagellates after feeding of 2-C^{14}-sodium pyruvate. On the other hand, Tsukahara (1961) found that extracts of the organisms did freely oxidize all intermediates of the cycle, and he concluded that Krebs cycle reactions probably are of considerable importance to *Trichomonas vaginalis;* Kunitake *et al.* (1962) reported that the flagellates slowly metabolize glucose-U-C^{14} and succinate -2,3-C^{14} to CO_2 and amino acids. They also assume a functional Krebs cycle. It is possible that strain differences occur in this respect, as they do in respect to the previously mentioned production of hydrogen.

While the occurrence of a functional tricarboxylic acid cycle has not yet been demonstrated in parasites with the same strictness of proof as in vertebrate tissues or in bacteria, it is usually assumed that the following protozoa do possess one: the culture forms of most trypanosomids, the malarial parasites, and *Trichomonas gallinae.* It seems to be absent in some trichomonads, the blood-stream forms of the trypanosomes of the *brucei* group, and probably also those of the *lewisi* group. As to helminths, there is fair evidence for a functional cycle in the scoleces of *Echinococcus granulosus,* the small intestinal nematodes, the larvae of *Trichinella spiralis,* and in *Ditylenchus triformis.* On the other hand, it appears unlikely that such parasites as *Ascaris lumbricoides* have a complete cycle, but the evidence for a partial cycle is good. Its importance to the worm lies, as explained in a previous section, in the fact that the reaction sequence leads to succinic acid.

The assumption of a functional tricarboxylic acid cycle in some parasites does, of course, not imply correspondence in all details with the classical cycle of vertebrate tissues. As pointed out previously, acids belonging to the sequence are frequently excreted by parasites — in contrast to vertebrates — necessitating auxiliary reactions for the maintenance of the cycle. The excretion of Krebs cycle acids must be based on the relative activities of the enzymes leading to the production of these acids and those responsible for their transformation into the next compound in the sequence. However, whether quantitative enzyme deficiencies, or regulatory processes restricting the activity of certain enzymes are involved is a hitherto unresolved problem. It is certainly curious that succinic acid is often excreted in very large amounts, although the succinic dehydrogenase activity of parasite homogenates can be very pronounced in these cases. This may indicate the presence of regulatory mechanisms linked to the intactness of cellular organization.

X. CHARACTERISTICS OF KREBS CYCLE ENZYMES AND TERMINAL AEROBIC PROCESSES

The isocitric dehydrogenase of the culture form of *Trypanosoma cruzi* (Agosin and Weinbach, 1956) and of *Ascaris* eggs (Oya *et al.,* 1963) are both TPN-linked and in neither case was there an indication for a DPN-linked enzyme. The *Trypanosoma cruzi* enzyme was purified about 50-fold, the purified preparations catalyzing formation of oxalosuccinic acid from isocitric acid as well as formation of α-ketoglutaric acid from oxalosuccinic acid. Both these reactions required Mn^{++}. The dehydrogenase has a pH optimum of 7.4 and a K_m of $<3.1 \times 10^{-5} M$. Distinct differences between mammalian and protozoan enzyme were observed in respect to substrate affinity (1.25×10^{-4} and $1.25 \times 10^{-5} M$, respectively), the greater affinity of the *cruzi* enzyme for Mn^{++} and its absolute dependency on that metal.

The succinic dehydrogenase is generally connected closely to the respiratory chain forming the succinoxidase system. Of the relevant protozoan systems only that of the culture form of *Trypanosoma cruzi* has been studied in some detail. The dehydrogenase (Agosin and von Brand, 1955) is essentially particle-bound, functioning most effectively with brilliant cresyl blue as electron carrier, while cytochrome c is ineffective in this respect. Of inorganic substances only Ca^{++} proved stimulating. The enzyme was readily inhibited by low concentrations of malonate; in contrast to intact flagellates, the inhibition was not relieved by even fairly high concentrations of succinate. The succinoxidase system itself differs in some respect from the corresponding mammalian system. *Trypanosoma cruzi* has no cytochrome c, but only cytochrome b (Baernstein and Tobie, 1951). Although it has a cytochrome reductase, it is unable to oxidize cytochrome c. Obviously then, the terminal oxidase cannot be a cytochrome c oxidase. Seaman (1953c) is of the opinion that the electron transport involves cytochrome b and the so-called Slater factor, leading to an unknown carrier, possibly a flavoprotein.

Better known is the succinoxidase system of *Ascaris lumbricoides* which has been studied intensively by Bueding who summarized his and his co-workers studies in two stimulating papers (Bueding, 1962, 1963). The enzyme system is localized in the mitochondria, but it could be solubilized by means of deoxycholate, allowing a subsequent 45-fold purification by fractionation with ammonium sulfate (Kmetec and Bueding, 1961). Cytochrome oxidase as terminal oxidase has been ruled out since *Ascaris* adults contain neither appreciable amounts of cytochrome c or of cytochrome oxidase (Bueding and Charms, 1952). It is characteristic for the *Ascaris* system that it works more efficiently at high than at low oxygen tensions, that hydrogen peroxide rather than water is produced during succinate oxidation, and that the system is not inhibited by cyanide, azide, or antimycin A (Laser, 1944; Bueding *et al.*, 1955). It is probable therefore that the system reacts with atmospheric oxygen by means of a flavin-containing terminal oxidase which was found to be Mn^{++} activated. The view that flavin enzymes participate in the system is strongly supported by the observation that purified preparations contain flavin adenine dinucleotide as major component, while they contain only little flavin mononucleotide or riboflavin (Bueding, 1963).

The terminal oxidase of the succinoxidase system seems to be identical with the terminal enzyme of a DPNH-oxidizing system. Because the oxidase depends on rather high oxygen tension for effective functioning and because the oxygen tension in the natural environments of *Ascaris* is very low, Bueding (1962) assumes that under natural conditions the oxidation of both succinate and DPNH is insignificant and that the importance of the system lies in another direction. *Ascaris* degrades carbohydrate by phosphorylative glycolysis, but does not produce appreciable amounts of lactic acid. The question then arises by what means DPNH formed during glycolysis is reoxidized. Bueding (1962) points out that this can be accomplished by a reversal of the succinoxidase reaction. Some evidence for succinate production via reversed Krebs cycle reactions plus CO_2 fixation has been presented in the preceding section. It is sufficient here to emphasize that according to Kmetec and Bueding (1961) succinate is produced during anaerobic incubation with DPNH and fumarate of a purified particulate system isolated from *Ascaris* muscle suggesting that in the absence of oxygen electrons can be directed to fumarate. Therefore, in Bueding's (1962) words "the succinoxidase system of *Ascaris* can serve as an electron acceptor for succinate or as an electron donor to fumarate" (Fig. 5). In contrast to the mammalian succinoxidase the worm system reduces fumarate rapidly, but oxidizes

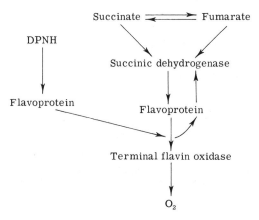

Fig. 5.   Succinoxidase system of *Ascaris lumbricoides*. (After Bueding, 1962.)

succinate only slowly at low oxygen tensions. This, according to Bueding (1962) can be considered as an adaptation to the normally predominantly anaerobic type of life led by *Ascaris*. It should be kept in mind that the regeneration of oxidized DPN is perhaps not the only biological function of the succinoxidase system. It has been observed that the dehydrogenation of DPNH is coupled, both aerobically and anaerobically, with phosphorylations (Chin and Bueding, 1954; Seidman and Entner, 1961) which lead to the production of energy-rich bonds in the form of ATP. This would seemingly point to the possibility that succinate formation is involved in supplying the energy for muscle contraction in *Ascaris*. Bueding (1963) cites as supporting evidence for this assumption the observation of Bueding *et al.* (1959) that piperazine produces both a reversible paralysis and a marked reduction in succinate production in *Ascaris*. Since, however, paralyzed muscle does incorporate lactate-C^{14} into succinate normally it appears that the muscle is paralyzed by piperazine, resulting in a lowered demand for succinate because of a lowered energy demand for muscular contraction.

E. Bueding (personal communication, 1965) is of the opinion that anaerobic dehydrogenation of DPNH, leading to the reduction of fumarate to succinate, may provide energy in the form of ATP not only in *Ascaris,* but in other organisms as well. He quotes the following evidence as pointing in this direction: The fact the CO_2 increases the survival *in vitro* of *Trichuris vulpis* and *Hymenolepis diminuta,* the observation that many anaerobic succinate-producing organisms require CO_2 for growth, and the finding of Quastel *et al.* (1925) that *Escherichia coli* grows anaerobically only in the presence of fumarate which is reduced to succinate during growth.

The remarkable success in elucidating the details of the succinoxidase system of *Ascaris* was due largely to the fact that it proved possible to dissociate various parts of the system by certain procedures. Thus the succinic dehydrogenase could be dissociated from the electron transport system by using acetone powders (Kmetec and Bueding, 1961) or by the action of lipase (Bueding *et al.,* 1955). The isolated succinic dehydrogenase reacted with phenazine methosulfate, but not with oxygen or methylene blue. The DPNH and succinate systems could be dissociated by heat treatment (Kmetec and Bueding, 1961), 10 minutes heating at 55°C inactivating the DPNH system by 99% but being without effect on the succinate system. The inactivation must therefore have taken place either at the level of the DPNH dehydrogenase or some intermediate electron transport site not involved in the succinate system.

Although not strictly a Krebs cycle enzyme, the enzyme catalyzing the oxidative decarboxylation of malate in *Ascaris* (Saz and Hubbard, 1957) may be mentioned here briefly since by virtue of its reverse reaction, fixation of CO_2 into pyruvate, it has close connection to the succinoxidase system. In contrast to a typical "malic enzyme" the *Ascaris* preparations did not catalyze the decarboxylation of oxaloacetic acid regardless of pH and the absence or presence of ATP. All other malic enzyme preparations so far studied decarboxylate oxaloacetic acid between pH 4 and 5. Another peculiarity of the worm enzyme is that it reacts both with TPN and DPN, but optimally with DPN.

The malate dehydrogenases of *Trypanosoma cruzi* (Baernstein, 1953b) and *Trichomonas vaginalis* (Baernstein, 1961), although both catalyzing the same reaction, differ from one another in various respects. The enzyme of the former flagellate can be inhibited by iodoacetic acid, that of the latter not. However, the facts that *p*-chloromercuribenzoate inhibits the *vaginalis* enzyme and that the inhibition can be reversed by dimercaptopropanol indicates that it too requires functional SH-groups. The trichomonad enzyme could be purified partially. It proved to be strictly bound to DPN and L($-$) malate, no activity resulting with TPN or D($+$) malate. The substrate concentration, allowing half-maximal activity of the *cruzi* and *vaginalis* enzymes, respectively, were 2.5×10^{-5} M and 2×10^{-5} M for oxaloacetic acid and $1.4 \times 10^{-2} 2$ M and 1×10^{-3} M, respectively, for malate.

A terminal oxidation not connected with Krebs cycle reactions in any way has been found in trypanosomes. It has been known for a long time (literature in von Brand, 1951) that the blood-stream form of the *brucei* trypanosomes consume large amounts of oxygen despite a respiration insensitive to cyanide and that the sugar degradation ceases essentially at the pyruvate stage. Evidently then the oxygen consumption cannot be related to the functioning of any Krebs cycle enzyme that some of these organisms still have in an apparently nonfunctional form (Ryley, 1962). Furthermore, it cannot involve a typical cytochrome system. The question how DPNH, formed during the incomplete glycolysis characterizing these forms, is reoxidized received some clarification through Fulton and Spooner (1959). They observed that in contrast to most known flavoenzymes, the oxidase of the blood-stream form of *Trypanosoma rhodesiense* does not lead to the formation of hydrogen peroxide. The relevant mechanisms were then clarified by Grant and Sargent (1960), and Grant *et al.* (1961), who showed that the largest part of the oxygen consumption can be explained by a substrate specific L-α-glycerophosphate oxidase system which is coupled to a DPN-linked L-α-glycerophosphate dehydrogenase. The two enzymes catalyze the following steps:

(1) L-α-Glycerophosphate + 1/2 O_2 $\longrightarrow$ dihydroxyacetonephosphate + H_2O

(2) Dihydroxyacetonephosphate + DPNH + H^+ $\longrightarrow$ L-α-glycerophosphate + DPN$^+$

In sum: DPNH + 1/2 O_2 $\longrightarrow$ DPN$^+$ + H_2O

The link to glycolysis proper can then be visualized as follows:

(1) 2 L-α-Glycerophosphate $+ O_2 \longrightarrow 2$ triosephosphate $+ 2\ H_2O$

(2) Triosephosphate $+$ DPNH $+ H^+ \longrightarrow$ L-α-glycerophosphate $+$ DPN$^+$

(3) Triosephosphate $+$ DPN$^+ + H_3PO_4 \longrightarrow 1,3$-diphosphoglyceric acid $+$ DPNH $+ H^+$

In sum: L-α-Glycerophosphate $+ O_2 \longrightarrow 1,3$-diphosphoglyceric acid $+ H_2O$

So far only the properties of one component of the system, the dehydrogenase, have been studied in some detail by Grant and Sargent (1960, 1961). It was strictly specific for the L form of α-glycerophosphate and is completely inactive with glycerol or β-glycerophosphate as substrates. The most effective electron acceptors were phenazin methosulfate and 2,6-dichlorophenol-indophenol. K_m for substrate and electron acceptors, respectively, was 9.0 and 0.34 μM. The enzyme has functional SH-groups. Baernstein (1963) has pointed out that the above system does not explain the absence of hydrogen peroxide as end product. The latter cannot react with pyruvic acid, since in that case one would expect the formation of large amounts of CO_2 and acetate, which are not produced to any extent by the trypanosomes of the *brucei* group. Nor can H_2O_2 be decomposed by catalase or peroxidase, since these enzymes do not occur in the flagellates. This phase of the problem then needs further clarification.

It is interesting to note, and well in agreement with what is known about their metabolism, that the glycerophosphate system is by far more active in the blood-stream forms of the *brucei* group than in those of the *congolense, vivax,* and *lewisi* groups and that it is least active in the culture forms of various trypanosomidae. Curiously enough among the latter, species were found in which the above system was inhibited by cyanide and Antimycin A, while in others it was not (Grant *et al.*, 1961).

REFERENCES

Abou Akkada, A. R., and Howard, B. H. (1960) *Biochem. J.* **76**, 445–451.

Abou Akkada, A. R., and Howard, B. H. (1961) *Biochem. J.* **78**, 512–517.

Adler, S. (1953). *Acta Med. Orient.* **12**, 204–205.

Agosin, M. (1957). *Exptl. Parasitol.* **6**, 586–593.

Agosin, M., and Aravena, L. C. (1959a). *Exptl. Parasitol.* **8**, 10–30.

Agosin, M., and Aravena, L. C. (1959b). *Biochim. Biophys. Acta* **34**, 90–102.

Agosin, M., and Aravena, L. C. (1960). *Exptl. Parasitol.* **10**, 28–38.

Agosin, M., and Brand, T. von (1954). *Exptl. Parasitol.* **3**, 517–524.

Agosin, M., and Brand, T. von (1955). *Exptl. Parasitol.* **4**, 548–563.

Agosin, M., and Repetto, Y. (1963). *Comp. Biochem. Physiol.* **8**, 245–261.

Agosin, M., and Weinbach, E. C. (1956). *Biochim. Biophys. Acta* **21**, 117–126.

Alt, H. L., and Tischer, O. A. (1931). *Proc. Soc. Exptl. Biol. Med.* **29**, 222–224.

Andrews, J., and Brand, T. von (1938). *Am. J. Hyg.* **28,** 138–147.

Armer, J. M. (1944). *J. Parasitol.* **30,** 131–142.

Asami, K. (1956). *Keio J. Med.* **5,** 169–190.

Baba, T., Nagata, K., and Nakajima, T. (1957). *Gunma J. Med. Sci.* **6,** 22–30.

Baernstein, H. D. (1953a). *Ann. N.Y. Acad. Sci.* **56,** 982–994.

Baernstein, H. D. (1953b). *Exptl. Parasitol.* **2,** 380–396.

Baernstein, H. D. (1954). *Federation Proc.* **13,** 177.

Baernstein, H. D. (1959). *J. Parasitol.* **45,** 491–498.

Baernstein, H. D. (1961). *J. Parasitol.* **47,** 279–284.

Baernstein, H. D. (1963). *J. Parasitol.* **49,** 12–21.

Baernstein, H. D., and Rees, C. W. (1952). *Exptl. Parasitol.* **1,** 215–228.

Baernstein, H. D., and Tobie, E. J. (1951). *Federation Proc.* **10,** 159.

Baernstein, H. D., Rees, C. W., and Reardon, L. V. (1954). *Am. J. Trop. Med. Hyg.* **3,** 839–848.

Bailey, R. W. (1958). *New Zealand J. Agr. Res.* **1,** 825–833.

Bailey, R. W., and Clarke, R. T. J. (1963). *Nature* **199,** 1291–1292.

Bailey, R. W., and Howard, B. H. (1963a). *Biochem. J.* **86,** 446–452.

Bailey, R. W., and Howard, B. H. (1963b). *Biochem. J.* **87,** 146–151.

Bailey, R. W., Clarke, R. T. J., and Wright, D. E. (1962). *Biochem. J.* **83,** 517–523.

Ball, E. G., McKee, R. W., Anfinsen, C. B., Cruz, W. O., and Geiman, Q. M. (1948). *J. Biol. Chem.* **175,** 547–571.

Bauchop, T. (1962). *Biochim. Biophys. Acta* **59,** 742–743.

Becker, C. E., and Geiman, Q. M. (1955). *Exptl. Parasitol.* **4,** 493–501.

Bellelli, L., and Bonacci, S. (1961). *Arch. Ital. Sci. Med. Trop. Parassitol.* **42,** 543–556.

Benham, R. S., and Havens, I. (1958). *J. Infect. Diseases* **102,** 121–142.

Berntzen, A. K. (1962). *J. Parasitol.* **48,** 785–797.

Blacklock, D. B., Gordon, R. M., and Fine, J. (1930). *Ann. Trop. Med. Parasitol.* **24,** 5–54.

Blanchard, L., and Dinulescu, G. (1932). *Compt. Rend. Soc. Biol.* **110,** 343–344.

Bovarnick, M. R., Lindsay, A., and Hellerman, L. (1946). *J. Biol. Chem.* **163,** 523–533.

Bowman, I. B. R., Brand, T. von, and Tobie, E. J. (1960a). *Exptl. Parasitol.* **10,** 274–283.

Bowman, I. B. R., Grant, P. T., and Kermack, W. O. (1960b). *Exptl. Parasitol.* **9,** 131–136.

Bowman, I. B. R., Grant, P. T., Kermack, W. O., and Ogston, D. (1961). *Biochem. J.* **78,** 472–478.

Bowman, I. B. R., Tobie, E. J., and Brand, T. von (1963). *Comp. Biochem. Physiol.* **9,** 105–114.

Bragg, P. D., and Reeves, R. E. (1962). *Exptl. Parasitol.* **12,** 393–400.

Brand, T. von (1932). *Z. Parasitenk.* **4,** 753–775.

Brand, T. von (1933a). *Z. Vergleich. Physiol.* **18,** 562–596.

Brand, T. von (1933b). *Z. Vergleich. Physiol.* **19,** 587–614.

Brand, T. von (1934). *Z. Vergleich. Physiol.* **21,** 220–235.

Brand, T. von (1937). *J. Parasitol.* **23,** 68–72.

Brand, T. von (1940). *J. Parasitol.* **26,** 301–307.

Brand, T. von (1946). "Anaerobiosis in Invertebrates," Biodynamica Monographs No. 4. Biodynamica, Normandy, Missouri.

Brand, T. von (1950). *J. Parasitol.* **36,** 178–192.

Brand, T. von (1951). *In* "Biochemistry and Physiology of Protozoa" (A. Lwoff, ed.), Vol. 1, pp. 177–234. Academic Press, N. Y.

Brand, T. von (1952). "Chemical Physiology of Endoparasitic Animals." Academic Press, New York.

Brand, T. von (1963). *Ergeb. Mikrobiol., Immunitaetsforsch. Exptl. Therapie* **36,** 1–58.

Brand, T. von, and Agosin, M. (1955). *J. Infect. Diseases* **97**, 274–279.
Brand, T. von, and Bowman, I. B. R. (1961). *Exptl. Parasitol.* **11**, 267–297.
Brand, T. von, and Jahn, T. L. (1942). *In* "An Introduction to Nematology" (J. R. Christie, ed.), Section 2, Part 2, pp. 356–371. Chitwood, Babylon, New York.
Brand, T. von, and Mercado, T. I. (1961). *J. Parasitol.* **47**, 459–463.
Brand, T. von, and Simpson, W. F. (1944). *J. Parasitol.* **30**, 121–129.
Brand, T. von, and Simpson, W. F. (1945). *Proc. Soc. Exptl. Biol. Med.* **60**, 368–371.
Brand, T. von, and Tobie, E. J. (1948). *J. Cell. Comp. Physiol.* **31**, 49–68.
Brand, T. von, and Tobie, E. J. (1959). *J. Parasitol.* **45**, 204–208.
Brand, T. von, Tobie, E. J., Kissling, R. E., and Adams, G. (1949). *J. Infect. Diseases* **85**, 5–16.
Brand, T. von, Baernstein, H. D., and Mehlman, B. (1950). *Biol. Bull.* **98**, 266–276.
Brand, T. von, Weinstein, P. P., Mehlman, B., and Weinbach, E. C. (1952). *Exptl. Parasitol.* **1**, 245–255.
Brand, T. von, Tobie, E. J., Mehlman, B., and Weinbach, E. C. (1953). *J. Cell. Comp. Physiol.* **41**, 1–22.
Brand, T. von, Weinbach, E. C., and Tobie, E. J. (1955). *J. Cell. Comp. Physiol,* **45**, 421–434.
Brand, T. von, Bowman, I. B. R., Weinstein, P. P., and Sawyer, T. K. (1963). *Exptl. Parasitol.* **13**, 128–133.
Brand, T. von, McMahon, P., Gibbs, E., and Higgins, H. (1964). *Exptl. Parasitol.* **15**, 410–429.
Braune, R. (1914). *Arch Protistenk.* **32**, 111–116.
Bryant, C., and Smith, M. J. H. (1963). *Comp. Biochem. Physiol.* **9**, 189–194.
Bryant, C., and Williams, J. P. G. (1962). *Exptl. Parasitol.* **12**, 372–376.
Bueding, E. (1949a). *J. Exptl. Med.* **89**, 107–130.
Bueding, E. (1949b). *Physiol. Rev.* **29**, 195–218.
Bueding, E. (1949c). *Federation Proc.* **8**, 188–189.
Bueding, E. (1950). *J. Gen. Physiol.* **33**, 475–495.
Bueding, E. (1951). *J. Biol. Chem.* **191**, 401–418.
Bueding, E. (1953). *J. Biol. Chem.* **202**, 505–512.
Bueding, E. (1962). *Federation Proc.* **21**, 1039–1046.
Bueding, E. (1963). *In* "Control Mechanisms in Respiration and Fermentation" (B. Wright, ed.), Ronald Press, New York.
Bueding, E., and Charms, B. (1952). *J. Biol. Chem.* **196**, 615–627.
Bueding, E., and Farrow, G. W. (1956). *Exptl. Parasitol.* **5**, 345–349.
Bueding, E., and Mackinnon, J. A. (1955). *J. Biol. Chem.* **215**, 507–513.
Bueding, E., and Mansour, J. M. (1957). *Brit. J. Pharmacol. Chemotherapy* **12**, 159–165.
Bueding, E., and Oliver-Gonzalez, J. (1950). *Brit. J. Pharmacol.* **5**, 62–64.
Bueding, E., and Orrell, S. A. (1961). *J. Biol. Chem.* **236**, 2854–2857.
Bueding, E., and Yale, H. W. (1951). *J. Biol. Chem.* **193**, 411–423.
Bueding, E., Peters, L., and Waite, J. F. (1947). *Proc. Soc. Exptl. Biol. Med.* **64**, 111–113.
Bueding, E., Ruppender, H., and Mackinnon, J. (1954). *Proc. Natl. Acad. Sci. U.S.* **40**, 773–777.
Bueding, E., Entner, N., and Farber, E. (1955). *Biochim. Biophys. Acta* **18**, 305–306.
Bueding, E., Saz, H. J., and Farrow, G. W. (1959). *Brit. J. Pharmacol. Chemotherapy* **14**, 497–500.
Bueding, E., Kmetec, E., Swartzwelder, C., Abadie, S., and Saz, H. J. (1961). *Biochem. Pharmacol.* **5**, 311–322.
Cailleau, R. (1937). *Ann. Inst. Pasteur* **59**, 137–172.
Capella, J. A., and Kaufman, H. E. (1964). *Am. J. Trop. Med. Hyg.* **13**, 664–666.

Cavier, R. (1951). *Bull. Soc. Chim. Biol.* **33**, 1391–1400.
Cavier, R., and Savel, J. (1952). *Compt. Rend.* **234**, 2562–2564.
Cavier, R., and Savel, J. (1953). *Compt. Rend.* **237**, 99–101.
Chakravarty, N., Sánchez, M., and Ercoli, N. (1962). *Proc. Soc. Exptl. Biol. Med.* **110**, 517–521.
Chang, S. L. (1948). *J. Infect. Diseases* **82**, 109–116.
Chapman-Andresen, C., and Holter, H. (1955). *Exptl. Cell Res. Suppl.* **3**, 53–63.
Chatterjee, A. N., and Ghosh, J. J. (1958). *Ann. Biochem. Exptl. Med. (Calcutta)* **18**, 69–76.
Chatterjee, A. N., and Ghosh, J. J. (1959). *Ann. Biochem. Exptl. Med. (Calcutta)* **19**, 37–50.
Chatterjee, A. N., Ray, J. C., and Ghosh, J. J. (1958). *Nature* **182**, 109–110.
Chen, G., and Geiling, E. M. K. (1945). *J. Infect. Diseases* **77**, 139–143.
Chen, G., and Geiling, E. M. K. (1946). *Proc. Soc. Exptl. Biol. Med.* **63**, 486–487.
Chin, C., and Bueding, E. (1954). *Biochim. Biophys. Acta* **13**, 331–337.
Christophers, S. R., and Fulton, J. D. (1938). *Ann. Trop. Med. Parasitol.* **82**, 43–75.
Citri, N. (1954). Thesis, Hebrew University of Jerusalem.
Clausen, J. K. (1955). *J. Gen. Microbiol.* **12**, 496–502.
Colas-Belcour, J., and Lwoff, A. (1925). *Compt. Rend. Soc. Biol.* **93**, 1421–1422.
Cole, B. A. (1950). *Proc. Helminthol. Soc. Wash., D.C.* **17**, 65–74.
Coleman, G. S. (1962). *J. Gen. Microbiol.* **28**, 271–281.
Coleman, R. M., and Brand, T. von. (1957). *J. Parasitol.* **43**, 263–270.
Colucci, A. V., Orrell, S. A., Saz, H. J., and Bueding, E. (1964). *Federation Proc.* **23**, 320.
Cook, S. F. (1932). *Biol. Bull.* **63**, 246–257.
Cook, S. F. (1943). *Physiol. Zool.* **16**, 123–128.
Cook, S. F., and Smith, R. E. (1942). *J. Cell. Comp. Physiol.* **19**, 211–219.
Cosgrove, W. B. (1959). *Can. J. Microbiol.* **5**, 573–578.
Cosgrove, W. B. (1963). *Exptl. Parasitol.* **13**, 173–177.
Costello, L. C., and Brown, H. (1962). *Exptl. Parasitol.* **12**, 33–40.
Costello, L. C., and Grollman, S. (1959). *Exptl. Parasitol.* **8**, 83–89.
Crowley, K., and Warren, L. G. (1963). *J. Protozool.* **49**, No. 5, Sec. 2, 52–53.
Crowther, S., Fulton, J. D., and Joyner, L. P. (1954). *Biochem. J.* **56**, 182–185.
Daugherty, J. W. (1956). *J. Parasitol.* **42**, 17–20.
Daugherty, J. W., and Taylor, D. (1956). *Exptl. Parasitol.* **5**, 376–390.
Dawes, B., and Muller, R. (1957). *Nature* **180**, 1217.
De Ley, J., and Vercruysse, R. (1955). *Biochim. Biophys. Acta* **16**, 615–616.
Dobell, C., and Laidlaw, P. P. (1926). *Parasitology* **18**, 283–318.
Dogiel, V. A. (1925). *Trav. Soc. Naturalistes Leningrad* **54**, 67–93 [not seen, quoted in Westphal, A. (1934)].
Doran, D. J. (1957). *J. Protozool.* **4**, 182–190.
Doran, D. J. (1958). *J. Protozool.* **5**, 89–93.
Dropkin, V. H. (1963). *Nematologica* **9**, 444–454.
Dunagan, T. T. (1962). *Proc. Helminthol. Soc. Wash., D.C.* **29**, 131–135.
Dunagan, T. T. (1964). *Proc. Helminthol. Soc. Wash., D.C.* **31**, 166–172.
Eadie, J. M., and Oxford, A. E. (1955). *J. Gen. Microbiol.* **12**, 298–310.
Earl, P. R. (1959). *Ann. N.Y. Acad. Sci.* **77**, 163–175.
Ellison, T., Thomson, W. A. B., and Strong, F. M. (1960). *Arch. Biochem. Biophys.* **91**, 247–254.
Enigk, K. (1938). *Z. Parasitenk.* **10**, 386–414.
Entner, N. (1957). *Arch. Biochem. Biophys.* **71**, 52–61.
Entner, N. (1958). *J. Parasitol.* **44**, 638.

Entner, N., and Anderson, H. H. (1954). *Exptl. Parasitol.* **3**, 234–239.
Entner, N., and Gonzalez, C. (1959). *Exptl. Parasitol.* **8**, 471–479.
Entner, N., and Hall, N. D. (1955). *Exptl. Parasitol.* **4**, 92–99.
Epps, W., Weiner, M., and Bueding, E. (1950). *J. Infect. Diseases* **87**, 149–151.
Esch, G. W. (1964). *J. Parasitol.* **50**, 72–76.
Fairbairn, D. (1954). *Exptl. Parasitol.* **3**, 52–63.
Fairbairn, D. (1960). *In* "Nematology" (J. N. Sasser and W. R. Jenkins, eds.), pp. 267–296.
    Univ. of North Carolina Press, Chapel Hill, North Carolina.
Fairbairn, D., Wertheim, G., Harpur, R. P., and Schiller, E. L. (1961). *Exptl. Parasitol.*
    11, 248–263.
Farber, E., and Bueding, E. (1956). *J. Histochem. Cytochem.* **4**, 357–362.
Fauré-Fremiet, E. (1913). *Arch. Anat. Microscop.* **15**, 435–757.
Faust, E. C., and Read, T. R. (1959). *Am. J. Trop. Med. Hyg.* **8**, 293–303.
Fenyvessy, B. von, and Reiner, L. (1924). *Z. Hyg. Infektionskrankh.* **102**, 109–119.
Fenyvessy, B. von, and Reiner, L. (1928). *Biochem. Z.* **202**, 75–80.
Fernando, M. A. (1963). *Exptl. Parasitol.* **13**, 90–97.
Fernando, M. A., and Wong, H. A. (1964). *Exptl. Parasitol.* **15**, 284–292.
Fischer, A. (1924). *Biochem. Z.* **144**, 224–228.
Fisher, F. M. (1964). *J. Parasitol.* **50**, 803–804.
Flury, F. (1912). *Arch. Exptl. Pathol. Pharmakol.* **67**, 275–392.
Flury, F., and Leeb, F. (1926). *Klin. Wochschr.* **5**, 2054–2055.
Fraser, D. M., and Kermack, W. O. (1957). *Brit. J. Pharmacol.* **12**, 16–23.
Friedl, F. E. (1961). *J. Parasitol.* **47**, 244–247.
Fulton, J. D. (1939). *Ann. Trop. Med. Parasitol.* **33**, 217–227.
Fulton, J. D., and Joyner, L. P. (1949). *Trans. Roy. Soc. Trop. Med. Hyg.* **43**, 273–286.
Fulton, J. D., and Spooner, D. F. (1956). *Exptl. Parasitol.* **5**, 59–76.
Fulton, J. D., and Spooner, D. F. (1959). *Exptl. Parasitol.* **8**, 137–162.
Fulton, J. D., and Spooner, D. F. (1960). *Exptl. Parasitol.* **9**, 293–301.
Fulton, J. D., and Stevens, T. S. (1945). *Biochem. J.* **39**, 317–320.
Geiger, A., Kligler, I. J., and Comaroff, R. (1930). *Ann. Trop. Med. Parasitol.* **24**, 319–327.
Geigy, R., Huber, M., Weinman, D., and Wyatt, G. R. (1959). *Acta Trop.* **16**, 255–262.
Gerzeli, G. (1955). *Riv. Parassitol.* **16**, 209–215.
Gilmour, D. (1940). *Biol. Bull.* **79**, 297–308.
Glaessner, K. (1908). *Zentr. Bakteriol. Parasitenk., Abt. I: Orig.* **47**, 351–362.
Glocklin, V. C., and Fairbairn, D. (1952). *J. Cell. Comp. Physiol.* **39**, 341–356.
Glowazky, F. (1937). *Z. Hyg. Infektionskrankh.* **119**, 741–752.
Goffart, H., and Heiling, A. (1962). *Nematologica* **7**, 173–176.
Goil, M. M. (1957). *Z. Parasitenk.* **18**, 36–39.
Goil, M. M. (1961). *Parasitology* **51**, 335–337.
Goldberg, E. (1957). *Exptl. Parasitol.* **6**, 367–382.
Goldberg, E. (1958). *J. Parasitol.* **44**, 363–370.
Goldberg, E., and Nolf, L. O. (1954). *Exptl. Parasitol.* **3**, 275–284.
Graff, D. J. (1964). *J. Parasitol.* **50**, 230–234.
Grant, P. T., and Fulton, J. D. (1957). *Biochem. J.* **66**, 242–250.
Grant, P. T., and Sargent, J. R. (1960). *Biochem. J.* **76**, 229–236.
Grant, P. T., and Sargent, J. R. (1961). *Biochem. J.* **81**, 206–214.
Grant, P. T., Sargent, J. R., and Ryley, J. F. (1961). *Biochem. J.* **81**, 200–206.
Grembergen, G. van (1944). *Enzymologia* **11**, 268–281.
Grembergen, G. van (1949). *Enzymologia* **13**, 241–257.
Guevara Pozo, D., and Monteoliva, M. (1959). *Rev. Iberica Parasitol.* **19**, 105–111.
Gutierrez, J. (1955). *Biochem. J.* **60**, 516–522.

Gutierrez, J. (1956). *J. Protozool.* **3**, 39–42.

Gutierrez, J., and Davis, R. E. (1962). *Appl. Microbiol.* **10**, 305–308.

Guttman, H. N. (1963). *Exptl. Parasitol.* **14**, 129–142.

Hallman, F. A., and DeLamater, J. N. (1953). *Exptl. Parasitol.* **2**, 170–173.

Hallman, F. A., Michaelson, J. B., Blumenthal, H., and DeLamater, J. N. (1954). *Am. J. Hyg.* **59**, 128–131.

Hammen, C. S., and Lum, S. C. (1962). *J. Biol. Chem.* **237**, 2419–2422.

Harnisch, O. (1932). *Z. Vergleich. Physiol.* **17**, 365–386.

Harpur, R. P. (1963). *Can. J. Biochem. Physiol.* **41**, 1673–1689.

Harpur, R. P., and Waters, W. R. (1960). *Can. J. Biochem. Physiol.* **38**, 1009–1020.

Harvey, S. C. (1949). *J. Biol. Chem.* **179**, 435–453.

Heald, P. J., and Oxford, A. E. (1953). *Biochem. J.* **53**, 506–512.

Hilker, D. M., and White, A. G. C. (1959). *Exptl. Parasitol.* **8**, 539–548.

Hilker, D. M., Sherman, H. J., and White, A. G. C. (1957). *Exptl. Parasitol.* **6**, 459–464.

Hopkins, C. A. (1950). *J. Parasitol.* **36**, 384–390.

Hopkins, C. A. (1952). *Exptl. Parasitol.* **1**, 196–213.

Hopkins, D. L., and Warner, K. L. (1946). *J. Parasitol.* **32**, 175–189.

Hoshino, M., and Suzuki, H. (1956). *Fukushima J. Med. Sci.* **3**, 51–56.

Howard, B. H. (1959a). *Biochem. J.* **71**, 671–675.

Howard, B. H. (1959b). *Biochem. J.* **71**, 675–680.

Huang, F. Y., and Chu, C. H. (1962). *Sheng Wu Hua Hsueh Yu Shing Wu Wu Li Hsueh Pao* **2**, 286–294; *Chem. Abstr.* **59**, 14333 (1963).

Hungate, R. E. (1939). *Ecology* **20**, 230–245.

Hungate, R. E. (1942). *Biol. Bull.* **83**, 303–319.

Hungate, R. E. (1943a). *Ann. Entomol. Soc. Am.* **36**, 730–739.

Hungate, R. E. (1943b). *Biol. Bull.* **84**, 157–163.

Hunter, F. R. (1960). *Exptl. Parasitol.* **9**, 271–280.

Hunter, N. W. (1955). *Physiol. Zool.* **28**, 302–307.

Ichii, S., Matsumoto, K., and Sugiura, K. (1959). *Kiseichugaku Zasshi* **8**, 19–21.

Ikeda, T. (1955). *Gunma J. Med. Sci.* **4**, 279–284.

Issekutz, B. von (1933). *Arch. Exptl. Pathol. Pharmakol.* **173**, 479–498.

Ivanov, I. I., and Jakovlev, G. (1943). *Biokhimiya* **8**, 229–233.

Jones, C. A., Swartzwelder, C., and Abadie, S. H. (1955). *J. Parasitol.* **41**, No. 6, Sect. 2, 48–49.

Kaneko, M. (1956). *Kiseichugaku Zasshi* **5**, 88–91.

Karlson, P. (1961). "Kurzes Lehrbuch der Biochemie." Thieme, Stuttgart.

Kemnitz, G. von (1914). *Verhandl. Deut. Zool. Ges.* **24**, 294–307.

Kemnitz, G. von (1916). *Z. Biol.* **67**, 129–244.

Khabir, P. A., and Manwell, R. D. (1955). *J. Parasitol.* **41**, 595–603.

Kidder, G. W., and Dutta, B. N. (1958). *J. Gen. Microbiol.* **18**, 621–638.

Kilejan, A. (1963). *J. Parasitol.* **49**, 862–863.

Kligler, I. J. (1926). *Trans. Roy. Soc. Trop. Med. Hyg.* **19**, 330–335.

Kmetec, E., and Bueding, E. (1961). *J. Biol. Chem.* **233**, 584–591.

Kobert, R. (1903). *Arch. Ges. Physiol.* **99**, 116–186.

Krueger, F. (1936). *Zool. Jahrb., Abt. Allgem. Zool. Physiol.* **57**, 1–56.

Krummacher, O. (1919). *Z. Biol.* **69**, 293–321.

Krusberg, L. R. (1960). *Phytopathology* **50**, 9–22.

Kudicke, R., and Evers, E. (1924). *Z. Hyg. Infektionskrankh.* **101**, 317–326.

Kun, E., and Bradin, J. L. (1953). *Biochim. Biophys. Acta* **11**, 312–313.

Kun, E., Bradin, J. L., and Dechary, J. M. (1956). *Biochim. Biophys. Acta* **19**, 153–159.

Kunitake, G., Stitt, C., and Saltman, P. (1962). *J. Protozool.* **9**, 371–373.

Kupferberg, A. B. (1955). *Intern. Record Med. Gen. Pract. Clin.* **168**, 709–717.

Kupferberg, A. B., Singher, H. O., Lampson, G., Levy, L., and Romano, A. H. (1953). *Ann. N.Y. Acad. Sci.* **56**, 1006–1015.

Laser, H. (1944). *Biochem. J.* **38**, 333–338.

Laurie, J. S. (1957). *Exptl. Parasitol.* **6**, 245–260.

Laurie, J. S. (1959). *Exptl. Parasitol.* **8**, 188–197.

Laurie, J. S. (1961). *Comp. Biochem. Physiol.* **4**, 63–71.

Lee, D. L. (1958). *Parasitology* **48**, 437–447.

Lee, D. L., Rothman, A. H., and Senturia, J. B. (1963). *Exptl. Parasitol.* **14**, 285–295.

Lindblom, G. P. (1961). *J. Protozool.* **8**, 139–150.

Loran, M. R., Kerner, M. W., and Anderson, H. H. (1956). *Exptl. Cell Res.* **10**, 241–245.

McKee, R. W., Ormsbee, R. A., Anfinsen, C. B., Geiman, Q. M., and Ball, E. G. (1946). *J. Exptl. Med.* **84**, 569–582.

Magliocca, R. (1963). *Studi Sassaresi, Sez. I* **41**, 234–239.

Maier, J., and Coggeshall, L. T. (1941). *J. Infect. Diseases* **69**, 87–96.

Mancilla, R., and Agosin, M. (1960). *Exptl. Parasitol.* **10**, 43–50.

Mansour, T. E. (1959a). *Biochim. Biophys. Acta* **34**, 456–464.

Mansour, T. E. (1959b). *J. Pharmacol.* **126**, 212–216.

Mansour, T. E. (1962). *J. Pharmacol. Exptl. Therapy* **135**, 94–101.

Mansour, T. E., and Bueding, E. (1953). *Brit. J. Pharmacol.* **8**, 431–434.

Mansour, T. E., and Bueding, E. (1954). *Brit. J. Pharmacol.* **9**, 459–462.

Manwell, R. D., and Feigelson, P. (1949). *Proc. Soc. Exptl. Biol. Med.* **70**, 578–582.

Manwell, R. D., and Loeffler, C. A. (1961). *J. Parasitol.* **47**, 285–290.

Margolin, S. (1930). *Biol. Bull.* **59**, 301–305.

Markov, G. S. (1939). *Compt. Rend. Acad. Sci. URSS* **25**, 93–96.

Marshall, P. B. (1948a). *Brit. J. Pharmacol.* **3**, 1–7.

Marshall, P. B. (1948b). *Brit. J. Pharmacol.* **3**, 8–14.

Massey, V., and Rogers, W. P. (1949). *Nature* **163**, 909.

Massey, V., and Rogers, W. P. (1950). *Australian J. Sci. Res.* **B3**, 251–264.

Medina, H., Amaral, D., and Bacila, M. (1955). *Arquiv. Biol. Tecnol. Inst. Biol. Pesquisas Tecnol.* **10**, 103–119.

Meier, W. (1931). *Z. Biol.* **91**, 459–474.

Mercado, T. I. (1947). Master's Thesis, Catholic University, Washington, D.C.

Monteoliva, M. (1961). *Rev. Iberica Parasitol.* **21**, 339–344.

Monteoliva, M., and Guevara Pozo, D. (1958). *Rev. Iberica Parasitol.* **18**, 107–115.

Morgan, G. T., and McAllan, J. W. (1962). *Nematologica* **8**, 209–215.

Morita, Y. (1938). *J. Orient. Med.* **28**, 38 (English summary).

Mould, D. L., and Thomas, G. J. (1958). *Biochem. J.* **69**, 327–337.

Moulder, J. W. (1947). *Science* **106**, 168–169.

Moulder, J. W. (1948a). *J. Infect. Diseases* **83**, 33–41.

Moulder, J. W. (1948b). *J. Infect. Diseases* **83**, 42–49.

Moyle, V., and Baldwin, E. (1952). *Biochem. J.* **51**, 504–510.

Myuge, S. G. (1957). *Zool. Zh.* **36**, 620–622.

Myuge, S. G. (1960). *Conf. Sci. Problems Plant Prod., Budapest, 1960,* pp. 333–338.

Nakamura, M., and Baker, E. E. (1956). *Am. J. Hyg.* **64**, 12–22.

Nakamura, M., Hrenoff, A. K., and Anderson, H. H. (1953). *Am. J. Trop. Med. Hyg.* **2**, 206–211.

Newton, B. A. (1957). *J. Gen. Microbiol.* **17**, 708–717.

Ninomiya, H., and Suzuoki, Z. (1952). *J. Biochem. (Tokyo)* **39**, 321–331.

Noguchi, H. (1926). *J. Exptl. Med.* **44**, 327–337.

Nomura, H. (1957). *J. Keio Med. Assoc.* **34**, 75–88.

Oesterlin, M. (1937). *Z. Vergleich. Physiol.* **25**, 88–91.

Oxford, A. E. (1951). *J. Gen. Microbiol.* **5**, 83–90.

Oxford, A. E. (1955). *Exptl. Parasitol.* **4**, 569–605.

Oxford, A. E. (1958). *New Zealand J. Agr. Res.* **1**, 809–824.

Oya, H., Costello, L. C., and Smith, W. (1963). *Exptl. Parasitol.* **14**, 186–192.

Pandya, G. T. (1961). *Z. Parasitenk.* **20**, 466–469.

Passey, R. F., and Fairbairn, D. (1957). *Can. J. Biochem. Physiol.* **35**, 511–525.

Pennoit-DeCooman, E. (1940). *Ann. Soc. Roy. Zool. Belg.* **71**, 76–77.

Pennoit-DeCooman, E., and Grembergen, G. van (1942). *Verhandel. Koninkl. Vlaam. Acad. Wetenschap. Belg., Kl. Wetenschap.* **4**, No. 6, 7–77.

Phifer, K. (1958). *Exptl. Parasitol.* **7**, 269–275.

Phifer, K. (1960a). *J. Parasitol.* **46**, 51–62.

Phifer, K. (1960b). *J. Parasitol.* **46**, 137–144.

Phifer, K. (1960c). *J. Parasitol.* **46**, 145–153.

Plastridge, W. N. (1943). *J. Bacteriol.* **45**, 196–197.

Plunkett, A. (1946). Master's Thesis, Catholic University, Washington, D.C.

Quastel, J. H., Stephenson, M., and Whetham, M. D. (1925). *Biochem. J.* **19**, 304–317.

Quinn, L. Y., Burroughs, W., and Christiansen, W. C. (1962). *Appl. Microbiol.* **10**, 583–592.

Rathbone, L. (1955). *Biochem. J.* **61**, 574–579.

Rathbone, L., and Rees, K. R. (1954). *Biochim. Biophys. Acta* **15**, 126–133.

Raw, I. (1959). *Rev. Inst. Med. Trop. Sao Paulo* **1**, 192–194.

Read, C. P. (1951). *Exptl. Parasitol.* **1**, 1–18.

Read, C. P. (1952). *Exptl. Parasitol.* **1**, 353–362.

Read, C. P. (1953). *Exptl. Parasitol.* **2**, 341–347.

Read, C. P. (1956). *Exptl. Parasitol.* **5**, 325–344.

Read, C. P. (1957a). *J. Parasitol.* **43**, 385–394.

Read, C. P. (1957b). *Exptl. Parasitol.* **6**, 288–293.

Read, C. P. (1961a). *J. Parasitol.* **47**, 1015–1016.

Read, C. P. (1961b). In "Comparative Physiology of Carbohydrate Metabolism in Hetero-thermic Animals" (A. W. Martin, ed.), pp. 3–34. Univ. of Washington Press, Seattle, Washington.

Read, C. P., and Rothman, A. H. (1957). *Exptl. Parasitol.* **6**, 280–287.

Read, C. P., and Rothman, A. H. (1955). *Am. J. Hyg.* **61**, 249–260.

Read, C. P., and Rothman, A. H. (1958a). *Exptl. Parasitol.* **7**, 217–223.

Read, C. P., and Rothman, A. H. (1958b). *Exptl. Parasitol.* **7**, 191–197.

Read, C. P., and Simmons, J. E. (1963). *Physiol. Rev.* **43**, 263–305.

Read, T. R., and Faust, E. C. (1958). *J. Parasitol.* **44**, Suppl., 23–24.

Regendanz, P. (1930). *Zentr. Bakteriol. Parasitenk., Abt. I: Orig.* **118**, 175–186.

Reichenow, E. (1937). *Proc. 12th Intern. Congr. Zool., Lisbon, 1935,* Vol. 3, pp. 1955–1968. Casa Portuguesa, Lisbon.

Reid, W. M. (1942). *J. Parasitol.* **28**, 319–340.

Reid, W. M. (1945). *J. Parasitol.* **31**, 406–410.

Reiner, L., Smythe, C. V., and Pedlow, J. T. (1936). *J. Biol. Chem.* **113**, 75–88.

Rhodes, M. B., Marsh, C. L., and Kelley, G. W. (1964). *Exptl. Parasitol.* **15**, 403–409.

Robinson, D. L. H. (1956). *J. Helminthol.* **29**, 193–202.

Rogers, W. P. (1940). *J. Helminthol.* **18**, 143–154.

Rogers, W. P. (1958). *Nature* **181**, 1410–1411.

Rogers, W. P., and Lazarus, M. (1949). *Paristology* **39**, 302–314.

Rothman, A. H. (1959). *J. Parasitol.* **45**, 379–383.

Roy, D. N. (1937). *Parasitology* **29**, 150–162.

Ryley, J. F. (1951). *Biochem. J.* **49**, 577–585.
Ryley, J. F. (1953). *Nature* **171**, 747.
Ryley, J. F. (1955a). *Biochem. J.* **59**, 353–361.
Ryley, J. F. (1955b). *Biochem. J.* **59**, 361–369.
Ryley, J. F. (1956). *Biochem. J.* **62**, 215–222.
Ryley, J. F. (1962). *Biochem. J.* **85**, 211–223.
Saz, H. J., and Gerzon, K. (1962). *Exptl. Parasitol.* **12**, 204–210.
Saz, H. J., and Hubbard, J. A. (1957). *J. Biol. Chem.* **225**, 921–933.
Saz, H. J., and Vidrine, A. (1959). *J. Biol. Chem.* **234**, 2001–2005.
Saz, H. J., and Weil, A. (1960). *J. Biol. Chem.* **235**, 914–918.
Saz, H. J., and Weil, A. (1962). *J. Biol. Chem.* **237**, 2053–2056.
Saz, H. J., Vidrine, A., and Hubbard, J. A. (1958). *Exptl. Parasitol.* **7**, 477–490.
Schimmelpfennig, G. (1903). *Arch. Wiss. Prakt. Tierheilk.* **29**, 332–376.
Schulte, H. (1917). *Arch. Ges. Physiol.* **166**, 1–44.
Schulze, P. (1924). *Z. Morphol. Oekol. Tiere* **2**, 643–666.
Schwabe, C. W. (1957). *Am. J. Hyg.* **65**, 325–337.
Schwabe, C. W. (1959). *Am. J. Trop. Med. Hyg.* **8**, 20–28.
Schwabe, C. W., Koussa, M., and Acra, A. N. (1961). *Comp. Biochem. Physiol.* **2**, 161–172.
Schwartz, J. B. (1961). *J. Protozool.* **8**, 9–12.
Seaman, G. R. (1953a). *Exptl. Parasitol.* **2**, 236–241.
Seaman, G. R. (1953b). *Exptl. Parasitol.* **2**, 366–373.
Seaman, G. R. (1953c). *Exptl. Parasitol.* **2**, 236–241.
Seaman, G. R. (1956). *Exptl. Parasitol.* **5**, 138–148.
Seaman, G. R. (1957). *J. Biol. Chem.* **228**, 149–161.
Searle, D. S., and Reiner, L. (1940). *Proc. Soc. Exptl. Biol. Med.* **43**, 80–82.
Searle, D. S., and Reiner, L. (1941). *J. Biol. Chem.* **141**, 563–572.
Seidman, I., and Entner, N. (1961). *J. Biol. Chem.* **236**, 915–919.
Senft, A. W., and Senft, D. G. (1962). *J. Parasitol.* **48**, 551–554.
Shaw, J. J., Voller, A., and Bryant, C. (1964). *Ann. Trop. Med. Parasitol.* **58**, 17–24.
Sherman, I. W. (1961). *J. Exptl. Med.* **114**, 1049–1062.
Silverman, M., Ceithaml, J., Taliaferro, L. G., and Evans, E. A. (1944). *J. Infect. Diseases* **75**, 212–230.
Slater, W. K. (1925). *Biochem. J.* **19**, 604–610.
Slater, W. K. (1928). *Biol. Rev. Cambridge Phil. Soc.* **3**, 303–328.
Smith, W., Costello, L. C., and Oya, H. (1963). *J. Parasitol.* **49**, No. 5, Sect. 2, 51.
Speck, J. F., and Evans, E. A. (1945). *J. Biol. Chem.* **159**, 71–96.
Speck, J. F., Moulder, J. W., and Evans, E. A. (1946). *J. Biol. Chem.* **164**, 119–144.
Stannard, J. N., McCoy, O. R., and Latchford, W. B. (1938). *Am. J. Hyg.* **27**, 666–682.
Stephenson, W. (1947a). *Parasitology* **38**, 116–122.
Stephenson, W. (1947b). *Parasitology* **38**, 140–144.
Sugden, B. (1953). *J. Gen. Microbiol.* **9**, 44–53.
Sugden, B., and Oxford, A. E. (1952). *J. Gen. Microbiol.* **7**, 145–153.
Suzuoki, Z., and Suzuoki, T. (1951a). *J. Biochem.* **38**, 237–254.
Suzuoki, Z., and Suzuoki, T. (1951b). *Nature* **168**, 610.
Szwejkowska, G. (1929). *Bull. Intern. Acad. Polon. Sci., Cl. Sci. Math. Nat.* **B1928**, 489–519.
Takuma, I., Inoue, C., and Kawamitsu, C. (1958a). *Nagasaki Igakkai Zasshi* **33**, Suppl., 111–114.
Takuma, I., Kawamitsu, K., and Inoue, C. (1958b). *Nagasaki Igakkai Zasshi* **33**, Suppl., 105–110.

Tatchell, R. J. (1958). *Parasitology* **48**, 448–458.
Taylor, A. E. R. (1963). *Exptl. Parasitol.* **14**, 304–310.
Teras, J. (1963). *In* "Progress in Protozoology" (J. Ludvik *et al.*, eds.), pp. 572–576. Czech. Acad. Sci., Prague.
Thorsell, W. (1963). *Acta Chem. Scand.* **17**, 2129–2131.
Threadgold, L. T. (1963). *Quart. J. Microscop. Sci.* **104**, 505–512.
Thurston, J. P. (1958). *Parasitology* **48**, 149–164.
Tobie, E. J., Brand, T. von, and Mehlman, B. (1950). *J. Parasitol.* **36**, 48–54.
Toryu, Y. (1936). *Sci. Rept. Tohoku Imp. Univ., Fourth Ser.* **10**, 687–696.
Tracey, M. V. (1958). *Nematologica* **3**, 179–183.
Trager, W. (1932). *Biochem. J.* **26**, 1793–1771.
Trager, W. (1934). *Biol. Bull.* **66**, 182–190.
Trager, W. (1957). *J. Protozool.* **4**, 269–276.
Trier, H. J. (1926). *Z. Vergleich. Physiol.* **4**, 305–330.
Trussell, R. E., and Johnson, G. (1941). *Proc. Soc. Exptl. Biol. Med.* **47**, 176–178.
Tsukahara, T. (1957). *Niigata Igaku-kai Zasshi* **71**, 418–425.
Tsukahara, T. (1961). *Japan. J. Microbiol.* **5**, 157–169.
Ueno, Y. (1960). *J. Biochem.* **48**, 161–168.
Ueno, Y., Oya, H., and Bando, T. (1960). *J. Biochem.* **47**, 771–776.
Umbreit, W. W. (1952). "Metabolic Maps." Burgess, Minneapolis, Minnesota.
Usuelli, F. (1930). *Wiss. Arch. Landwirtsch.* **B3**, 4–19.
van Grembergen, G., *see* Grembergen, G. van.
Vernberg, W. B., and Hunter, W. S. (1956). *Exptl. Parasitol.* **5**, 441–448.
Vernberg, W. B., and Hunter, W. S. (1960). *Exptl. Parasitol.* **9**, 42–46.
Vernberg, W. B., and Hunter, W. S. (1963). *Exptl. Parasitol.* **14**, 311–315.
Visintin, B. (1941). *Riv. Biol. Coloniale (Rome)* **4**, 27–44.
von Brand, T., *see* Brand, T. von.
von Fenyvessy, B., *see* Fenyvessy, B. von.
von Issekutz, B., *see* Issekutz, B. von.
von Kemnitz, G., *see* Kemnitz, G. von.
Waechter, J. (1934). *Z. Biol.* **95**, 497–501.
Waitz, J. A. (1963). *J. Parasitol.* **49**, 285–293.
Waitz, J. A., and Schardein, J. L. (1964). *J. Parasitol.* **50**, 271–277.
Ward, H. L. (1952). *J. Parasitol.* **38**, 493–494.
Wardle, R. A. (1937). *Can. J. Res.* **D15**, 117–126.
Warren, L. G. (1961). *J. Parasitol.* **47**, Suppl., 29.
Warren, L. G. (1963). *J. Parasitol.* **49**, No. 5, Sect. 2, 52.
Warren, L. G., and Guevara, A. (1962). *Rev. Biol. Trop., Univ. Costa Rica* **10**, 149–159.
Warren, L. G., and Guevara, A. (1964). *J. Protozool.* **11**, 107–108.
Warren, L. G., and Kitzman, W. B. (1963). *J. Parasitol.* **49**, 808–813.
Warren, L. G., and Manwell, R. D. (1954). *Exptl. Parasitol.* **3**, 16–24.
Warren, L. G., and Patrzek, D. (1963). *Acta Cient. Venezolana* Suppl. 1, 127–134.
Watkins, W. M. (1953). *Biochem. J.* **54**, xxxii.
Watkins, W. M. (1956). *Biochem. J.* **64**, 21P–22P.
Watkins, W. M. (1959). *Biochem. J.* **71**, 261–274.
Watkins, W. M. (1962). *Immunology* **5**, 245–266.
Watkins, W. M., and Morgan, W. T. (1955). *Nature* **175**, 676–677.
Weatherly, N. F., Hansen, M. F., and Moser, H. C. (1963). *Exptl. Parasitol.* **14**, 37–48.
Weineck, E. (1934). *Arch. Protistenk.* **82**, 169–202.
Weinland, E. (1901). *Z. Biol.* **42**, 55–90.
Weinland, E. (1904). *Z. Biol.* **45**, 113–116.

Weinland, E. (1910). *In* "Handbuch der Biochemie" (C. Oppenheimer, ed.), 1st ed., Vol. 4, Sect. 2, pp. 446–528. Fischer, Jena.

Weinland, E., and Brand, T. von (1926). *Z. Vergleich Physiol.* **4**, 212–285.

Weinland, E., and Ritter, A. (1902). *Z. Biol.* **43**, 490–502.

Weinman, D. (1957). *Trans. Roy. Soc. Trop. Med. Hyg.* **51**, 560–561.

Weinman, D. (1960). *Nature* **186**, 166.

Weinstein, P. P. (1953). *Am. J. Hyg.* **58**, 352–376.

Weinstein, P. P., and Jones, M. F. (1959). *Ann. N.Y. Acad. Sci.* **77**, 137–162.

Wellerson, R., and Kupferberg, A. B. (1962). *J. Protozool.* **9**, 418–424.

Wellerson, R., Doscher, G. E., and Kupferberg, A. B. (1959). *Ann. N.Y. Acad. Sci.* **83**, 253–258.

Wellerson, R., Doscher, G. E., and Kupferberg, A. B. (1960). *Biochem. J.* **75**, 562–565.

Wendel, W. B. (1943). *J. Biol. Chem.* **148**, 21–34.

Westphal, A. (1934). *Z. Parasitenk.* **7**, 71–117.

Whitlock, B., and Strong, F. M. (1963). *Arch. Biochem. Biophys.* **103**, 459–460.

Williams, P. P., Davis, R. E., Doetsch, R. N., and Gutierrez, J. (1961). *Appl. Microbiol.* **9**, 405–409.

Wilson, P. A. G., and Fairbairn, D. (1961). *J. Protozool.* **8**, 410–416.

Wirtschafter, S. K. (1954). *J. Parasitol.* **40**, 360–362.

Wirtschafter, S. K., and Jahn, T. L. (1956). *J. Protozool.* **3**, 83–85.

Wirtschafter, S. K., Saltman, P., and Jahn, T. L. (1956). *J. Protozool.* **3**, 86–88.

Wright, D. E. (1960). *Arch. Biochem. Biophys.* **86**, 251–254.

Yonesawa, T. (1953). *Med. Bull. Kagoshima Univ.* Spec. No. Dec. 1953, pp. 4–6.

Yorke, W., Adams, A. R. D., and Murgatroyd, F. (1929). *Ann. Trop. Med. Parasitol.* **23**, 601–618.

Zeledon, R. (1960a). *J. Parasitol.* **46**, 541–551.

Zeledon, R. (1960b). *Rev. Biol. Trop., Univ. Costa Rica* **8**, 25–33.

Zinovev, V. P. (1957). *Zool. Zh.* **36**, 617–620 [not seen, quoted in Fairbairn, D. (1960)].

Chapter 4

CARBOHYDRATES III.
HOST-PARASITE CARBOHYDRATE
RELATIONSHIPS

I. DISTURBANCES OF THE HOST'S CARBOHYDRATE METABOLISM DURING PROTOZOAN INFECTIONS

Disturbances in the carbohydrate metabolism of the host occur rather frequently during protozoan infections. Usually they find their expression in abnormalities in the blood sugar level and polysaccharide reserves, while other facets of the problem, such as the alimentary blood sugar curve, or glycogen synthesizing capacity of the liver have been studied less frequently. Comparative data on relevant findings are presented in Table XXIX.

Many studies have been done on experimental animals infected with pathogenic trypanosomes, sparked by a rather acrimonious controversy in regard to origin and significance of the typical terminal hypoglycemia that arose as soon as the first papers dealing with these topics appeared (Schern, 1925; Regendanz and Tropp, 1927).

It had been suggested originally that the pathogenic trypanosomes consume so much sugar in the blood-stream that the carbohydrate reserves of the host would become exhausted. Such a severe strain would be put on the liver that its function would break down and the animals would die in the end of what was called "glycopryvic intoxication." In other words, it was assumed that practically the entire pathological syndrome would result directly from the glucose consumption of the parasites. This view, first proposed by Schern (1925, 1928) was subsequently accepted by several workers (von Fenyvessy, 1926; Scheff, 1928, 1932; Knowles and Das Gupta, 1927–28; Schern and Artagaveytia-Allende, 1936) and has found adherents even in recent years (Hoppe and Chapman, 1947; Bouisset *et al.* 1956).

Although it is true that the rate of glucose consumption of the pathogenic African trypanosomes is very high, the above theory is unsatisfactory as an explanation for the damage sustained by the host, because

157

TABLE XXIX

BLOOD SUGAR AND GLYCOGEN RESERVES IN PROTOZOAN INFECTIONS

Host	Parasite	Blood sugar	Liver glycogen	Muscle glycogen	References
Man	*Leishmania donovani*	Normal or hypoglycemia in adults, hyperglycemia in children			Banerjee and Saha (1923); Auricchio (1924); Mukherjee et al. (1957).
Dog	*Leishmania donovani*	Normal			Stein and Wertheimer (1942)
Rat	Trypanosomes of the *lewisi* group	Usually normal; occasionally terminal hypoglycemia		Normal (total body glycogen)	Regendanz and Tropp (1927); Regendanz (1929a); Linton (1929); Molomut (1947); von Brand et al. (1949)
Various small and large warm-blooded animals	Trypanosomes of the *evansi, brucei,* and *congolense* groups	Usually normal during greater part of infection with pronounced terminal hypoglycemia; rarely hyperglycemia during part of infection	Terminally usually very low; occasionally total depletion	Usually somewhat lowered; sometimes normal or even increased	Scherm (1925, 1928); von Fenyvessy (1926); Regendanz and Tropp (1927); Dubois and Bouckaert (1927); Cordier (1927); Bruynoghe et al. (1927); Knowles and Das Gupta (1927/28); Zotta and Radacovici (1929a,b); Scheff (1928, 1932); Regendanz (1929b); Linton (1930); Locatelli (1930); von Brand and Regendanz (1931); Tubangui and Yutuc (1931); von Brand et al. (1932); Krijgsman (1933); von Jancso and von Jancso (1935a,b); Poindexter (1935); Browning (1938); French (1938); Hudson (1944); Hoppe and Chapman (1947); Bouisset et al. (1956); Kawamitsu (1958).
Man	*Trypanosoma gambiense*	Normal			Walravens (1931); Wormall (1932)

158

Host	Parasite	Blood sugar			References
Man	*Plasmodium vivax; P. malariae, P. falciparum*	Frequently hyperglycemia in pyrexic stages; sometimes normal in all stages; sometimes hypoglycemia			DeLangen and Schut (1917); Yoshida and Ko (1920); Massa (1927); Ruge (1929, 1935); Petersen (1926); Rudolf and Marsh (1927); Sinton and Hughes (1924); Williams (1927); T. A. Hughes and Malik (1930); Sinton and Kehar (1931); Zaun (1935); Gall and Steinberg (1947); Birnbaum (1954); Devakul (1960)
Monkey	*Plasmodium knowlesi*	Hypoglycemia	Decreased	Decreased	Fulton (1939); Singh *et al.* (1956); Devakul and Maegraith (1958).
Rat	*Plasmodium berghei*	Hypoglycemia	Decreased	Decreased	Mercado (1952); Mercado and von Brand (1954); Chatterji and Sen Gupta (1957)
Dog	*Babesia canis*	Normal	Decreased		Maegraith *et al.* (1957)
Duck	*Plasmodium lophurae*	Terminal hypoglycemia			Marvin and Rigdon (1945)
Chicken	*Eimeria tenella*	Hyperglycemia	Normal or increased	Normal or decreased	Pratt (1940, 1941); Waxler (1941)
Sheep	*Eimeria ninae-kohl-yakimovi; E. faurei*	Hyperglycemia			Shumard (1957)
Rat	*Haemobartonella muris*	Terminal hypoglycemia			Linton (1929); Regendanz (1929a); Hoffenreich (1932); von Brand *et al.* (1932)

159

it cannot be reconciled with the following facts. In the first place the terminal hypoglycemia cannot be due to total exhaustion of the carbohydrate reserves since it can be relieved temporarily by injections of adrenaline (Regendanz, 1929b; Regendanz and Tropp, 1927; Krijgsman, 1933) and since the blood sugar level returns to normal even in fasting animals after administration of trypanocidal drugs (Scheff, 1932). Actually these observations point rather to an involvement of such organs as the suprarenals, pancreas, or thyroid (Bellelli and Caraffa, 1956; Lippi and Benedetto, 1958). The assumption of adrenal involvement especially is probably correct since Nyden (1948) found the ascorbic acid content of the adrenals markedly reduced in rats infected with *Trypanosoma hippicum,* and Takagi (1956) found a lipid depletion of the adrenals of mice infected with *Trypanosoma gambiense* and *Trypanosoma evansi.* It may also be significant in this connection that injections of adrenocorticotropic hormone did not relieve the terminal hypoglycemia of rats parasitized by *Trypanosoma equiperdum,* but this finding is not conclusive since cortisone also failed to raise the blood sugar level (von Brand, *et al.* 1951).

In the second place, identical symptoms, terminal hypoglycemia and lowered glycogen reserves, occur in small laboratory animals like rats where the parasites reach concentrations of 2 to 3 billion per ml blood and in rabbits where so few parasites develop that they can often be found only with difficulty in the peripheral blood (von Brand and Regendanz, 1931). It is clearly inconceivable that the few trypanosomes existing at any one time in a rabbit could exhaust the carbohydrate reserves of the host by their sugar consumption alone. Finally, the feeding of sugar to trypanosome-infected animals does perhaps slightly prolong the lives of the hosts, but only for short periods and does not prevent the development of the terminal hypoglycemia (Cordier, 1927; Angolotti and Carda, 1929; Bruynoghe *et al.,* 1927; J. Andrews *et al.,* 1930; Hoppe and Chapman, 1947; Bouisset *et al.,* 1956).

In discussing the possible role of the trypanosomes' glucose consumption as a factor in pathogenesis it should be kept in mind that the main metabolic end product of the carbohydrate metabolism of pathogenic African trypanosomes is pyruvic acid. This acid, however, regardless of whether it is produced in the host's own metabolism or by the parasite, is readily metabolized by the tissues of the host (Coleman and von Brand, 1957; Grant and Fulton, 1957). The "loss of sugar" sustained by the host is then, at least from a caloric standpoint, more fictional than real since the host loses only the energy released during the glucose-pyruvate sequence, but salvages the much greater amount of energy resulting from complete oxidation of pyruvate.

It is not surprising, in view of the serious objections raised against the glucose consumption theory of trypanosome injury, that alternate explanations have been discussed. One of them is the possibility that asphyxiation of the host is involved, either brought about by the oxygen consumption of the parasites directly (Scheff and Rabati, 1938), or by changes in the hemoglobin/oxygen relationships induced by lactic acid supposedly produced by the flagellates (Kligler *et al.*, 1929), or finally by agglutination of trypanosomes in the vessels of heart and lung which would prevent proper aeration of the blood (J. Andrews *et al*, 1930). This theory is unacceptable because it does not explain how rabbits with their few parasites could become asphyxiated by any of the above mechanisms, and in the case of Kligler and co-workers' (1929) theory because the parasites do not produce appreciable amounts of lactic acid. It is true, on the other hand, that the lactic acid level of the host's blood is increased, at least during the terminal stages of an infection. This has been demonstrated repeatedly by direct determinations of the blood lactate, or by less convincing indirect methods (lowering of blood pH, or alkaline reserve) (Kligler and Geiger, 1928; Scheff, 1928; Kligler *et al.*, 1929; Dominici, 1930; Linton, 1930; J. Andrews *et al.*, 1930; von Brand *et al.*, 1932; Krijgsman, 1933). It is clear that the source for the increased lactate must be sought in the tissues of the host and not in the parasites directly. It is therefore an indication for a metabolic disturbance, but Krijgsman (1936) has emphasized that the accumulation of lactic acid is not high enough to cause injury to the host or to produce asphyxiation.

Still another theory, the view that increased serum potassium levels (Zwemer and Culbertson, 1939) could be involved in producing the trypanosome injuries, is insufficient to explain the observed facts, because, as already mentioned in Chapter 1, potassium-resistant rats die as quickly of an infection as non-resistant ones (Scheff and Thatcher, 1949).

This leaves the assumption that one or more hitherto unrecognized metabolic end products of the trypanosomes, usually designated as toxins, are responsible for the injurious action of the flagellates. This assumption is favored by several authors (Reichenow, 1921; Regendanz and Tropp, 1927; Zotta and Radacovici, 1929a; Locatelli, 1930; von Brand and Regendanz, 1931; Krijgsman, 1933, 1936; von Brand, 1938; French, 1938). It must be realized, however, that it has not been possible so far to demonstrate trypanosome toxins in a convincing manner. Some investigators (Laveran, 1913; Laveran and Roudsky, 1913) reported killing mice by the injection of large doses (0.12 to 0.15 gm) of dried *Trypanosoma gambiense* or *Trypanosoma brucei*, while others obtained completely negative results (Braun and Teichmann, 1912; Kligler *et al.*, 1929; J. Andrews *et al.*, 1930; Fiennes, 1950). These differences may be explained, at least partially, by the observations of Schilling and Rondoni

(1913) and Schilling *et al.* (1938), who reported that killed trypanosomes become toxic only 1 hour after death, but that the toxic action is again lost after 18 hours' storage. This would seem to indicate that an actively toxic principle was obtained only during a certain stage of the autolytic decomposition processes.

More recently Tokura (1935) reported toxic manifestations in experimental animals after injection of dried or lysed pathogenic trypanosomes. The most concrete evidence has been presented by Kawamitsu (1958). He observed 3 to 5 hours after injection into rats of emulsions of heat-killed *Trypanosoma gambiense,* but not *Trypanosoma lewisi,* a distinct hypoglycemia and lowering of the glycogen reserves of the liver, that is, the symptoms appear to have simulated rather closely those observed during an actual infection. The active principle was destroyed by alkali and acid and by heating for 30 minutes to 100°C, but not by heating for a similar period to 60 to 80°C.

Indirect evidence that toxic influences are at work during trypanosomiasis has often been reported. Reichenow (1921) pointed out that the body temperature of infected humans is frequently normal when there are many parasites in the blood, but that it usually rises upon the destruction of large numbers of flagellates as a result of antibody formation. This observation corroborates the assumption that the parasites contain endotoxins. On the other hand, the pronounced metabolic disturbances in experimental animals during the later stages of an infection are better understood on the basis of exotoxins. Krijgsman (1936) thinks, without experimental proof, that the latter may be amines. Evidently, the whole question urgently requires a thorough reinvestigation.

Whatever the final explanation of the mechanism underlying the metabolic disturbances during trypanosomiasis will be, no doubt exists that the liver is involved. It has been shown by both quantitative chemical and by histochemical procedures that animals infected with pathogenic African trypanosomes form considerably less liver glycogen from orally administered carbohydrate than normal ones (von Brand and Regendanz, 1931; Mercado and von Brand, 1960). The intimate distribution of glycogen, as revealed by specific staining of histological sections, varied somewhat, depending upon the trypanosome species. In infections with *Trypanosoma equiperdum* glycogen deposition was seen chiefly in the periportal region of the liver lobules, while a centrilobular pattern was not rare in *Trypanosoma equinum* infections. In some animals, infected with either species, no special pattern of deposition was apparent (Mercado and von Brand, 1960). It was also found that starving infected rats formed little, and in the late stages of the disease, no glycogen at all from body proteins under the influence of cortisone (von Brand *et al.,* 1951). If fructose and Meticortelone were both given, an increased glycogen synthesis over that induced by fructose alone occurred, although not under all conditions studied, in infections with *Trypanosoma equinum* and *Trypanosoma congolense,* while neither fructose, Meticortelone, or a combination of both induced a higher degree of liver glycogen synthesis in *Trypanosoma equiperdum* infections (Mercado and von Brand, 1960).

Further evidence for hepatic damage can be seen in the facts that the alimentary blood sugar curve of infected animals is abnormal (von Brand and Regendanz, 1931; Scheff, 1932; Bell and Jones, 1946) (Fig. 6.), that the utilization of fructose in impaired (Schern and Citron, 1913), and that the aldolase level of the liver tissue is lowered, while that of the serum is increased (Sebastiani, 1959). Increases in serum levels of glutamic-oxalacetic, and glutamic-pyruvate transaminases (Lippi and Sebastiani, 1958), lactic dehydrogenase (Corso and Frugoni, 1961a), malic dehydrogenase, succinic dehydrogenase, and leucine-amino-peptidase activity (Corso and Frugoni, 1961b) point into the same direction. Insofar as human infections are concerned no gross disturbance of the carbohydrate metabolism has been noted (Walravens, 1931; Wormall, 1932),

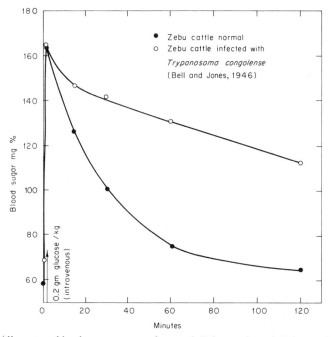

Fig. 6. Alimentary blood sugar curve of normal Zebu cattle and Zebu cattle infected with *Trypanosoma congolense* after intravenous administration of glucose. (After Bell and Jones, 1946.)

but the patients studied were not in the last stage of the disease. More recently Janssens *et al.* (1961) reported an increase in lactic dehydrogenase activity, but an approximately normal malic dehydrogenase level, of the cerebrospinal fluid in patients infected with *Trypanosoma gambiense.*

Trypanosoma cruzi, in contrast to the pathogenic African trypanosomes, has no distinct influence on the carbohydrate metabolism of the host. The latter's blood sugar and glycogen reserves remain essentially normal throughout the infection (von Brand *et al.,* 1949). Evidently, if *Trypanosoma cruzi* produces a toxin, it does not interfere with this phase of the host's metabolism. The presence of endotoxins in these parasites has been assumed on the basis of Roskin and Romanova's (1938), Klyueva and Roskin's (1946), and Coudert and Juttin's (1950) claims of having observed the regression of tumors after injections of extracts from the blood-stream or culture forms of the parasite into experimental animals, that is, they assume the flagellates have cancerolytic properties. Despite negative results reported by numerous other authors (Engel, 1944; Hauschka *et al.,* 1947; Cohen *et al.,* 1947; Brncic and Hoecker, 1949; Spain *et al.,* 1948; Belkin *et al.,* 1949; Talice, 1949) both the Russian (Roskin, 1963) and French (Coudert, 1961) groups maintain their views and use the trypanosome extracts clinically. Biochemically, the *Trypanosoma cruzi* extracts appear to reduce the aerobic glycolysis of tumor cells. They also seem to influence the distribution of DNA within the cells, since their acridine-yellow-induced fluorescence disappears without lowering their absolute amounts. RNA, on the other hand, seems to increase when large amounts of extract are provided (Michel-Brun, 1963; Coudert and Michel-Brun, 1963, 1964; Coudert *et al.,* 1964).

In malaria the evidence concerning disturbances of the carbohydrate metabolism of the host parallels to some extent that summarized for African trypanosomiasis, with the difference that more concrete evidence involving human cases is available. As indicated in Table XXIX the behavior of the blood sugar in humans is somewhat variable, but a transient hyperglycemia during the pyrexic stages has been observed so often that its occurrence cannot be doubted. Definite indications exist that human malaria affects the carbohydrate functions of the liver. Abnormalities in the blood sugar curve after administration of glucose or fructose have been described (Williams, 1927; Sinton and Hughes, 1924; Hughes and Malik, 1930), while, on the other hand, galactose tolerance tests gave approximately normal results in most cases (Lippincott *et al.,* 1946). Serum transaminases and lactic dehydrogenase are temporarily increased during the pyrexic stages of malaria, while aldolase remains essentially normal (Fuhrmann, 1962).

It has been suggested that the rise in blood sugar during malarial paroxysms is due to an excessive breakdown of liver glycogen (Sinton and Kehar, 1931). The underlying cause, if indeed a primary damage of the liver is involved, may be anoxia. Maegraith (1948) pointed out in this connection that anoxia induced by low oxygen content of the ambient atmosphere induces in rats a transient hyperglycemia which is followed by hypoglycemia. This is due to an initial stimulation of the adrenals resulting in the release of an excess of adrenalin which raises the blood sugar if enough liver glycogen is available, but may lead to hypoglycemia when the glycogen stores are exhausted. This sequence of events bears a marked similarity to that assumed by Sinton and Kehar (1931) as explaining corresponding phenomena in malaria.

There is good evidence that in human and animal malarias the adrenals are affected (Maegraith, 1954). At least in the later stages of the disease such signs of adrenal insufficiency as asthenia, peripheral vascular failure, or hypotension have been reported. In some chronic cases even pigmentation abnormalities of the skin and mucous membranes similar to those of Addison's disease have been observed (Paisseau and Lemaire, 1916; Junior and Brandao, 1937; Marañon, 1939).

As to animal malarias, in chickens infected with *Plasmodium gallinaceum* (Taylor *et al.*, 1956) and in rats infected with *Plasmodium berghei* (Highman *et al.*, 1954; Mercado and von Brand, 1957) but not in monkeys infected with *Plasmodium knowlesi* (Devakul and Maegraith, 1958), a lipid depletion of the suprarenals has been found. During the course of the chicken malaria the adrenals become hypertrophied (Nadel *et al.*, 1949) and show abnormalities in ascorbic acid content (to be reviewed in Chapter 8).

A rather clear-cut connection between adrenal dysfunction and carbohydrate metabolism has been described by Mercado and von Brand (1957). If Meticortelone is injected into noninfected starving rats, a certain amount of liver glycogen is synthesized, and similarly liver glycogen is deposited after feeding fructose to starving animals. If both Meticortelone and fructose are given to rats, the glycogen synthesis is clearly additive and corresponds closely to the sum of syntheses resulting from the separate treatments. On the other hand, in rats infected with *Plasmodium berghei*, the administration of both the hormone and fructose results in a definitely higher synthesis than that which would correspond to an addition of the glycogen synthesized under the influence of the single treatments. In malarial rats fed fructose glycogen synthesis is essentially restricted to the peripheral regions of the liver lobules (von Brand and Mercado, 1956), while a centrilobular lipid infiltration occurs (von Brand and Mercado, 1958). Upon administration of both Meticortelone and fructose the pattern of glycogen deposition is largely normalized (Mercado and von Brand, 1957), that is, the patchy glycogen distribution seen after fructose feeding has been replaced by a more uniform distribution. The glycogen-free centrilobular zone has become much narrower, indicating that the stimulus provided by the adrenal hormone restored the glycogenic functions of the liver cells. In principle similar observations have been reported in respect to the liver of *Macaccus mulatta* infected with *Plasmodium knowlesi* (Devakul and Maegraith, 1958). Evidently in these cases the affected liver cells were not damaged irreversibly. It does seem apparent that they were unable to respond adequately to the relatively weak normal adrenal stimulation, but did require the stronger artificial stimulus provided by hormone injection. It should be noted that the latter normalized only the glycogen picture. It was without demonstrable effect on the lipid infiltration, resulting in the unexpected situation that in an intermediate zone of the liver lobules the cells contained appreciable amounts of both glycogen and lipids.

Little is known so far about the intimate mechanisms bringing about the lowered glycogen synthesis in the malarious liver. Von Brand and Mercado (1956) studied the comparative glycogen synthesis resulting from the administration of identical amounts of various carbohydrates under standardized conditions (Table XXX). They found in all cases a definitely reduced synthesis, when the latter was expressed in milligram per unit weight rat. If, however, the relative rates are considered, a different picture emerged. Fructose was the best glycogen former. Upon setting the glycogen synthesis from other carbohydrates in relation to that obtained with fructose, no significant difference (with the possible exception of the synthesis due to mannose) between noninfected and infected rats was seen. This seems to indicate that the glycogenic functions of the liver are qualitatively essentially normal and that they are reduced only quantitatively. Further studies on the cellular level will be required to clarify the situation further.

While malaria parasites (Fig. 7) and African trypanosomes produce a hypoglycemia in their hosts, at least during the terminal stages of the infections, *Eimeria* species, on the contrary, produce an often pronounced hyperglycemia. This has been shown for the chicken parasite *Eimeria tenella* (Pratt, 1940; Waxler, 1941) and the ovine species *Eimeria ninae-kohl-yakimovi* and *Eimeria faurei* (Shumard, 1957), making it probable that a specific influence by the parasite, rather than a specialized response of a host species is at work. The glycogen stores of the chicken become depleted during the infection (Pratt, 1941). It had originally been assumed that the rise in blood sugar was a simple consequence of the severe hemorrhage characterizing the infection of chicken, but this explanation is by far too simple. Daugherty (1950) has found

TABLE XXX

GLYCOGEN FORMED IN THE LIVER OF NORMAL RATS AND RATS INFECTED WITH
Plasmodium berghei[a,b]

Compound	Liver glycogen (mg) synthesized/100 gm rat		Relative rate of synthesis	
	Noninfected	Infected	Noninfected	Infected
Fructose	132	74	100	100
Melezitose	118	52	89	70
Saccharose	57	25	43	37
Lactose	48	33	40	45
Glucose	46	29	36	39
Galactose	38	11	29	15
Mannose	24	2	18	3
Sorbose	20	12	15	16

[a] Three hours after oral administration of 500 mg of the specified compound.
[b] After von Brand and Mercado (1956).

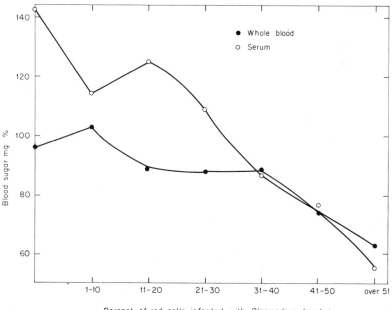

Fig. 7.   Blood sugar of rats infected with *Plasmodium berghei,* as related to parasite density. (After Mercado, 1952.)

that homogenates from ceca of infected chickens inhibited glycolysis of chicken brain *in vitro,* but did not interfere with the degradation of fructose-1,6-phosphate. They did, in contrast to homogenates of uninfected ceca, interfere with the esterification of inorganic phosphate. On the basis of these observations it seems probable that some phases of intermediate carbohydrate metabolism, especially the phosphorylative steps, are disturbed during coccidiosis (Daugherty and Herrick, 1952). Whether a similar disturbance occurs in liver coccidiosis has not yet been studied in detail. The only relevant observation consists in finding abnormal high blood sugar in a rabbit after oral administration of sugar (von Brand, 1952). It is possible that toxic substances produced by the parasites are responsible for the above pathological symptoms. Burns (1959) observed death of rabbits injected with extracts of *Eimeria tenella.* These observations were substantiated and extended by Rikimaru *et al.* (1961), who reported some results of special significance to the present discussion, namely, the fact that upon injection of the extracts a significant rise in blood sugar occurs which is followed by hypoglycemia and almost total depletion of blood glucose at time of death.

II. DISTURBANCES OF THE HOST'S CARBOHYDRATE METABOLISM DURING HELMINTHIC INFECTIONS

Disturbances in the host's carbohydrate metabolism as a consequence of helminthic infections have been studied in less detail than those found in trypanosomiasis or malaria. With the exception of nippostrongylosis, only more or less disconnected observations have been reported and they indicate that on the whole the disturbances that occur are less severe than those in the above protozoan infections. In addition to the data assembled in Table XXXI, it has been observed (Lewert and Lee, 1955) that hepatic cells in the vicinity of growing cysticerci of *Taenia taeniae- formis* lack glycogen, while the growing parasites accumulate progressively more polysaccharide. After they have become surrounded by a well-formed connective tissue capsule, the adjacent liver cells are again normal in respect to glycogen content. A somewhat different type of change has been found during experimental *Clonorchis* infections of rabbits. Here, especially during the period 40 to 50 days after infection, a decrease in liver polysaccharide was found which was most pronounced in the peripheral regions of the lobules. Most remarkable, however, was the appearance of polysaccharide granules in the previously polysaccharide-free epithelium of the proliferated bile ducts (Kuwamura, 1958). Liver involvement in this infection was probable only prior to Kuwamura's (1958) investigation. It had been reported (Uyeno, 1935; Kawai, 1937) that the sugar tolerance of infected rabbits was abnormal.

In schistosomiasis, the eggs of the worms produce extensive necrotic lesions in the liver. Therefore disturbances in the hepatic functions, including glycogen synthesis and detoxification mechanisms, should be expected to occur in severe cases. Glycosuria and even frank diabetes mellitus have been described from some human infections and the alimentary blood sugar curve was then highly abnormal (Day, 1924; Erfan and Camb, 1933; Seife and Lisa, 1950). It is evident that these conditions are due not only to liver damage, but to pancreas involvement as well. An infiltration of helminth eggs into the pancreas occurs (Seife and Lisa, 1950), but this alone cannot explain the diabetic condition, since the latter ceases rapidly after anthelminthic medication (Day, 1924; Erfan and Camb, 1933). In infections with *Schistosoma japonicum* the glycogen content of the liver was increased and the polysaccharide was uniformly distributed throughout the lobules. In the same infection an acid mucopolysaccharide of the hyaluronic acid type appeared in the walls of the portal vessels and around the egg lesions, while a different type of polysaccharide surrounded the eggs and also appeared in the egg-shells (Sawada *et al.*, 1956). In human infections with *Schistosoma japonicum* only slight abnormalities in sugar tolerance have been reported, only minor irregularities in the galactose test having been found in some, but not all, patients (Lippincott *et al.*, 1947). Similarly, only slight deviations from the norm have been found during sugar tolerance tests of humans parasitized by hookworms, but there were some indications pointing toward a lowered absorption (Saito, 1933; Firki and Ghalioungi, 1937; Sheehy *et al.*, 1962).

Very much more pronounced is this lowered absorption rate in infections with *Nippostrongylus muris*. It is of special interest that it was found exclusively in the jejunum, amounting there to only 20% of the normal rate. It was correlated to a decrease in alkaline phosphatase activity and reduced efflux of Na^+ from the mucosa. It is thus reasonable to assume that the "sodium pump" is implicated in the defective glucose absorption mechanism. In contrast to the jejunum, the glucose absorption of the entire intestine was normal (Symons, 1961). Symons and Fairbairn (1962, 1963) found the pancreatic secretion of amylase normal, but the concentration of the enzyme in the jejunal fluid was considerably lower than normal as a consequence of the sharply increased volume of jejunal fluid in the infected animals. On the other hand, the maltase activity of the brush border of the jejunal mucosa was reduced at least by 50% in infected animals.

In contrast to the faulty absorption of carbohydrates, their intermediate metabolism is essentially normal, at least in the liver. Gallagher and Symons (1959) found normal rates of anaerobic glycolysis, normal oxidation of tricarboxylic acid cycle intermediates, and normal oxidative

TABLE XXXI
BLOOD SUGAR AND GLYCOGEN RESERVES IN HELMINTHIC INFECTIONS

Host	Parasite	Blood sugar	Liver glycogen	Muscle glycogen	References
Rabbit	*Clonorchis sinensis*	Sometimes hyper-glycemia, some-times hypoglycemia			Uyeno (1935); Kawai (1937)
Sheep, rabbit	*Fasciola hepatica*	Normal or slight hypoglycemia			Balian (1940); Goldbergiene (1962)
Sheep	*Paramphistomum microbothrium*	Normal or slight hyperglycemia			Lengy (1962)
Man	*Schistosoma mansoni*	Normal, sometimes hyper- or hypo-glycemia			Day (1924); Erfan and Camb (1933); Pons (1937); Seife and Lisa (1950)
Sheep	*Schistomosa bovis*	Hyperglycemia			Lengy (1962)
Australorbis glabratus	*Schistosoma mansoni*			Decreased (total body glycogen)	von Brand and Files (1947)
Helisoma trivolvis	*Glyptelmins pennsylvaniensis*		Decreased		Snyder and Cheng (1961); Cheng and Snyder (1962); Cheng (1963b)

Echinostoma revolutum	*Physa occidentalis*		Decreased (total body glycogen)	Hurst (1927)
Trichinella spiralis	Man, dog, rabbit	Normal, sometimes hypoglycemia		Augustine (1936); Harwood *et al.* (1937); Pierce *et al.* (1939); Hartman *et al.* (1940); Hatieganu and Fodor (1942)
Ascaris lumbricoides	Man	Sometimes hypoglycemia		Frank (1944)
Hookworms	Man	Normal		Donomae (1927)
Ancylostoma caninum	Dog	Normal	Normal	von Brand and Otto (1938)

phosphorylation in liver homogenates or mitochondrial preparations. The anaerobic glycolysis of jejunal tissues proved also normal, but the oxidation of citrate and succinate occurred at 2 to 3 times the normal rate. This increase was related to an uncoupling of oxidative phosphorylation which was traced back to the large amount of calcium present in the gut wall of the parasites. Use of ethylenediaminetetraacetic acid while preparing the jejunal mitochondria resulted in preparations oxidizing both citrate and succinate at normal rates and showing normal P/O ratios. It is then unlikely that the above mechanism can be operative *in vivo*. Furthermore, Gallagher and Symons (1959) consider it as unlikely that a toxin produced by the worms is involved in the pathogenesis of nippostrongylosis.

Infections with *Trichinella spiralis* seem not to interfere materially with the carbohydrate metabolism of the host (Table XXXI); a normal sugar tolerance curve has been found in infected rabbits (Augustine, 1936). It is rather curious that according to Lewis (1928) *Trichinella* larvae invade primarily glycogen-poor muscles. Similarly unexplained is the finding of Zarzycki (1956) that, at least according to histochemical evidence, the glycogen content of muscles of mice first increases after being invaded by larvae. However, beginning with the eleventh day after invasion, the glycogen of the muscle fibers diminishes and they eventually become glycogen-free.

When *Ascaris* larvae migrate through the liver, the glycogen content of the parasitic foci proper is very low, but that of the surrounding liver tissue, though variable, proved essentially normal (Münnich, 1958, 1959–1960). On the other hand, however, Kawazoe (1961) found a decrease in the host's liver glycogen and its blood sugar, and M. F. Andrews *et al.* (1961) reported an increase in serum glutamic-pyruvic and glutamic-oxalacetic transaminase, as well as aldolase, indicative of organ damage.

Insofar as invertebrates are concerned, the influence of parasitism on the carbohydrate metabolism of the host has so far only been studied in molluscs infected with larval trematodes. These infections lead generally to a lowering of the polysaccharide content of the invaded organ (Table XXXI). Cheng and Snyder (1962) observed that paralleling the disappearance of hepatopancreatic glycogen from the snail, an increase in glycogen occurred within the bodies of the cercariae of *Glyptelmins pennsylvaniensis* which developed in sporocysts. They found that the presence of the parasites led to glycogen depletion, not only in the host cells directly in contact with the sporocysts, but also at some distance of the latter. They consider it as possible that the parasites secrete an "activating substance" which would stimulate the glycolytic system of the host cells. According to Cheng (1963b) larval trematodes can secure carbohydrates from their hosts from three sources and utilize them for glycogen synthesis: the hepatopancreas, (Cheng and Snyder, 1963), the musculature (Hurst, 1927; Cheng and Snyder, 1962), or the host's blood sugar. The latter source is especially probable in cases like those of the cercariae of *Gorgodera amplicava* which accumulate glycogen while parasitizing the glycogen-free gills of *Musculium partumeium* (Cheng, 1963a).

III. DISTURBANCES OF THE HOST'S CARBOHYDRATE METABOLISM DURING ARTHROPOD INFECTIONS

Carcinus specimens parasitized by *Sacculina* seem not to store appreciable amounts of glycogen in their subcutaneous tissues as do normal crabs, at least before a molt. Smith (1913) assumes that this failure is responsible for the inability of sacculinized crabs to molt, but whether this assumption is completely justified remains to be established. It should be remembered that in insects at least the molting process is governed by hormonal processes. Smith (1913) furthermore found that normal animals kept the glycogen content of their hepatopancreas fairly constant even during prolonged starvation, while in sacculinized specimens a progressive depletion occurred. He assumes that the former replenish the liver glycogen from the subcutaneous stores, but that the latter are unable to do so. The influence of the purely ectoparasitic *Gyge* on the glycogen stores of its host, *Upogebia,* apparently is of a different nature. Somewhat more glycogen was found in parasitized specimens than in normal ones (T. E. Hughes, 1940).

IV. HOST DIETARY CARBOHYDRATES AND PARASITES

It has been indicated in preceding sections that parasites derive their carbohydrates from the host's intestinal contents, its tissues, or body fluids. The question whether this constitutes such a serious withdrawal of food material as to adversely affect the nutritional state of the host can legitimately be raised. While the carbohydrates are singled out here, the following discussion is essentially valid also for the other major groups of food materials.

The question as to the importance of food robbery by parasites in the economy of the host has in the past often been answered affirmatively. The modern attitude is one of scepticism. The weight relations between parasites and hosts are in most instances such that even a parasite with a very high rate of metabolism withdraws only an insignificant fraction of the normal daily caloric food intake of its host. Of course exceptionally heavy worm burdens occur occasionally. Hall (1917) described thus the case of an individual harboring 11 lb of *Ascaris*. But even this mass of worms would have consumed only about 8% of a normal 2500 calorie diet (von Brand, 1948). Furthermore, in caloric terms this figure is probably considerably too high. *Ascaris* excretes volatile fatty acids which may well be utilized by the host, forming then a parallel to the proved utilization of the pyruvic acid produced by the African pathogenic trypanosomes (Coleman and von Brand, 1957). Similar calculations and assumptions are probably justified in other cases, such as the parasitization of mice by larval *Taenia taeniaeformis,* where the worm burden can amount to 10% or more of the total weight of the host.

Even more extreme cases can be found among parasitized invertebrates. The dry substance of the external sac of *Peltogaster* (to which its root system would have to be added) may reach values of 15%, or occasionally even more, of the total dry weight of the host crab (Reinhard and von Brand, 1944). In snails infected with larval trematodes so much host tissue is frequently replaced by parasite tissue that the latter should amount to a significant proportion of the former. However, metabolic determinations on normal *Australorbis* and snails parasitized by *Schistosoma mansoni* are not favorable to the view that food robbery is of major importance (von Brand and Files, 1947).

It could be argued that the cases of retarded growth related to parasitism were due to undernourishment of the host because of food robbery by the parasites. It is of course true that parasitism often interferes with growth both of warm-blooded hosts (e.g., Spindler, 1947) and of cold-blooded hosts (e.g., Cross, 1935). However, there is no indication that food robbery by the parasites is responsible; rather such factors as diminished absorption, interference with digestion, anorexia, and similar factors have to be incriminated (Stewart, 1933; Shearer and Stewart, 1933; J. S. Andrews *et al.,* 1944; J. S. Andrews, 1938; Gordon, 1957, 1958; Cauthen and Landram, 1958; Bremner, 1961). It should also be kept in mind that in other instances, both with protozoa or helminths as parasites, and vertebrates or invertebrates as hosts, stimulation rather than retardation of growth of the host has been observed (Wesenberg-Lund, 1934; Rothschild, 1941; Whitlock, 1949; Lincicome *et al.,* 1960; Lincicome and Shepperson, 1963; Lincicome, 1963; Mueller, 1962, 1965a,b).

There is good evidence that a host diet rich in carbohydrates benefits many parasites. Hegner and Eskridge (1937) found it favorable to intestinal amoebas of the rat; Sassuchin (1931) and Armer (1944) reported similar observations for cockroach protozoa, as did Mowry and Becker (1930) for rumen ciliates, and Westphal (1939) for the human parasites

Chilomastix and *Enteromonas*. Curiously, no corresponding beneficial influence was found in the case of tadpole trichomonads. In mixed infections of *Tritrichomonas augusta* and *Tritrichomonas batracharum* the former disappeared when the hosts were kept on a high carbohydrate diet, but not on a high protein diet (Cairns, 1956).

Insofar as parasitic worms are concerned, by far the greatest amount of information is available for tapeworms, chiefly as a result of the investigations of C. P. Read and his co-workers. It had been reported, previous to their work, that *Raillietina cesticillus* and *Hymenolepis diminuta* thrive best when the host's diet contained a high proportion of carbohydrate (Reid, 1942; Chandler, 1943). Read and Rothman (1957a) found that rats parasitized by *Hymenolepis diminuta* and placed on a carbohydrate-deficient diet for 2 weeks lose a high proportion of the worms; the remainder cease to produce eggs and weigh only about 15% as much as control worms kept in adequately fed host animals. Both worm size and reproductive rate were directly related to the quantity of carbohydrate ingested by the rats, up to 3.0 gm starch/rat/day. Above this level no further beneficial effect was noticed (Read *et al.*, 1958).

Hymenolepis diminuta appears especially sensitive to carbohydrate deficiencies in the host's diet; *Hymenolepis citelli* and *Hymenolepis nana* are less so (Read and Rothman, 1958a). It is of considerable interest that this differential sensitivity could be correlated with differences in growth patterns (Read, 1959, 1961). *Hymenolepis diminuta* grows at a nearly constant rate as long as the host lives, while *Hymenolepis nana* grows only for 10 to 12 days, after which time it becomes senescent and dies at about 25 days of age. Only during its growth period has the worm a definite requirement for host dietary carbohydrate. *Hymenolepis citelli* has growth characteristics intermediate between those of the above two species, and characteristically its carbohydrate requirements are also intermediate. Less is known about other species; it has, however, been established that *Oochoristica* from rodents and *Lacistorhynchus* from dogfish also require carbohydrate for growth or maintenance (Read, 1957). Further supporting the discussed relationship is the fact that *Schistocephalus*, which matures sexually and dies within a few days after reaching the final host, appears not to be affected by the host's dietary carbohydrates (Hopkins, 1950, 1951).

Little is known about the possible occurrence of similar relationships in other groups of worms. The only parallel to tapeworms found so far is the acanthocephalan *Moniliformis dubius*, whose growth is arrested and whose body size decreases upon maintenance in a host on a carbohydrate-deficient diet (Read and Rothman, 1958b). The observation that *Ascaridia galli* is rapidly lost from the host when the latter is starved (Reid, 1945a,b) may indicate a similar sensitivity in roundworms, but the influence of a low carbohydrate diet has not yet been established in this case.

A host diet can be quantitatively or qualitatively inadequate for a parasite. In preceding sections the spectra of utilizable carbohydrates have been discussed for various parasites and these data need not to be repeated here. It must be emphasized, however, that if a host diet contains as sole carbohydrate a compound not utilized by a parasite, the influence on the latter will approximate that of carbohydrate deprivation. This is not surprising; a good example is fructose and *Hymenolepis diminuta* (Read and Rothman, 1957b). However, the physiological processes of the host cannot be neglected; they may be of importance in modifying the ability of a parasite to benefit from a given carbohydrate. It has thus been found that glucose in the diet is less favorable to *Hymenolepis diminuta* than starch. As Read (1959) pointed out this seemingly paradoxical finding can be explained on the assumption that less glucose than starch reaches the actual site of the worms, because a large proportion of this sugar is absorbed already in the upper parts of the intestine, while starch has first to be degraded before being ready for absorption by the intestinal mucosa. In an even more difficult position in the above respect than parasites of the small intestine are those parasitizing the large intestine; it is significant that Westphal (1939) found a beneficial influence of a carbohydrate diet on the flagellates *Chilomastix* and *Enteromonas* only if the carbohydrates were given to the host in a form that is not rapidly digested and absorbed, for example, in the form of lentils.

Other interactions between carbohydrates in the diet and host physiology influencing parasites do occur. It has thus been observed that one dietary carbohydrate, lactose, or milk has an unfavorable action on several intestinal parasites: rumen ciliates (Eberlein, 1895), intestinal nematodes (Ackert and Riedel, 1946; Shorb and Spindler, 1947; Spindler *et al.*, 1944), and cestodes (Hager, 1941). It is probable that in these cases indirect influences cause the damage. As Read (1950) has pointed out a diet high in lactose changes the intestinal pH and oxidation reduction potential, the intestinal emptying time, the vitamin synthesis by intestinal bacteria, and probably many other factors that may influence parasites. It must be stressed, however, that not all intestinal parasites react in the same way to whatever changes are brought about by a milk diet. Thus the latter seems not to be inimical to *Haemonchus contortus, Ostertagia* sp., or *Trichostrongylus* spp. (Gordon, 1960). Even a beneficial action of lactose has been reported. According to Greenberg and Taylor (1950) a high proportion of lactose or galactose in the diet favors the establishment of infections with *Entamoeba histolytica* in the rat, an abnormal host.

Tissue or blood parasites normally will be less susceptible to influences emanating from the host diet than intestinal parasites, at least insofar as influences induced by dietary carbohydrates are concerned. The well-known inhibitory influence of a milk diet on rodent malaria (Maegraith *et al.*, 1952; Raffaele and Carrescia, 1954; Ramakrishnan *et al.*, 1953; Jacobi and Kretschmar, 1962; and others) is not evident in all cases, perhaps due to strain differences, perhaps due to differences in experimental design (Galliard *et al.*, 1954; Corradetti *et al.*, 1955; Ramakrishnan *et al.*, 1956). At any rate it cannot be ascribed to the lactose content of the milk. While it is probable that a pure milk diet induces a *p*-aminobenzoic acid deficiency severe enough to account for the reduced severity of the malarial infection (Hawking, 1953; Raffaele and Carrescia, 1954; Hawking and Terry, 1957), this may not be the only factor involved. Fulton and Spooner (1955) and Sautet *et al.* (1956) do not assume such a specific influence of the milk diet. The former assume that milk does not contain all the necessary components required for the growth of the malarial parasites, while the latter are inclined to ascribe the action of milk to the latter's vitamins and minerals which are partially lacking in the normal diet; i.e., in their view it is not the milk but the normal diet that is incomplete.

V.   CARBOHYDRATE METABOLISM OF PARASITES AND CHEMOTHERAPY

Several antiparasitic drugs exert their primary action by interfering with some phase of the carbohydrate metabolism of parasites, a fact which is not surprising in view of the enormous importance carbohydrates play in the metabolism of parasites. Active compounds have been found to interfere with the carbohydrate metabolism at different levels, especially with the absorption of carbohydrates and their intracellular utilization.

The former mechanism lies at the root of the chemotherapeutic activity of alkyldibenzylamines against schistosomes. Under their influence the worms consume much less glucose than normally, but their lactic acid production is not reduced to the same degree. The source for the lactate eliminated must be intracellular glycogen of which more is mobilized than before exposure (Bueding and Swartzwelder, 1957; Bueding, 1959, 1962). Furthermore, alkyldibenzylamines do not inhibit hexokinase, or interfere with the rate of glycolysis of homogenates or extracts of the worms, nor do they stimulate their phosphorylase, phosphoglucomutase, or ATPases. Bueding (1959, 1962) therefore concludes that the point of attack is the glucose transport mechanism.

A somewhat similar line of reasoning has been employed by Bueding *et al.* (1961) to prove a corresponding mechanism in the case of the anthelminthic activity of a cyanine dye, dithiazanine, against *Trichuris vulpis.* The drug inhibits the glucose uptake at low concentrations which do not inhibit mobility of the worms. The dye does not inhibit hexokinase activity, but under its influence the total carbohydrate content as well as the free glucose decrease sharply. It is then assumed that the primary action is against glucose absorption. A consequence of its inhibition is a decrease in the concentration of energy-rich phosphate bonds; finally, the energy required for survival becomes inadequate and the worms die.

Little is known about the occurrence of corresponding mechanisms in protozoan chemotherapy. Ghosh and Chatterjee (1961) found that the antibiotic nystatin inhibits the oxidative utilization of various carbohydrates very markedly, while at very low concentrations some stimulation was observed. Anaerobic endogenous metabolism was stimulated even at concentrations of the drug inhibiting aerobic metabolism. In cell-free preparations nystatin did not interfere with hexokinase, glucose -6-phosphate dehydrogenase, isocitric dehydrogenase, cytochrome oxidase, ATPase, or transaminase. Its activity therefore seems not to be related to enzyme inhibition, but may rest on the induction of permeability changes, i.e., it may interfere with the absorption of substrates.

Many more drugs appear to interfere with some phase of intracellular carbohydrate utilization than with absorption from the environment. In other words, in many cases the activity is due to enzyme inhibition. Undoubtedly, however, many drugs are not specific in the sense that they inhibit just a single enzyme. In this respect trivalent arsenicals are a good example. Chen (1948) and Marshall (1948a) have shown that the hexokinase of *Trypanosoma equiperdum* and *Trypanosoma evansi* is very sensitive to this class of compounds. Blocking the enzyme effectively interrupts glucose utilization according to the glycolytic pathway. Since the African trypanosomes are absolutely dependent for their energy requirements on glycolytic processes, it seems likely that the trypanocidal activity of trivalent arsenicals can be explained largely by this inhibition of one of the glycolytic key enzymes. Arsenicals are sulfhydryl inhibitors and it can be expected that their activity is not limited to hexokinase. Indeed Thurston (1958) has shown that organic arsenicals, such as neoarsphenamine or reduced Stovarsol thioglycollate, inhibit almost to the same extent when *Trypanosoma equiperdum* metabolizes glycerol rather than glucose. Since glycerol utilization does not involve hexokinase, this enzyme cannot be the only one susceptible to arsenic inhibition. In fact it can be expected that most, if not all, enzymes requiring functional SH-groups for their activity will be inhibited by these arsenicals. It is curious, however, that according to Thurston (1958) sodium arsenite acts differently from the organic arsenicals mentioned above; it may be specifically active against hexokinase.

It thus becomes necessary to examine the criteria proving drug activity by inhibition of specific enzymes. They have been elaborated by Hunter and Lowry (1956) and their application to a concrete example dealing with parasites, the inhibition of schistosome phosphofructokinase by antimonials, has been discussed by Bueding (1959) (see also Mansour and Bueding, 1954; Bueding and Mansour, 1957) whose paper the following exposition closely follows. Four relevant criteria are available. (1) The enzyme should be inhibited in the intact cell. That the phosphofructokinase of schistosomes is inhibited in the living worms can be deduced from the fact that upon incubation of worms in low concentrations of potassium antimonyl tartrate or upon administration of subcurative doses of stibophen to the host an accumulation of fructose-6-phosphate and a reduction in concentration of fructose-1, 6-diphosphate occurs within the worm bodies. (2) The inhibition of the enzyme should quantitatively explain the effects of the drug. Since a consequence of phosphofructokinase inhibition is a reduced rate of glycolysis in schistosomes and since these parasites depend on glycolysis for their energy requirements, inhibition of the enzyme may well account for the death of the worms. (3) Enzyme inhibition should occur with drug concentrations no greater than necessary to produce drug action. Reduction of parasite survival *in vitro* from 30 days to 8 hours by exposure to antimonials in concentrations producing an inhibition of phosphofructokinase of more than 50% is in agreement with this point. (4) If an isolated enzyme is inhibited by a concentration as low as that producing an effect in the intact cell, it must be established that other cell constituents do not bind a substantial fraction of the drug. Since the drug inhibits phosphofructokinase activity of crude schistosome extracts to the same degree as purified enzyme preparations, it seems unlikely that other cell constituents of the worms cells bind significant amounts of antimonials. While thus a good case can be made for causal connection between inhibition of phosphofructokinase and schistosomicidal activity of trivalent antimonials, Bueding (1959) emphasizes that the available evidence does not exclude the possibility that the drugs may also be active against other mechanisms essential for survival of the parasites. More recently E. Bueding (personal communication, 1965) found that the phosphofructokinase inhibition produced by antimonials is reversible both *in vitro* and *in vivo*. The drug (potassium antimony tartrate), administered in a single dose to infected animals, brings about a shift of the schistosomes to the liver. As a result of drug-induced enzyme inhibition he found in worms recovered from this organ a marked increase in concentration of hexosemonophosphate and a reduction in the levels of hexosediphosphate and triosephosphate. After some time the worms return to their normal habitat, the mesenteric or portal veins, and in these worms the concentrations of the phosphate esters are approximately normal, a clear indication that the phosphofructokinase was no longer inhibited.

Antimonials are active not only against schistosomes but they have proved effective against trypanosomes and especially leishmanias as well. The mode of action in these latter infections has been studied less intensively than in schistosomiasis. It was established a long time ago that pentavalent antimonials are transformed into trivalent compounds within the bodies of the hosts and that these latter are essentially responsible for the parasiticidal activity (Voegtlin and Smith, 1920), paralleling the metabolic fate of pentavalent arsenicals (Ehrlich, 1909; Voegtlin et al., 1923, 1924; Voegtlin, 1925; Crawford and Levvy, 1947). This view is supported by the observation (Chen and Geiling, 1945) that pentavalent antimonials are much less effective in vitro than trivalent compounds in inhibiting the glucose consumption of Trypanosoma equiperdum and by the similar finding (Fulton and Joyner, 1949) in respect to the inhibition of the oxygen consumption of Leishmania donovani. Trivalent antimonials inhibit the hexokinase of trypanosomes (Chen et al., 1945; Chen, 1948) and in parallel to arsenicals this may be sufficient to explain their trypanocidal activity, but the point has not yet been established with certainty. In the case of the culture form of Leishmania tropica at any rate a different type of interference with glucose metabolism has been reported recently by Voller et al. (1963). They observed that the trivalent fouadin, and, only at high concentrations, the pentavalent pentostan reduced the rate of glucose uptake rather drastically. Analysis of the utilization of C^{14}-glucose showed that the entry of radiocarbon into the Krebs cycle was reduced, accompanied by an increase in concentration of by-products (glycerate, dihydroxy acetone) and end products (lactate, alanine) of the glycolytic sequence. The exact point of attack of the drugs is not known; authors are inclined to incriminate inhibition of pyruvate decarboxylation.

Whether other trypanocidal drugs interfere seriously with the carbohydrate metabolism of the flagellates is uncertain. What is known about their enzyme-inhibiting activities is derived mostly from nontrypanosome material, as the surveys presented by Williamson (1962) and Hawking (1963) show. Undecanediamidine, a straight-chain compound, stimulated in Marshall's (1948a) experiments the glucose consumption of Trypanosoma evansi slightly; it had no apparent influence on the phosphorylated intermediates, but decreased pyruvate production. The drug is thought to attack somewhere in the dehydrogenase system. Stilbamidine, an aromatic compound, did not interfere with oxygen and glucose consumption, but did change the levels of phosphorylated intermediates (Marshall, 1948a). This effect, however, may be only secondary and the main chemotherapeutic activity of the compound may be related to inhibition of protein synthesis or to interference with nucleoproteins.

Bayer 205 (suramin) inhibits strongly a variety of enzyme systems of different provenience *in vitro* (Quastel, 1931; Beiler and Martin, 1948; Town and Wormall, 1949; Wills and Wormall, 1949) and the view has been expressed (Town *et al.,* 1949) that it eliminates trypanosomes by interference with some of their metabolic enzymes. However, the drug when used *in vitro* has no distinct influence on either respiration or glycolysis of trypanosomes (von Fenyvessy and Reiner, 1928; von Issekutz, 1933a,b). Only after long exposure to the drug are respiration and glycolysis reduced and, in contrast to untreated controls, glycerol is accumulated in anaerobic incubates (Glowazky, 1937). However, it should be recalled (see previous sections) that according to more recent studies, pathogenic African trypanosomes normally produce glycerol under lack of oxygen. The mode of action of suramin is then essentially unknown. The possibility of slow penetration or change to a more active compound within the host's body may have to be taken into account. According to Wills and Wormall (1949), suramin almost certainly cannot penetrate through the cell wall of yeast.

In respect to antimalarial drugs, a few relevant data are available for quinine. It does not inhibit glycolysis *in vitro* at approximately therapeutic concentrations ($6 \times 10^{-6} M$), but at higher concentrations ($10^{-3} M$) both aerobic and anaerobic glycolysis of *Plasmodium gallinaceum* are affected (Silverman *et al.,* 1944). It has been reported (Moulder, 1948, 1949) that the oxidation of pyruvate is strongly inhibited in parasites taken from chickens previously treated with quinine. Moulder interpreted his results as probably indicating interference of conversion of pyruvate into a reactive two carbon particle. This mechanism may, however, not represent the sole point of attack of quinine. Marshall (1948b) found, besides inhibition of pyruvate oxidation, an inhibitory effect on the hexokinase, phosphoglyceraldehyde dehydrogenase, and lactic dehydrogenase of *Plasmodium gallinaceum.* He points out that trivalent arsenicals, which specifically inhibit sulfhydryl enzymes, are inactive against malarial parasites probably because alternate metabolic pathways exist or because various substrates can be utilized. Quinine, on the other hand, in his opinion can interrupt metabolic sequences at various points and is therefore also active against a metabolically versatile organism.

Of the newer antimalarial drugs Atabrine (quinacrine, mepacrine) has received most attention. The compound inhibits enzymes which have flavin as prosthetic group or as coenzymes. Its activity is, however, not completely restricted to flavo enzymes (Wright and Sabine, 1944; Haas,

1944; Bovarnick *et al.*, 1946a,b; Hellerman *et al.*, 1946) and it may inhibit the synthesis of an essential flavine (Ball *et al.*, 1948). Atabrine inhibits several glycolytic enzymes, specifically hexokinase (Speck and Evans, 1945; Marshall, 1948b; Fraser and Kermack, 1957), 6-phospho-fructokinase, and triose phosphate dehydrogenase (Marshall, 1948b; Bowman *et al.*, 1961), as well as lactic dehydrogenase (Speck and Evans, 1945). The recent experiments of Bowman *et al.* (1961) have shown that in *Plasmodium berghei* 6-phosphofructokinase is much more sensitive to Atabrine inhibition than hexokinase. These authors assume that the 6-phosphofructokinase reaction governs the rate of glucose utilization by *Plasmodium berghei.* Interference with this reaction by Atabrine would increase the intracellular concentration of glucose-6-phosphate, which in turn would inhibit in a noncompetitive manner the hexokinase reaction.

A last group of potential antimalarials, the naphthoquinones, may be mentioned briefly, although they are of no practical value in human malaria therapy. Some members of this group, especially the hydro-xynaphthoquinones, strongly inhibit the respiration of malarial parasites (Wendel, 1946; Fieser and Heyman, 1948) due chiefly to an inhibition of succinic dehydrogenase brought about by an interference with the inter-action of cytochrome b with cytochrome c (Ball *et al.*, 1947). The activity of naphthoquinones varies greatly from species to species be-cause of differential inactivation by the serum albumin of various mam-malian species (Heyman and Fieser, 1948). In schistosomes these com-pounds are active against glycolytic processes, but here too inactivation by serum restricts the usefulness in practical chemotherapy (Bueding and Peters, 1951).

Another drug inhibiting succinate production by a parasite is piperazine (Bueding *et al.*, 1959). It is well known that *Ascaris* produces normally large quantities of succinic acid both under aerobic and anaerobic con-ditions (Bueding and Farrow, 1956). Under the influence of piperazine the production of succinate is greatly reduced. Because piperazine has a paralyzing action on *Ascaris,* probably because it acts as myoneural blocking agent, the question of the relations between paralyzing action and reduced succinate production arises. Bueding and Swartzwelder (1957) pointed out that at the state of knowledge existing then two alter-native explanations are possible. It is possible that the utilization of succinate is connected with the energy requirements of the worms for muscular contraction. Suppression of muscular activity by piperazine would lower the energy requirements of the muscle, thereby inducing a decreased production of succinate. Alternatively, it would appear possible that the *Ascaris* muscle requires at the myoneural junction chemical reactions associated with the production of succinate. Such reactions, e.g., the formation of CoA or succinyl CoA may be necessary to allow the stimulatory action of acetylcholine to take place in the normal muscle. Subsequently (Bueding *et al.*, 1959) it was found that piperazine does not affect the incorporation of 2-C^{14}-lactate into succinate. Evidently, the inhibition of succinate production by the drug is the result, not the cause, of the paralysis. It appears likely that the primary effect of piperazine is an inhibition of the effects of acetylcholine, resulting ultimately in paralysis.

REFERENCES

Ackert, J. E., and Riedel, B. B. (1946). *J. Parasitol.* **32,** Suppl., 15.

Andrews, J., Johnson, C. M., and Dormal, V. J. (1930). *Am. J. Hyg.* **12,** 381–400.

Andrews, J. S. (1938). *J. Agr. Res.* **57,** 349–361.

Andrews, J. S., Kauffman, W., and Davis, R. E. (1944). *Am. J. Vet. Res.* **5,** 22–29.

Andrews, M. F., McIlvain, P. K., and Eveleth, D. F. (1961). *Am. J. Vet. Res.* **22,** 1026–1029.

Angolotti, E., and Carda, P. (1929). *Med. Paises Calidos* **2,** 431–435.

Armer, J. M. (1944). *J. Parasitol.* **30,** 131–142.

Augustine, D. L. (1936). *Am. J. Hyg.* **24,** 170–176.

Auricchio, L. (1924). *Pediatria (Napoli)* **32,** 704–711.

Balian, B. (1940). *Nuova Vet.* **18,** No. 6, 14–22, and No. 7, 10–16.

Ball, E. G., Anfinsen, C. B., and Cooper, O. (1947). *J. Biol. Chem.* **168,** 257–270.

Ball, E. G., McKee, R. W., Anfinsen, C. B., Cruz, W. O., and Geiman, Q. M. (1948). *J. Biol. Chem.* **175,** 547–571.

Banerjee, D. N., and Saha, J. C. (1923). *Calcutta Med. J.* **17,** 109–114.

Beiler, J. M., and Martin, C. J. (1948). *J. Biol. Chem.* **174,** 31–35.

Belkin, M., Tobie, E. J., Kahler, J., and Shear, M. J. (1949). *Cancer Res.* **9,** 560.

Bell, F. R., and Jones, E. R. (1946). *Ann. Trop. Med. Parasitol.* **40,** 199–208.

Bellelli, L., and Caraffa, V. (1956). *Giorn. Mal. Infettive Parassit.* **8,** 521–523.

Birnbaum, D. (1954). *Harefuah* **47,** No. 3, 1–4.

Bouisset, L., Harant, H., and Ruffié, J. (1956). *Ann. Parasitol. Humaine Comp.* **31,** 331–349.

Bovarnick, M. R., Lindsay, A., and Hellerman, L. (1946a). *J. Biol. Chem.* **163,** 523–533.

Bovarnick, M. R., Lindsay, A., and Hellerman, L. (1946b). *J. Biol. Chem.* **163,** 535–551.

Bowman, I. B. R., Grant, P. T., Kermack, W. O., and Ogston, D. (1961). *Biochem. J.* **78,** 472–478.

Brand, T. von (1938). *Quart. Rev. Biol.* **13,** 41–50.

Brand, T. von (1948). *Proc. 4th Intern. Congr. Trop. Med. Malaria, Washington, D.C., 1948* Vol. 2, pp. 984–991. Government Printing Office, Washington, D.C.

Brand, T. von (1952). *"Chemical Physiology of Endoparasitic Animals."* Academic Press, New York.

Brand, T. von, and Files, V. S. (1947). *J. Parasitol.* **33,** 476–482.

Brand, T. von, and Mercado, T. I. (1956). *Exptl. Parasitol.* **5**, 34–37.

Brand, T. von, and Mercado, T. I. (1958). *Am. J. Hyg.* **67**, 311–320.

Brand, T. von, and Otto, G. F. (1938). *Am. J. Hyg.* **27**, 683–689.

Brand, T. von, and Regendanz, P. (1931). *Biochem. Z.* **242**, 451–468.

Brand, T. von, Regendanz, P., and Weise, W. (1932). *Zentr. Bakteriol. Parasitenk., Abt I: Orig.* **125**, 461–468.

Brand, T. von, Tobie, E. J., Kissling, R. E., and Adams, G. (1949). *J. Infect. Diseases* **85**, 5–16.

Brand, T. von, Tobie, E. J., and Mehlman, B. (1951). *Am. J. Hyg.* **54**, 76–81.

Braun, H., and Teichmann, E. (1912). "Versuche sur Immunisierung der Trypanosomen." Jena (not seen). Quoted Index Catalogue *Med. Vet. Parasitol.* (1937). Part 2, p. 507.

Bremner, K. C. (1961). *Australian J. Agr. Res.* **12**, 498–512.

Brncic, D., and Hoecker, G. (1949). *Bol. Inform. Parasitol. Chilenas* **4**, 42–43.

Browning, P. (1938). *J. Pathol. Bacteriol.* **46**, 323–329.

Bruynoghe, R., Dubois, A., and Bouckaert, J. P. (1927). *Bull. Acad Roy. Med. Belg.* [5] **7**, 142–156.

Bueding, E. (1959). *J. Pharm. Pharmacol.* **11**, 385–392.

Bueding, E. (1962). *Biochem. Pharmacol.* **11**, 17–28.

Bueding, E., and Farrow, G. W. (1956). *Exptl. Parasitol.* **5**, 345–349.

Bueding, E., and Mansour, J. M. (1957). *Brit. J. Pharmacol.* **12**, 159–165.

Bueding, E., and Peters, L. (1951). *J. Pharmacol. Exptl. Therap.* **101**, 210–229.

Bueding, E., and Swartzwelder, C. (1957). *Pharmacol. Rev.* **9**, 329–365.

Bueding, E., Saz, H. J., and Farrow, G. W. (1959). *Brit. J. Pharmacol.* **14**, 497–500.

Bueding, E., Kmetec, E., Swartzwelder, C., Abadie, S., and Saz, H. J. (1961). *Biochem. Pharmacol.* **5**, 311–322.

Burns, W. C. (1959). *J. Parasitol.* **45**, 38–46.

Cairns, J. (1956). *Notulae Naturae* **292**, 1–4.

Cauthen, G. E., and Landram, J. F. (1958). *Am. J. Vet. Res.* **19**, 811–814.

Chandler, A. C. (1943). *Am. J. Hyg.* **37**, 121–130.

Chatterji, A., and Sen Gupta, P. C. (1957). *Bull. Calcutta Sch. Trop. Med.* **5**, 169–170.

Chen, G. (1948). *J. Infect. Diseases* **82**, 226–230.

Chen, G., and Geiling, E. M. K. (1945). *J. Infect. Diseases* **77**, 139–143.

Chen, G., Geiling, E. M. K., and Mac Hatton, R. M. (1945). *J. Infect. Diseases* **76**, 152–154.

Cheng, T. C. (1963a). *Proc. Helminthol. Soc. Wash., D.C.* **30**, 101–107.

Cheng, T. C. (1963b). *Ann. N.Y. Acad. Sci.* **113**, 289–321.

Cheng, T. C., and Snyder, R. W. (1962). *Trans. Am. Microscop. Soc.* **81**, 209–228

Cheng, T. C., and Snyder, R. W. (1963). *Trans. Am. Microscop. Soc.* **82**, 343–346.

Cohen, A. L., Borsook, H., and Dubnoff, J. W. (1947). *Proc. Soc. Exptl. Biol. Med.* **66**, 440–444.

Coleman, R. M., and Brand, T. von (1957). *J. Parasitol.* **43**, 263–270.

Cordier, G. (1927). *Compt. Rend. Soc. Biol.* **96**, 971–973.

Corradetti, A., Tentori, L., and Verolini, F. (1955). *Rend. Ist. Super. Sanita* **18**, 256–260.

Corso, P., and Frugoni, G. (1961a). *Arch. Ital. Sci. Med. Trop. Parassitol.* **42**, 145–151.

Corso, P., and Frugoni, G. (1961b). *Arch. Ital. Sci. Med. Trop. Parassitol.* **42**, 453–460.

Coudert, J. (1961). *Anais Congr. Intern. Doenca Chagas, Rio de Janeiro 1959* Vol. 2, 447–457.

Coudert, J., and Juttin, P. (1950). *Compt. Rend. Soc. Biol.* **144**, 847–849.

Coudert, J., and Michel-Brun, J. (1963). *Proc. Intern. 7 Congr. Med. Trop. Malaria, Rio de Janeiro 1963,* Vol. 2, p. 240. Rio de Janeiro.

Coudert, J., and Michel-Brun, J. (1964). *Compt. Rend. Soc. Biol.* **158**, 68–71.

Coudert, J., Michel-Brun, J., and Ambroise-Thomas, P. (1964). *Compt. Rend. Soc. Biol.* **158,** 72–75.

Crawford, T. B. B., and Levvy, G. A. (1947). *Biochem. J.* **41,** 333–336.

Cross, S. X. (1935). *J. Parasitol.* **21,** 267–273.

Daugherty, J. W. (1950). *J. Parasitol.* **36,** Suppl. 42.

Daugherty, J. W., and Herrick, C. A. (1952). *J. Parasitol.* **38,** 298–304.

Day, H. B. (1924). *Trans. Roy. Soc. Trop. Med. Hyg.* **18,** 121–130.

DeLangen, C. D., and Schutt, H. (1917). *Geneesk. Tijdschr. Ned.-Indie* **57,** 330 [not seen, quoted in Maegraith (1948)].

Devakul, K. (1960). *Trans. Roy. Soc. Trop. Med. Hyg.* **54,** 87.

Devakul, K., and Maegraith, B. G. (1958). *Ann. Trop. Med. Parasitol.* **52,** 366–375.

Dominici, A. (1930). *Boll. Ist. Sieroterap. Milan.* **9,** 438–441.

Donomae, I. (1927). *Japan. J. Med. Sci., Part 8* **1,** 385–412.

Dubois, A., and Bouckaert, J. P. (1927). *Compt. Rend. Soc. Biol.* **96,** 431 -433.

Eberlein, R. K. (1895). *Z. Wiss. Zool.* **59,** 233–304.

Ehrlich, P. (1909). *Ber.* **42,** 17–47.

Engel, R. (1944). *Klin. Wochschr.* **23,** 127–129.

Erfan, M., and Camb, H. (1933). *J. Trop. Med. Hyg.* **36,** 348–349.

Fenyvessy, B. von (1926). *Biochem. Z.* **173.** 289–297.

Fenyvessy, B. von, and Reiner, L. (1928). *Biochem. Z.* **202,** 75–80.

Fiennes, R. N. T. W. (1950). *Ann. Trop. Med. Parasitol.* **44,** 42–54.

Fieser, L. F., and Heyman, H. (1948). *J. Biol. Chem.* **176,** 1363–1370.

Firki, M. M., and Ghalioungi, P. (1937). *Lancet* **I,** 800–802.

Frank, L. L. (1944). *Am. J. Digest. Diseases* **11,** 195–197.

Fraser, D. M., and Kermack, W. O. (1957). *Brit. J. Pharmacol.* **12,** 16–23.

French, M. H. (1938). *J. Comp. Pathol. Therap.* **51,** 269–281.

Fuhrmann, G. (1962). *Z. Tropenmed. Parasitol.* **13,** 53–67.

Fulton, J. D. (1939). *Ann. Trop. Med. Parasitol.* **33,** 217–227.

Fulton, J. D., and Joyner, L. P. (1949). *Trans. Roy. Soc. Trop. Med. Hyg.* **43,** 273–286.

Fulton, J. D., and Spooner, D. F. (1955). *Indian J. Malariol.* **9,** 161–176.

Gall, E. A., and Steinberg, A. (1947). *J. Lab. Clin. Med.* **32,** 508–525.

Gallagher, C. H., and Symons, L. E. A. (1959). *Australian J. Exptl. Biol. Med. Sci.* **37,** 421–432.

Galliard, H., Lapierre, J., and Murard, J. (1954). *Bull. Soc. Pathol. Exotique* **47,** 885–895.

Ghosh, B. K., and Chatterjee, A. N. (1961). *Ann. Biochem. Exptl. Med. Calcutta* **21,** 307–322.

Glowazky, F. (1937). *Z. Hyg. Infektionskrankh.* **119,** 741–752.

Goldbergiene, M. (1962). *Acta Parasitol. Lithuanica* **4,** 55–64.

Gordon, H. McL. (1957). *Advan. Vet. Sci.* **3,** 287–351.

Gordon, H. McL. (1958). *Proc. Australian Soc. Animal Prod.* **2,** 59–68.

Gordon, H. McL. (1960). *Proc. Australian Soc. Animal Prod.* **3,** 93–104.

Grant, P. T., and Fulton, J. D. (1957). *Biochem. J.* **66,** 242–250.

Greenberg, J., and Taylor, D. J. (1950). *J. Parasitol.* **36,** Suppl., 21.

Haas, E. (1944). *J. Biol. Chem.* **155,** 321–331.

Hager, A. (1941). *Iowa State Coll. J. Sci.* **15,** 127–153.

Hall, M. C. (1917). *In* "A Handbook of Practical Treatment" (J. H. Musser and T. C. Kelly, eds.), Vol. 4, pp. 389–419. Saunders, Philadelphia, Pennsylvania.

Hartman, E., Foote, M., and Pierce, H. B. (1940). *Am. J. Hyg.* **31,** Sect. D, 74–75.

Harwood, P. D., Spindler, L. A., Cross, S. X., and Cutler, J. T. (1937). *Am. J. Hyg.* **25,** 362–371.

Hatieganu, J., and Fodor, O. (1942). *Wien. Klin. Wochschr.* **55,** 807–809.

Hauschka, T. S., Saxe, L. H., and Blair, M. (1947). *J. Natl. Cancer Inst.* **7**, 189–197.

Hawking, F. (1953). *Brit. Med. J.* **I**, 1201–1202.

Hawking, F. (1963). *In* "Experimental Chemotherapy" (R. J. Schnitzer and F. Hawking, eds.), Vol. 1, pp. 129–256. Academic Press, New York.

Hawking, F., and Terry, R. J. (1957). *Z. Tropenmed. Parasitol.* **8**, 151–156.

Hegner, R., and Eskridge, L. (1937). *J. Parasitol.* **23**, 105–106.

Hellerman, L., Bovarnick, M. R., and Porter, C. C. (1946). *Federation Proc.* **5**, 400–405.

Heyman, H., and Fieser, L. F. (1948). *J. Pharmacol. Exptl. Therap.* **94**, 97–111.

Highman, B., Greenberg, J., and Coatney, G. R. (1954). *Riv. Parassitol.* **15**, 449–459.

Hoffenreich, F. (1932). *Arch. Schiffs- u. Tropen-Hyg.* **36**, 141–144.

Hopkins, C. A. (1950). *J. Parasitol.* **36**, 384–390.

Hopkins, C. A. (1951). *Exptl. Parasitol.* **1**, 196–213.

Hoppe, J. O., and Chapman, C. W. (1947). *J. Parasitol.* **33**, 509–516.

Hudson, J. R. (1944). *J. Comp. Pathol. Therap.* **54**, 108–119.

Hughes, T. A., and Malik, K. S. (1930). *Indian J. Med. Res.* **18**, 249–257.

Hughes, T. E. (1940). *J. Exptl. Biol.* **17**, 331–336.

Hunter, F. E., and Lowry, O. H. (1956). *Pharmacol. Rev.* **8**, 89–135.

Hurst, C. T. (1927). *Univ. California (Berkeley) Publ. Zool.* **29**, 321–404.

Issekutz, B. von (1933a). *Arch. Exptl. Pathol. Pharmakol.* **173**, 479–498.

Issekutz, B. von (1933b). *Arch. Exptl. Pathol. Pharmakol.* **173**, 499–507.

Jacobi, K., and Kretschmar, W. (1962). *Z. Trop. Med. Parasitol.* **13**, 286–304.

Jancso, N. von, and Jancso, H. von (1935a). *Z. Immunitaetsforsch.* **84**, 471–504.

Jancso, N. von, and Jancso, H. von (1935b). *Z. Immunitaetsforsch.* **86**, 1–30.

Janssens, P. G., Karcher, D., Van Sande, M., Lowenthal, A., and Ghysels, G. (1961). *Bull. Soc. Pathol. Exotique* **54**, 322–331.

Junior, P., and Brandao, P. P. (1937). *Brasil-Med.* **51**, 1047–1058.

Kawai, T. (1937). *J. Formosan Med. Assoc.* **36**, 604–605 (English summary).

Kawamitsu, K. (1958). *Nagasaki Igakkai Zassi* **33**, No. 11, Suppl., 22–39.

Kawazoe, Y. (1961). *Japan. J. Parasitol.* **10**, 145–151.

Kligler, I. J., and Geiger, A. (1928). *Proc. Soc. Exptl. Biol. Med.* **26**, 229–230.

Kligler, I. J., Geiger, A., and Comaroff, R. (1929). *Ann. Trop. Med. Parasitol.* **23**, 325–335.

Klyueva, N. G., and Roskin, G. (1946). *Am. Rev. Soviet Med.* **4**, 127–129.

Knowles, R., and Das Gupta, B. M. (1927–1928). *Indian J. Med. Res.* **15**, 997–1057.

Krijgsman, B. J. (1933). *Z. Parasitenk.* **6**, 1–22.

Krijgsman, B. J. (1936). *Z. Vergleich. Physiol.* **23**, 663–711.

Kuwamura, T. (1958). *Shikoku Acta Med.* **12**, 28–57.

Laveran, C. L. A. (1913). *Bull. Soc. Pathol. Exotique* **6**, 693–698.

Laveran, C. L. A., and Roudsky, D. (1913). *Bull. Soc. Pathol. Exotique* **6**, 176–181.

Lengy, J. (1962). *Refuah Vet.* **19**, 115–111 (sic).

Lewert, R. M., and Lee, C. L. (1955). *J. Infect. Diseases* **97**, 177–186.

Lewis, J. H. (1928). *Zentr. Bakteriol. Parasitenk., Abt. I: Orig.* **107**, 114–126.

Lincicome, D. R. (1963). *Ann. N.Y. Acad. Sci.* **113**, 360–380.

Lincicome, D. R., Rossan, R. N., and Jones, W. C. (1960). *J. Parasitol.* **46**, Sect. 2, 42.

Lincicome, D. R., and Shepperson, J. R. (1963). *J. Parasitol.* **49**, 31–34.

Linton, R. W. (1929). *Ann. Trop. Med. Parasitol.* **23**, 307–313.

Linton, R. W. (1930). *J. Exptl. Med.* **52**, 103–111.

Lippi, M., and Benedetto, A. (1958). *Arch. Ital. Sci. Med. Trop. Parassitol.* **39**, 446–451.

Lippi, M., and Sebastiani, A. (1958). *Arch. Ital. Sci. Med. Trop. Parassitol.* **39**, 145–154.

Lippincott, S. W., Marble, A., Ellerbrook, L. D., Hesselbrock, W. B., Engstrom, W. W., and Gordon, H. H. (1946). *J. Lab. Clin. Med.* **31**, 991–998.

Lippincott, S. W., Paddock, F. K., Rhees, M. C., Hesselbrock, W. B., and Ellerbrook, L. D. (1947). *Arch Internal. Med.* **79,** 62-76.

Locatelli, P. (1930). *Compt. Rend. Soc. Biol.* **105,** 449-451.

Maegraith, B. G. (1948). "Pathological Processes in Malaria and Blackwater Fever." Thomas, Springfield, Illinois.

Maegraith, B. G. (1954). *Ann. Rev. Microbiol.* **8,** 273-288.

Maegraith, B. G., Deegan, T., and Jones, E. S. (1952). *Brit. Med. J.* **II,** 1382-1384.

Maegraith, B. G., Gilles, H. M., and Devakul, K. (1957). *Z. Tropenmed. Parasitol.* **8,** 485-514.

Mansour, T. E., and Bueding, E. (1954). *Brit. J. Pharmacol. Chemotherap.* **9,** 459-462.

Marañon, G. (1939). *Brasil-Med.* **53,** 93-95.

Marshall, P. B. (1948a). *Brit. J. Pharmacol.* **3,** 8-14.

Marshall, P. B. (1948b). *Brit. J. Pharmacol.* **3,** 1-7.

Marvin, H. N., and Rigdon, R. H. (1945). *Am. J. Hyg.* **42,** 174-178.

Massa, M. (1927). *Pathologica (Genova)* **19,** 535-541.

Mercado, T. I. (1952). *Am. J. Trop. Med. Hyg.* **1,** 932-935.

Mercado, T. I., and Brand, T. von (1954). *Exptl. Parasitol.* **3,** 259-266.

Mercado, T. I., and Brand, T. von (1957). *Am. J. Hyg.* **66,** 20-28.

Mercado, T. I., and Brand, T. von (1960). *J. Infect. Diseases* **106,** 95-105.

Michel-Brun, J. (1963). Thesis, University of Lyon.

Molomut, N. (1947). *J. Immunol.* **56,** 139-141.

Moulder, J. W. (1948). *J. Infect. Diseases* **83,** 262-270.

Moulder, J. W. (1949). *J. Infect. Diseases* **85,** 195-204.

Mowry, M. A., and Becker, E. R. (1930). *Iowa State Coll. J. Sci.* **5,** 35-60.

Mueller, J. F. (1962). *J. Parasitol.* **48,** Sect. 2, 45.

Mueller, J. F. (1965a). *J. Parasitol.* **51,** 523-531.

Mueller, J. F. (1965b). *J. Parasitol.* **51,** 537-540.

Münnich, H. (1958). *Naturwiss.* **45,** 551-552.

Münnich, H. (1959-1960). *Wiss. Z. Humboldt-Univ. Berlin, Math.-Naturw.Reihe* **9,** 389-403.

Mukherjee, K. L., Ghosh, S., and Sen Gupta, P. C. (1957). *Bull. Calcutta Sch. Trop. Med.* **5,** 16-17.

Nadel, E. M., Taylor, D. J., Greenberg, J., and Josephson, E. S. (1949). *J. Natl. Malaria Soc.* **8,** 70-79.

Nyden, S. J. (1948). *Proc. Soc. Exptl. Biol. Med.* **69,** 206-210.

Paisseau, G., and Lemaire, H. (1916). *Presse Med.* **24,** 545-547.

Petersen, W. F. (1926). *Proc. Soc. Exptl. Biol. Med.* **23,** 753-754.

Pierce, H. B., Hartman, E., Simcox, W. J., Aitken, T., Meservey, A. B., and Farnham, W. B. (1939). *Am. J. Hyg.* **29,** Sect. D, 75-81.

Poindexter, H. A. (1935). *J. Parasitol.* **21,** 292-301.

Pons, J: A. (1937). *Puerto Rico J. Public Health Trop. Med.* **13,** 171-254.

Pratt, I. (1940). *Trans. Am. Microscop. Soc.* **59,** 31-37.

Pratt, I. (1941). *Am. J. Hyg.* **34,** Sect. C, 54-61.

Quastel, J. H. (1931). *Biochem. J.* **25,** 1121-1127.

Raffaele, G., and Carrescia, P. M. (1954). *Riv. Malariol.* **33,** 47-62.

Ramakrishnan, S. P., Prakash, S., and Krishnaswami, A. K. (1953). *Indian J. Malariol.* **7,** 61-65.

Ramakrishnan, S. P., Prakash, S., and Sen Gupta, G. P. (1956). *Indian J. Malariol.* **10,** 175-182.

Read, C. P. (1950). *Rice Inst. Pamphlet* **27,** No. 2, 1-94.

Read, C. P. (1957). *Exptl. Parasitol.* **6**, 288–293.

Read, C. P (1959). *Exptl. Parasitol.* **8**, 365–382.

Read, C. P. (1961). *In* "Comparative Physiology of Carbohydrate Metabolism in Hetero-thermic Animals" (A. W. Martin, ed.), pp. 3–34. Univ. of Washington Press, Seattle, Washington.

Read, C. P., and Rothman, A. H. (1957a). *Exptl. Parasitol.* **6**, 1–7.

Read, C. P., and Rothman, A. H. (1957b). *Exptl. Parasitol.* **6**, 294–305.

Read, C. P., and Rothman, A. H. (1958a). *Exptl. Parasitol.* **7**, 217–223.

Read, C. P., and Rothman, A. H. (1958b). *Exptl. Parasitol.* **7**, 191–197.

Read, C. P., Schiller, E. L., and Phifer, K. O. (1958). *Exptl. Parasitol.* **7**, 198–216.

Regendanz, P. (1929a). *Ann. Trop. Med. Parasitol.* **23**, 523–527.

Regendanz, P. (1929b). *Arch. Schiffs- u. Tropen-Hyg.* **33**, 242–251.

Regendanz, P., and Tropp, C. (1927). *Arch. Schiffs- u. Tropen-Hyg.* **31**, 376–385.

Reichenow, E. (1921). *Z. Hyg. Infektionskrankh.* **94**, 266–385.

Reid, W. M. (1942). *J. Parasitol.* **28**, 319–340.

Reid, W. M. (1945a). *Am. J. Hyg.* **41**, 150–155.

Reid, W. M. (1945b). *J. Parasitol.* **31**, 406–410.

Reinhard, E. G., and Brand, T. von (1944). *Physiol. Zool.* **17**, 31–41.

Rikimaru, M. T., Galysh, F. T., and Shumard, R. F. (1961). *J. Parasitol.* **47**, 407–412.

Roskin, G., (ed.) (1963). "Cruzin and Cancer Therapeutics." Acad. Sci. U.S.S.R., Moscow (in Russian).

Roskin, G., and Romanova, K. G. (1938). *Bull. Biol. Med. Exptl. URSS* **6**, 118–120.

Rothschild, M. (1941). *Parasitology* **33**, 406–415.

Rudolf, G. deM., and Marsh, R. G. B. (1927). *J. Trop. Med. Hyg.* **30**, 57–63.

Ruge, H. (1929). *Arch. Schiffs- u. Tropen-Hyg.* **33**, 567–587.

Ruge, H. (1935). *Arch. Schiffs- u. Tropen-Hyg.* **39**, 14–19.

Saito. Y. (1933). *Mitt. Med. Ges. Okayama* **45**, 2709 (not seen, Reviewed in *Helminthol. Abstr.* (1933) **2**, 194).

Sassuchin, D. N. (1931). *Arch. Protistenk.* **70**, 681–686.

Sautet, J. J., Gevaudan, P., Vuillet, J., and Caporali, J. (1956). *Med. Trop. (Marseille)* **16**, 654–662.

Sawada, T., Hara, K., Takagi, K., Nagazawa, Y., and Oka, S. (1956). *Am. J. Trop. Med. Hyg.* **5**, 847–859.

Scheff, G. (1928). *Biochem. Z.* **200**, 309–330.

Scheff, G. (1932). *Biochem. Z.* **248**, 168–180.

Scheff, G., and Rabati, F. (1938). *Biochem. Z.* **298**, 101–109.

Scheff, G., and Thatcher, J. S. (1949). *J. Parasitol.* **35**, 35–40.

Schern, K. (1925). *Zentr. Bakteriol. Parasitenk., Abt. I: Orig.* **96**, 356–365 and 440–454.

Schern, K. (1928). *Biochem. Z.* **193**, 264–268.

Schern, K., and Artagaveytia-Allende, R. (1936). *Z. Immunitaetsforsch.* **89**, 21–63.

Schern, K., and Citron, H. (1913). *Deut. Med. Wochschr.* **39**, 1356–1357.

Schilling, C., and Rondoni, P. (1913). *Z. Immunitaetsforsch.* **18**, 651–665.

Schilling, C., Schreck, H., Neumann, H., and Kunert, H. (1938). *Z. Immunitaetsforsch.* **87**, 47–71.

Sebastiani, A. (1959). *Arch. Ital. Sci. Med. Trop. Parassitol.* **40**, 513–516.

Seife, M., and Lisa, J. R. (1950). *Am. J. Trop. Med.* **30**, 769–772.

Shearer, G. D., and Stewart, J. (1933). *Univ. Cambridge, Inst. Animal Pathol. Rept. Director* **3**, 87–97.

Sheehy, T. W., Meroney, W. H., Cox, R. S., and Soler, J. E. (1962). *Gastroenterology* **42**, 148–156.

Shorb, D. A., and Spindler, L. A. (1947). *Proc. Helminthol. Soc. Wash., D.C.* **14**, 30–34.
Shumard, R. F. (1957). *J. Parasitol.* **43**, 548–554.
Silverman, M., Ceithaml, J., Taliaferro, L. G., and Evans, E. A. (1944). *J. Infect. Diseases* **75**, 212–230.
Singh, J., Basu, P. C., Ray, A. P., and Nair, C. P. (1956). *Indian J. Malariol.* **10**, 101–113.
Sinton, J. A., and Hughes, T. A. (1924). *Indian J. Med. Res.* **12**, 409–422.
Sinton, J. A., and Kehar, N. D. (1931). *Records Malaria Survey India* **2**, 287–304.
Smith, G. (1913). *Quart. J. Microscop. Sci.* **59**, 267–295.
Snyder, R. W., and Cheng, T. C. (1961). *J. Parasitol.* **47**, Sect. 2, 52.
Spain, D. M., Molomut, N., and Warshaw, L. J. (1948). *Proc. Soc. Exptl. Biol. Med.* **69**, 134–136.
Speck, J. F., and Evans, E. A. (1945). *J. Biol. Chem.* **159**, 71–81.
Spindler, L. A. (1947). *Proc. Helminthol. Soc. Wash., D.C.* **14**, 58–63.
Spindler, L. A., Zimmerman, H. E., and Hill, C. H. (1944). *Proc. Helminthol. Soc. Wash., D.C.* **11**, 9–12.
Stein, L., and Wertheimer, E. (1942). *Ann. Trop. Med. Parasitol.* **36**, 17–37.
Stewart, J. (1933). *Univ. Cambridge, Inst. Animal Pathol., Rept. Director* **3**, 58–76.
Symons, L. E. A. (1961). *Australian J. Biol. Sci.* **14**, 165–171.
Symons, L. E. A., and Fairbairn, D. (1962). *Federation Proc.* **21**, 913–918.
Symons, L. E. A., and Fairbairn, D. (1963). *Exptl. Parasitol.* **13**, 284–304.
Takagi, K. (1956). *Gumma J. Med. Sci.* **5**, 190–208.
Talice, R. V. (1949). *Trans. Roy. Trop. Med. Hyg.* **43**, 107–109.
Taylor, D. J., Greenberg, J., Josephson, E. S., and Nadel, E. M. (1956). *Acta Endocrinol.* **22**, 173–178.
Thurston, J. P. (1958). *Parasitology* **48**, 165–183.
Tokura, N. (1935). *Igaku Kenkyu* **9**, No. 6, 1–14 [not seen, quoted in Kawamitsu (1958)].
Town, B. W., and Wormall, A. (1949). *Biochem. J.* **44**, xxxviii.
Town, B. W., Wills, E. D., and Wormall, A. (1949). *Nature* **163**, 735–736.
Tubangui, M. A., and Yutuc, L. M. (1931). *Philippine J. Sci.* **45**, 93–107.
Uyeno, H. (1935). *Mitt. Med. Ges. Okayama* **47**, 673–691.
Voegtlin, C. (1925). *Physiol. Rev.* **5**, 63–94.
Voegtlin, C., and Smith, H. W. (1920). *Public Health Rept. (U.S.)* **35**, 2264–2273.
Voegtlin, C., Dyer, H. A., and Leonard, C. S. (1923). *Public Health Rept. (U.S.)* **38**, 1882–1912.
Voegtlin, C., Dyer, H. A., and Miller, D. W. (1924). *J. Pharmacol. Exptl. Therap.* **23**, 55–86.
Voller, A., Shaw, J. J., and Bryant, C. (1963). *Ann. Trop. Med. Parasitol.* **57**, 404–408.
von Brand, T., *see* Brand, T. von
von Fenyvessy, B., *see* Fenyvessy, B. von
von Issekutz, B., *see* Issekutz, B. von
von Jancso, N., *see* Jancso, N. von
Walravens, P. (1931). *Ann. Soc. Belg. Med. Trop.* **11**, 213–218.
Waxler, S. H. (1941). *Trans Am. Microscop. Soc.* **60**, 453–460.
Wendel, W. B. (1946). *Federation Proc.* **5**, 406–407.
Wesenberg-Lund, C. (1934). *Kgl. Danske Videnskab. Selskabs, Skrifter, Naturvidenskab. math. Afdel.* [9] **5**, No. 3, 1–223.
Westphal, A. (1939). *Z. Hyg. Infektionskrankh.* **122**, 146–158.
Whitlock, J. H. (1949). *Cornell Vet.* **39**, 146–182.
Williams, R. G. (1927). *Lancet* **II**, 1071–1073.
Williamson, J. (1962). *Exptl. Parasitol.* **12**, 323–367.

Wills, E. D., and Wormall, A. (1949). *Biochem J.* **44,** xxxix.

Wormall, A. (1932). *Biochem. J.* **26,** 1777–1787.

Wright, C. I., and Sabine, J. C. (1944). *J. Biol. Chem.* **155,** 315–320.

Yoshida, T., and Ko, K. (1920). *J. Formosan Med. Assoc.* Nos. 206 and 207 [not seen, quoted in Maegraith (1948)].

Zarzycki, J. (1956). *Med. Weterynar. (Poland)* **12,** 328–332.

Zaun, F. (1935). *Arch. Schiffs- u. Tropen-Hyg.* **39,** 363–373.

Zotta, G., and Radacovici, E. (1929a). *Arch. Roumaines Pathol. Exptl. Microbiol.* **2,** 55–80.

Zotta, G., and Radacovici, E. (1929b). *Compt. Rend. Soc. Biol.* **102,** 129–130.

Zwemer, R. L., and Culbertson, J. T. (1939). *Am. J. Hyg.* **29,** Sect. C, 7–12.

Chapter 5

LIPIDS

I. INTRODUCTORY REMARKS

Our knowledge of lipid relationships of parasites is being revolutionized by the recent application to parasitological problems of such newer isolation and separation techniques as column, thin layer, and especially gas chromatography or the newer rigorous identification techniques, such as infrared or ultraviolet spectroscopy. They have found their way into parasitology during the last decade and while they have not yet made all older data obsolete, they tend at least to make them obsolescent. Great future strides in the field of parasite lipid chemistry undoubtedly lie ahead.

The term "lipids" includes true fats (triglycerol esters of fatty acids), waxes, sterols, and other higher alcohols, as well as phospho- and glycolipids. In other words, lipids are a heterogeneous group of compounds which undoubtedly fulfill a variety of physiological functions. For instance, higher fatty acids, or their triglycerides, in many organisms represent important energy reserves, while in some anaerobically living parasites they appear to be essentially waste products. On the other hand, such structural lipids as sterols or phospholipids are probably equally important to all animal parasites, even though their exact physiological role is not too well understood.

II. CHEMISTRY OF LIPIDS

The total amount of lipid occurring in various species of parasites is quite variable (Table XXXII) and there is no indication that the type of habitat has a significant influence on the degree of lipid accumulation. Fractionation of lipids has been carried out in the case of several parasites (Table XXXIII) and it is noteworthy that phospholipids and unsaponifiable matter often account for a relatively high percentage of the total lipids.

The chemical constitution of the phospholipids has received detailed attention only in recent years. On the whole (Table XXXIV) it appears

TABLE XXXII
LIPID CONTENT OF SOME PARASITES[a]

Species	Lipids in per cent of		References
	Fresh tissues	Dry tissues	
Flagellates			
Crithidia fasciculata	2.99		Cosgrove (1959)
Trypanosoma cruzi, culture form	3.12	20.1	von Brand et al. (1959)
Sporozoa			
Goussia gadi	3.6	22.0	Panzer (1913)
Eimeria acervulina (oocyst)		14.4	Wilson and Fairbairn (1961)
Plasmodium knowlesi		28.8	Morrison and Jeskey (1947)
Ciliates			
Entodinium simplex		6.3	Williams et al. (1963)
Isotricha intestinalis		9.1	Williams et al. (1963)
Isotricha prostoma		7.7	Gutierrez et al. (1962)
Trematodes			
Fasciola gigantica	2.81	12.9	Goil (1958)
Fasciola hepatica	1.9–2.4	12.2–13.3	Flury and Leeb (1926); Weinland and von Brand (1926)
Gastrothylax crumenifer	0.38	1.36	Goil (1958)
Paramphistomum explanatum	1.16	4.5	Goil (1958)
Cestodes			
Diphyllobothrium latum	1.5–1.6	16.6–17.7	Smorodincev and Bebesin (1936b); Totterman and Kirk (1939)
Echinococcus granulosus, scoleces	2.0	13.6	Agosin et al. (1957)
Echinococcus granulosus, cyst membranes		1.3	Cmelik (1952)
Hymenolepis diminuta	9.5	9.5–34.6	Warren and Daugherty (1957); Roberts (1961); Goodchild and Vilar-Alvarez (1962)

TABLE XXXII (Continued)

LIPID CONTENT OF SOME PARASITES[a]

Species	Lipids in per cent of		References
	Fresh tissues	Dry tissues	
Moniezia expansa	3.4	30.1	von Brand (1933)
Taenia saginata	3.8	31.1	Cmelik and Bartl (1956)
Taenia taeniaeformis, adult	1.7–3.8	6.5–10.6	von Brand and Bowman (1961); McMahon (1961)
Taenia taeniaeformis, larval	0.9–2.3	3.1–6.9	von Brand and Bowman (1961); McMahon (1961)
Nematodes			
Ascaris lumbricoides ♀	1.6	8.9	Fairbairn (1955a); Cavier *et al.* (1958)
Ascaris lumbricoides ♂	1.3		Cavier *et al.* (1958)
Ascaridia galli ♀	1.34		Monteoliva (1960)
Ascaridia galli ♂	1.22		Monteoliva (1960)
Eustrongylides ignotus, larval	1.1	4.4	von Brand (1938)
Porrocaecum decipiens, larval		3.5	Fairbairn (1958)
Acanthocephala			
Macracanthorhynchus hirudinaceus ♀	0.9–1.5		von Brand (1939, 1940); Beames and Fisher (1964)
Macracanthorhynchus hirudinaceus ♂	1.7–2.1		von Brand (1940); Beames and Fisher (1964)
Arthropods			
Gastrophilus intestinalis, larval	5.2	16.2	von Kemnitz (1916)
Peltogaster paguri		26.6	Reinhard and von Brand (1944)

[a] Data on additional species of parasites, or additional data on species listed above will be found in the following papers: protozoa: Kligler and Olitzki (1936); Ikejiani (1947); cestodes: von Brand (1933); Smorodincev and Bebesin (1936a); Smorodincev *et al.* (1933); Salisbury and Anderson (1939); Reid (1942); nematodes: Weinland (1901); Flury (1912); Schulte (1917); von Brand (1934b); Smorodincev and Bebesin (1936c,d); Acanthocephala: Beames and Fisher (1964).

TABLE XXXIII

LIPID FRACTIONS ISOLATED FROM SOME PARASITES[a]

Species	Phospholipids	Unsaponifiable matter	Saturated acids	Unsaturated acids	Volatile acids	Nonvolatile acids	Glycerol	References
Protozoa								
Plasmodium knowlesi		16–32	36	41				Morrison and Jeskey (1947)
Trematodes								
Fasciola hepatica	30	19	4	12			2	von Brand (1928)
Gastrothylax crumenifer	16	25	5	20			2	Goil (1964)
Cestodes								
Hymenolepis diminuta	26	9	69					Fairbairn *et al.* (1961)
Moniezia expansa	15	7	8	51			4	von Brand (1933)
Nematodes								
Ascaridia galli ♀	10	22			10	49		Monteoliva (1960)
Ascaridia galli ♂	15	16			11	44		Monteoliva (1960)
Ascaris lumbricoides ♀, reproductive system	8	21			13	52		Fairbairn (1955a)
Ascaris lumbricoides, body wall	38	8			9	38		Fairbairn (1956)
Acanthocephala								
Macracanthorhynchus hirudinaceus ♀	27	24	2	32			2	von Brand (1939)
Macracanthorhynchus hirudinaceus ♀	47	21	30					Beames and Fisher (1964)
Macracanthorhynchus hirudinaceus ♂	46	38	16					Beames and Fisher (1964)
Moniliformis dubius ♀	19	10	63					Beames and Fisher (1964)
Moniliformis dubius ♂	9	8	64					Beames and Fisher (1964)

[a] Data on additional species of parasites, or additional data on species listed above will be found in the following papers: protozoa: Panzer (1913); cestodes: Faust and Tallqvist (1907); Tötterman and Kirk (1939); Cmelik and Bartl (1956); nematodes: Flury (1912); Schulz and Becker (1933); von Brand and Winkeljohn (1945); Fairbairn (1955b); Fairbairn and Passey (1955).

that the major phospholipid groups known from vertebrates occur also in parasites. Widely distributed are lecithins, characterized by their choline content and a P:N ratio of 1:1, and cephalins, which contain either ethanolamine or serine and have the same P:N ratio as the lecithins. The nitrogen-free inositides, and sphingomyelin, characterized by a P:N ratio of 1:2, are often, but not invariably, encountered, as are cardiolipins and plasmalogens. The latter are responsible for the histochemical aldehyde reaction known as plasmal reaction which has often been reported from parasites.

In view of the complex nature of phospholipids it would not be surprising if differences between parasitic species, or differences between parasites and free-living organisms would occur. Indeed, some indications to this effect have been reported. As shown in Table XXXIV, inositides have not been found in *Taenia taeniaeformis* and no sphingomyelin has been reported from *Hymenolepis diminuta*. Furthermore, McMahon (1961) found that the lecithin fraction of larval *Taenia taeniaeformis* migrates during paper electrophoresis at twice the rate of that of the adult worms. A hitherto unrecognized chemical difference must be responsible for this different behavior in the electrical field. Small amounts of lysolecithin and lysophosphatidylethanolamine have tentatively been identified only in *Hymenolepis diminuta* (Fairbairn *et al.,* 1961).

Of interest is also the older observation of Lesuk and Anderson (1941) that the lecithin fraction of larval *Taenia taeniaeformis* is largely a hydrolecithin, identified as dipalmitolecithin. The interest of this observation rests on the facts that hydrolecithin does not occur usually in animal tissues and that lecithins almost invariably contain one saturated and one unsaturated fatty acid per molecule.

It is probable that investigation with newer methods would reveal a more complex picture of the fatty acids contained in the phospholipids of *Taenia taeniaeformis* than indicated by the above work. In *Taenia saginata* Cmelik and Bartl (1956) found by paper chromatography that the phospholipids contain lauric, myristic, palmitic, and stearic acids, palmitic acid apparently being present in largest amounts. Gas chromatography revealed a still much more complicated picture. Beames (1964) investigated the fatty acids of various phospholipid fractions isolated from *Ascaris lumbricoides* and observed 30 to 31 different acids, varying in chain length from C_{12} to C_{20} (Table XXXV). Similarly complicated were the fatty aldehyde components of the plasmalogens. He found 21 different aldehydes which varied in chain length from C_{12} to C_{18}; they were partly saturated, partly unsaturated, branched or unbranched.

Another relevant observation has been reported from a protozoon, the culture form of *Trypanosoma cruzi* (von Brand, 1962). The fatty acids of

TABLE XXIV

PHOSPHOLIPIDS OF SOME PARASITES[a]

| Species | Cephalins | | Lecithins | Inositol phosphatides | Sphingomyelin | Cardiolipin | Plasmalogens | References |
	Phosphatidyl ethanolamine	Phosphatidyl serine	Phosphatidyl choline	Inositol	Sphingosine	Polyglycerol phosphatide	Ethanolamine, rarely serine or choline	
Flagellates								
Crithidia fasciculata	x		x	x		x		Hack *et al.* (1962b)
Crithidia luciliae	x		x	x		x		Hack *et al.* (1962b)
Herpetomonas culicis	x		x	x		x		Hack *et al.* (1962b)
Trypanosoma cruzi, culture form	x		x	x				Hack *et al.* (1962b)
Cestodes								
Diphyllobothrium latum	x		x					Tötterman and Kirk (1939)
Echinococcus granulosus			x					Kilejian *et al.* (1962)
Hymenolepis diminuta	x	x	x	x	—	x	x	Fairbairn *et al.* (1961)
Taenia saginata			x	x				Cmelik and Bartl (1956)

						Reference
Taenia taeniaeformis, adult and larval	x	x	x	—	x	McMahon (1961)
Nematodes						
Ascaridia galli	x	x	x		x	Monteoliva (1960)
Ascaris lumbricoides, various organs	x	x	x[b]	x[c]	x[b]	Rogers and Lazarus (1949); Fairbairn (1955a, 1956); Beames (1964).
Dirofilaria immitis	x	x	x			Hack *et al.* (1962a)
Acanthocephala						
Macracanthorhynchus hirudinaceus	x	x	x	x[d]	x	Beames and Fisher (1964)
Moniliformis dubius	x	x	x	x[d]	x	Beames and Fisher (1964)

[a] KEY: x = compound demonstrated; — = compound not found.
[b] Beames (1964) reported only suggestive evidence for the presence of inositol phosphatides and cardiolipins.
[c] Beames (1964) found sphingomyelin in lipids from muscle tissue, but not in those from reproductive systems.
[d] The evidence for the presence of sphingosine is only circumstantial.

TABLE XXXV

Fatty Acids Identified in Phospholipids of *Ascaris lumbricoides*[a,b,c]

Phospholipid	Chain length of fatty acid and degree of unsaturation															
	12 0	12 0 br.	13 0 br.	14 0	15 0 br.	15 0	16 2	16 1	16 0	17 1	17 0	18 2+3	18 1	18 0	20 3	20 0
Lecithin from muscle	x	x	x	x	x	x	x	x	x	x	x	x	x	x	x	x
Lecithin from female reproductive system	x	—	—	x	x	x	x	x	x	x	x	x	—	x	x	x
Choline plasmalogen from muscle	x	x	—	x	x	x	—	x	x	x	x	x	x	x	—	—
Choline plasmalogen from female reproductive system	x	x	x	x	x	x	—	x	x	x	x	x	—	x	—	x
Cephalin from muscle	x	x	—	x	x	x	—	x	x	x	x	x	x	x	—	x
Cephalin from female reproductive system	x	x	x	x	x	x	x	x	x	x	x	x	x	x	x	x
Cephalin plasmalogen from muscle	x	x	x	x	x	x	—	x	x	x	x	x	x	x	—	x
Cephalin plasmalogen from female reproductive system	x	x	x	x	x	x	—	x	x	x	x	x	x	x	—	x

[a] After Beames (1964).

[b] In addition to the acids listed, 14 acids varying in chain length from C_{13} to C_{20} were observed; they were, however, not characterized and are listed by Beames (1964) as unknown.

[c] KEY: x = acid has been found; — = acid has not been found; br. = branched.

the acetone-insoluble lipid fraction (Table XXXVI) contained 12 members ranging from C_{13} to C_{18}, consisting of branched and unbranched, saturated, mono-unsaturated and doubly unsaturated acids. Of interest was the occurrence of relatively large amounts of a C_{15} acid, since acids with uneven numbers of carbon atoms do not usually account for an appreciable percentage of the fatty acids deposited in animals. In *Ascaris*, for instance, fatty acids with 13, 15, or 17 carbon atoms account only for a small percentage of the total acids (Beames, 1964), at least of the phospholipids.

Glycolipids, that is, cerebrosides and gangliosides, are found in higher animals, especially in the nervous system. Cerebrosides, the only glycolipids so far described from parasites, are related structurally to sphingomyelins, but differ from these in that they contain one molecule of sugar, usually galactose, instead of phosphorylcholine. They have been found so far only in cestodes. A typical cerebroside, containing 47% fatty acid esters, 32% sphingosine, and 21.7% galactose, has been isolated from *Moniezia expansa* (Kent *et al.*, 1948). Larval *Taenia taeniaeformis*, on the other hand, contain an atypical compound. Their cerebroside fraction was studied by Lesuk and Anderson (1941) and proved to be essentially a hydrophrenosin, yielding upon hydrolysis galactose, phrenosinic acid (that is, probably, a mixture of α-hydroxy acids), and dihydrosphingosine. This last finding is especially interesting since all other hitherto known cerebrosides contain sphingosine instead. The wide distribution of cerebrosides in cestodes is attested to by the finding of corresponding fractions in *Diphyllobothrium latum* (Tötterman and Kirk, 1939) and *Hymenolepis diminuta* (Fairbairn *et al.*, 1961). The cerebroside fractions isolated from tapeworms are rather large, and it seems therefore somewhat unlikely that they could be confined to the somewhat rudimentary nervous system of these worms. However, nothing is known as yet concerning their localization in the bodies of cestodes.

The unsaponifiable lipid fraction of all parasites studied so far contains a larger or smaller proportion of sterols, with cholesterol the predominant compound; it has been reported from *Goussia gadi* (Panzer, 1913) and *Plasmodium knowlesi* (Morrison and Jeskey, 1947). While the evidence presented in these older papers is not entirely convincing, cholesterol has been identified conclusively as a lipid constituent of the culture form of *Trypanosoma cruzi*. It was characterized by such determinations as melting point, optical rotation, infrared absorption spectrum, and analogous properties of the acetate and dibromide (von Brand *et al.*, 1959). On the other hand, Halevy (1962), basing his conclusions on the Lieberman-Burchard colorimetric method, found no cholesterol, but an ergosterol-like sterol in the culture forms of four trypanosomids, among them

TABLE XXXVI

Fatty Acids Identified in Some Parasites[a]

Group headings: **Flagellates** (columns 1–8); **Ciliates** (9–10); **Sporozoa** (11); **Trematodes** (12); **Cestodes** (13–15); **Nematodes** (16); **Acanthocephala** (17–18)

Column key (with method shown):

1. Crithidia sp., Phospholipids (1) — G
2. Crithidia sp., Neutral lipids (1) — G
3. Leishmania enrietti, C. (2) — G
4. Leishmania tarentolae, C. (1) — G
5. Trypanosoma cruzi, C. (3) Acetone-soluble lipids — G
6. Trypanosoma cruzi, C. (3) Acetone-insoluble lipids — G
7. Trypanosoma lewisi B. (1) — G
8. Trypanosoma lewisi, C. (1) — G
9. Entodinium simplex (4) — P
10. Isotricha intestinalis (4) — P
11. Plasmodium knowlesi (5) — Ch
12. Fasciola hepatica (6) — Ch
13. Diphyllobothrium latum (7) — Ch
14. Moniezia expansa (8) — Ch
15. Taenia saginata (9) — Ch
16. Ascaris lumbricoides (10) — Ch
17. Macracanthorhynchus hirudinaceus (11) — G
18. Moniliformis dubius (11) — G

Chain Length	Unsaturation	1	2	3	4	5	6	7	8	9	10	11	12	13	14	15	16	17	18
8	0				x														
9	0				x														
10	0			x	x													(x)	x
10	1				x														(x)
11	0																		(x)
12	0			x	x	x												x	x
13	0					x													
14	0	x	x	x	x		x	x	x	x								x	x
14	1			x		x	x					x	x						x
15	0					x	x											(x)	x
15	1					x													
16	0	x	x	x	x	x	x	x	x	x	x		x	x	x	x	x	x	x
16	1			x	x	x	x	x	x									x	x
16	2					x	x												
17	0					x	x											(x)	x
18	0	x	x	x	x	x	x	x	x	x	x	x	x	x	x	x	x	x	x
18	1	x	x	x	x	x	x	x	x			x	x	x	x	x	x	x	x
18	2	x	x	x	x	x	x	x	x			x					x	}x	}x
18	3	x	x	x	x			x	x								x		
18	4				x														
20	0																	x	x
20	1																	x	x
20	2				x					x								x	x
20	3	x	x		x					x									
20	4	x			x					x	x							x	x
20	5									x	x								
22	4	x	x		x					x									
22	5	x	x		x					x	x								
22	6				x					x									

KEY: [a] C = culture form; B = bloodstream form; G = gas chromatography; P = paper chromatography; Ch = chemical fractionation.

(1) Korn et al. (1965); (2) Korn and Greenblatt (1963); (3) von Brand (1962); (4) Williams et al. (1963); (5) Morrison and Jeskey (1947); (6) von Brand (1933); (7) Faust and Tallqvist (1907); (8) von Brand (1933); (9) Cmelik and Bartl (1956); (10) Flury (1912); (11) Beames and Fisher (1964).

Trypanosoma cruzi and *Leishmania tropica.* The question was re-examined by Williamson (1963), who with more convincing methods than those employed by Halevy (1962), found no ergosterol, but both free and esterified cholesterol in the following parasites: blood and culture forms of *Trypanosoma rhodesiense* and *Trypanosoma lewisi,* the culture forms of *Trypanosoma cruzi, Leishmania donovani,* and *Strigomonas oncopelti,* as well as in the blood-stream form of *Plasmodium knowlesi.* However, Halevy and Girsy (1964) established unequivocally that the culture form of *Trypanosoma ranarum,* grown on a serum-free, yeast extract-containing medium, accumulated ergosterol, a finding possibly indicating that the medium on which trypanosomes are grown has a decisive influence on the type of sterol deposited. Finally, cholesterol seems to be the main sterol of *Trichomonas foetus* (Halevy, 1963).

It must be emphasized that cholesterol does not account for all the unsaponifiable substances occurring in some parasitic protozoa. Thus, higher unidentified alcohols have been reported from *Goussia gadi* by Panzer (1913) and von Brand *et al.* (1959) found in the culture form of *Trypanosoma cruzi* large amounts of unidentified waxlike substances as well as small amounts of a substance with an ultraviolet absorption spectrum characteristic of a 5,7-diene.

The older literature (von Brand, 1928, 1933, 1939, 1957; Salisbury and Anderson, 1939) shows that the unsaponifiable material isolated from various groups of helminths (trematodes, cestodes, Acanthocephala, and nematodes) contains sterols which were, however, not identified specifically. More precise data have recently become available. Cholesterol has been found in *Taenia saginata* (Cmelik and Bartl, 1956) and *Hymenolepis diminuta* (Fairbairn *et al.,* 1961); it seems to be accompanied by another sterol-like material in *Taenia saginata.* In *Taenia taeniaeformis* and *Moniezia expansa,* on the other hand, cholesterol accounted for 98 and 85%, respectively, of the total unsaponifiable material, that is, for surprisingly high fractions (Thompson *et al.,* 1960). The *Moniezia* sample contained, in addition to cholesterol, some 7-ketocholesterol which was probably formed during isolation or storage. Insofar as nematodes are concerned the only definite identification of sterols is owed to Fairbairn and Jones (1956). They proved the presence of cholesterol in lipids extracted from muscles and the female reproductive organs of *Ascaris lumbricoides.* Their material contained in addition small amounts of an unidentified saturated sterol.

Structurally related to steroids—both are isoprene derivatives—are the carotenes, yellow or reddish pigments of plant origin deposited secondarily in some parasites. Characteristic reactions have been observed in *Arhythmorhynchus* (Van Cleave and Rausch, 1950) and β-carotene, occasionally associated with chlorophyll derivatives and keto-carotenoids, has been identified in several larval trematodes (Nadakal, 1960). Carotenoid pigments are very characteristic for crustacea and it is therefore not surprising that they have been found in such parasites as *Sacculina* and *Parthenopea* (Lenel, 1954; Fox, 1953).

In contrast to what has been mentioned above for tapeworms, sterols represent quantitatively only a small fraction of the unsaponifiable lipids of *Ascaris* and *Parascaris*. This is due to the fact that they contain in addition to sterols unsaponifiable substances which in the older literature (Flury, 1912; Faure-Fremiet, 1913a; Schulz and Becker, 1933; von Brand and Winkeljohn, 1945) are described under the misleading term of ascaryl alcohol. The use of this term should be discontinued since recent studies of Polonsky *et al.* (1955), Fouquey *et al.* (1957), and Fouquey (1961) showed that "ascaryl alcohol" really consists of a mixture of at least three glycosides which received the names ascaroside A, B, and C. All three contain as carbohydrate moiety the hexose ascarylose which has been discussed in Chapter 2. One molecule of both ascarosides A and B contains one molecule of ascarylose, while one molecule of ascaroside C contains two molecules of the hexose. Ascaroside A, which corresponds to 20% of the total ascarosides, is probably not a uniform compound, but rather a mixture of homologous substances, since the carbons of the aglycone, a secondary monoalcohol, vary in number from 23 to 27. Ascarosides B (accounting for 67% of the total) and C (13% of the total) have the aglycone in common. It has been identified as 2,6-dihydroxyhentriacontane, a secondary dialcohol. The formulas of these unique compounds are shown in Fig. 8.

Ascarosides have been found in the muscles and the cuticle of female *Ascaris lumbricoides* (Fairbairn, 1956), as well as in male ascarids (von Brand and Winkeljohn, 1945; Cavier *et al.,* 1958). By far the highest concentration of the compounds, however, occurs within the eggs. In the nonfertilized *Ascaris* egg the ascarosides are esterified with acetic and propionic acids (Fouquey *et al.,* 1957) and are found within the cytoplasm. After fertilization they are utilized to form the vitelline membrane, or at least an important part of that membrane, accounting for at least 77% of its lipids (Fairbairn and Passey, 1955). Apparently the ascaroside esters of the oocyte yolk are hydrolyzed at the time of membrane formation, since the ascarosides in the membranes are not esterified (Fairbairn and Passey, 1955). The extreme resistance of the *Ascaris* egg to many unfavorable extraneous influences is probably due largely to the protective action of the lipid membrane (literature in Fairbairn, 1957). Vitelline membranes, consisting of lipids, often described on histochemical evi-

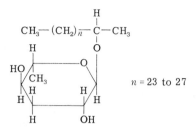

Ascaroside A

$n = 23$ to 27

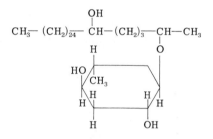

Ascaroside B

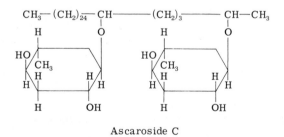

Ascaroside C

FIG. 8. Configuration of ascarosides A, B, and C. (After Fouquey, 1961.)

dence alone as sterol or wax, occur in many nematodes. It is possible that they contain ascarosides or related substances, but no analytical studies have been done yet on species other than *Ascaris* or *Parascaris*.

Older and newer observations on the lipid membrane of nematode eggs are recorded in the following papers: Fauré-Fremiet (1913a), Zawadowsky (1928), Wottge (1937), Chitwood (1938), Jacobs and Jones (1939), Monné and Hönig (1954a,b), Monné (1955), and Crites (1958).

Lower volatile fatty acids occur in abundance in *Parascaris* and *Ascaris* ether extracts, a fact known since Schimmelpfennig's (1903) and Flury's (1912) investigations. More recently, Fairbairn (1955a) reported relatively large amounts of volatile acids, ranging from C_2 to C_6 acids, from the female reproductive tract of *Ascaris,* where they occur in the form of glycerides. Similarly, volatile fatty acids occur in the male reproductive system of this nematode (Cavier *et al.,* 1958).

Data on higher fatty acids in parasites are summarized in Table XXXVI. They are in most cases derived from a study of the total lipids, that is, fatty acids bound to glycerol or sterols probably predominate, but those occurring in phospholipids are also included. Table XXXVI illustrates strikingly the much greater variety of fatty acids reported from gas chromatographic analyses than from studies utilizing the older methods. Actually, the variety of fatty acids is still greater than indicated by Table XXXVI. In most studies done with the help of gas chromatography several unidentified acids have been reported; a further complication is that the position of the double bonds varies in multiple unsaturated acids. As an example it may be mentioned that in *Leishmania tarentolae* two 18:3, two 20:3, three 20:4, and two 20:5 acids have been found, with certain variations occurring, depending upon the medium on which the flagellates were developed (Korn *et al.,* 1965). There can be little doubt that application of the newer analytical techniques would reveal more unsaturated acids in some of the helminths listed in Table XXXVI than shown there. This is indicated by the high iodine numbers reported for the fatty acids of *Taenia saginata* (Smorodincev and Bebesin, 1939) and *Hymenolepis diminuta* (Warren and Daugherty, 1957). A similar assumption is justified in the case of the protozoon *Goussia gadi* (Panzer, 1913). Finally, it can be hoped that the newer techniques will lead to the identification of the higher hydroxy acids occurring in relatively large amounts in *Moniezia expansa* (von Brand, 1933; Oesterlin and von Brand, 1934). It has not yet been established whether these acids occur as such, or as constituents of the cerebrosides mentioned in a previous paragraph.

Of special interest is the fact that the linolenic acid found in *Leishmania enrietti* is α-linolenic acid, since this form was heretofore thought to be characteristic of chlorophyll-containing higher and lower plants (Korn and Greenblatt, 1963).

A last group of lipids to be mentioned briefly are soaps. They account for approximately 20 and 16%, respectively, of the total lipids in *Goussia gadi* (Panzer, 1913) and *Fasciola hepatica* (von Brand, 1928), and have been demonstrated qualitatively in *Strongylus equinus* (Bondouy, 1910). Little information is available concerning their chemical constitution, but some indications exist that the fatty acids of the soaps may differ qualitatively or in their relative proportions from those of the glycerides. Thus, Panzer (1913) found the iodine number of the fatty acids bound as soaps lower than that of the other lipid fractions of *Goussia gadi* and von Brand (1928) reported the relatively low iodine number of 30 for the fatty acids isolated from the soaps of *Fasciola hepatica*.

III. DISTRIBUTION OF LIPIDS IN THE BODIES OF PARASITES

The occurrence of fatty materials in parasites has been studied frequently by means of more or less specific staining methods, e.g., osmic acid, Sudan III, and others. In evaluating these observations it must be kept in mind that all staining procedures show only a part, often only a small fraction, of the lipids extractable by chemical methods. It must be realized that negative observations, such as those by Armer (1944) on parasitic protozoa of cockroaches, do not indicate the actual absence of lipids. Despite their limitations, morphological data are of physiological interest because they permit a study of organisms or organs not available in sufficient quantity for chemical analysis.

No attempt has been made to collect all the morphological fat data relating to parasitic protozoa. In many instances the term "fat" is used quite loosely in the protozoological literature and is applied, without corroborating tests such as solubility studies or observations on staining characteristics, to granules that are highly refractive in the light microscope. Such data must be interpreted with caution.

Parasitic flagellates show a variable picture. Trypanosomids have few, if any, morphologically demonstrable lipid droplets (Gerzeli, 1955); trichomonads appear to have more inclusions positively stained by lipid reagents, especially in the posterior parts of their bodies (Nomura, 1957; Gerzeli, 1959; Wantland *et al.*, 1962); termite flagellates, finally, are reported as variable in this respect, depending upon the species studied (Lavette, 1964). *Joenia annectens* contains in the region of the parabasal apparatus a substance that according to histochemical evidence must be classified as a glycolipoprotein.

Little seems to have been published on the occurrence of histochemically demonstrable lipids in parasitic amoebae; *Endamoeba blattae* stores only small amounts (Sassuchin, 1928). Conditions are variable in sporozoa. Relatively little lipid has been found in *Toxoplasma* (Gerzeli, 1954b) or hemogregarines (Gerzeli, 1954a). On the contrary, fat droplets are seen frequently and sometimes in abundance in myxosporidia (Cohn, 1896; Doflein, 1898; Erdmann, 1917; Petruschewsky, 1932), gregarines, and coccidia (Joyet-Lavergne, 1926; Gurwitsch, 1927; Daniels, 1938; Patillo and Becker, 1955; Stein, 1963). It is of interest that in gregarines sexual differences have been reported, the female of an encysted pair having more lipids than the male. Similar in principle, lipid is found especially in the macrogametocytes and spores of *Eimeria* spp., while schizonts, merozoites, and microgametocytes are morphologically fat-free. Erythrocytic stages of *Plasmodium* spp. do not give lipid reactions, but the pre-erythrocytic stages of *Plasmodium cynomolgi* contain lipid, as do the oocysts (Das Gupta, 1960).

Parasitic ciliates show with some regularity, but not invariably, lipid inclusions (e.g., Cheissin, 1930). The "lipid bodies" of such forms as *Nyctotherus* or *Balantidium* are probably structures of mixed composition; besides lipids they also contain proteins and possibly other substances (Dutta, 1958a, 1959). *Opalina* and related species have been studied repeatedly (Kedrowsky, 1931; Dutta, 1958b; Sukhanova, 1963). In the case of *Opalina ranarum* a seasonal fat cycle has been recorded, a large accumulation of fat occurring in the fall which almost completely disappeared toward the end of the winter. There are apparently also variations in lipid content of various stages in the life cycle of this parasite.

For obvious anatomical reasons the distribution of lipids within organs of flatworms cannot be studied by quantitative chemical methods. The only point studied from a quantitative standpoint is the question as to whether a lipid gradient exists along the tapeworm strobila. Smorodincev and Bebesin (1935) have found in the head and neck region of *Taenia saginata* a fat content of 3.05% of the fresh tissues; while the figures for the middle region of the strobila and the gravid segments were 1.55% and 1.25%, respectively. On the contrary, Fairbairn *et al.* (1961) observed an increase in lipid content from 15% of the dry weight in the immature proglottids of *Hymenolepis diminuta* to 31% in the gravid proglottids. Fairbairn *et al.* (1961) furthermore observed that eggs isolated from the terminal proglottids contained only moderate amounts of lipids. The parenchyma therefore must have contained lipids well in excess of the 31% mentioned. The same type of gradient had been observed by histochemical methods in this worm and in *Raillietina cesticillus* by Hedrick (1958). Morphologically, the most important lipid storage organ of tapeworms generally is the parenchyma. Most other organs contain either no or only little lipid. The cuticle is often lipid-free, but a positive reaction was observed in the case of *Taenia taeniaeformis* (Waitz, 1963). Lipid droplets are often seen in the eggs. They are usually located between the embryo and the egg shell. In some instances, e.g., *Dipylidium caninum,* large fat droplets are observed in the lumen of the uterus. Peculiar to tapeworms is the fact that some lipid occurs in the calcareous corpuscles (von Brand *et al.,* 1960; Waitz, 1963) and that in some species rather close connections between lipids and excretory system exist. Thus, in *Echinococcus granulosus* (Coutelen, 1931) and *Moniezia expansa* (von Brand, 1933) fat droplets were found in the lumen of the excretory canals, and in *Hymenolepis diminuta* (Hedrick, 1958) rather heavy fat accumulations were observed around the canals. For further details concerning lipid distribution in cestode bodies, reference is made to the following papers: Schiefferdecker (1874), Brault and Loeper (1904), Arndt (1922), Pintner (1922), Smyth (1947, 1949), and Rao (1960).

The trematode species most often studied histochemically is *Fasciola hepatica* (Prenant, 1922; von Brand and Weinland, 1924; Vogel and von Brand, 1933; Stephenson, 1947; Reznik, 1963; Kublickiene, 1963; Pantelouris and Threadgold, 1963). General agreement exists that in adult liver flukes most of the morphologically demonstrable lipid occurs around and within the excretory system. Numerous fat droplets can be found embedded in the walls of the smaller excretory vessels while they are freely floating in the lumen of the larger ones. Their expulsion through the excretory pore could be observed under the microscope. Microchemical tests indicate that the droplets do not contain cholesterol, cholesterides, or lipins, but that they are probably triglycerides containing some unsaturated fatty acids. The absence of cholesterol is especially noteworthy because it indicates that no simple excretion of exogenous fat taken up with the food is involved. The environment of liver flukes is rich in cholesterol and the occurrence of this compound in the droplets would be expected if food lipids were involved. It is quite obvious that we are dealing with the excretion of fat presumably originating in the body of the worms themselves, as has been explained in a previous chapter, from the carbohydrate metabolism. Whether the finding of stearic acid both in the body and the cyst fluid of *Paragonimus ohirai* (Ogimoto, 1956) indicates excretion will require further study.

Evidently, then, a parallel exists between *Fasciola, Echinococcus,* and *Moniezia* in respect to the excretion of fat. It should be emphasized that in the case of tapeworms at least a part of the parenchymal fat can be considered as unexcreted waste product rather than as energy reserve. Von Brand (1952) and Fairbairn *et al.* (1961) have stressed the point that tapeworm segments are only ephemeral structures and that the lipids of the terminal proglottids are discarded at the time of expulsion. The view that fat deposits may represent waste products is not as unorthodox as may appear at first glance. Fats are undoubtedly less toxic than many other excreta and their excretion may not be as imperative as that of the more toxic end products.

It can be expected that excretion of fat as waste product will be found only in organisms that lead a predominantly anaerobic life. It is characteristic in this respect that the process is found only in the adult liver fluke. Its developmental stages, which probably can secure oxygen more or less readily, do not show it. Miracidiae, rediae, and cercariae of this species, and *Cercaria limnaea ovata* have some fat droplets within the tissues, but they are never found in the lumen of the excretory canals (Vogel and von Brand, 1933; Palm, 1962).

It is also worthy of attention that no fat excretion can be demonstrated in *Dicrocoelium dendriticum* (von Brand, 1934a), although it lives in exactly the same habitat as *Fasciola,* nor in *Clonorchis sinensis* (Takagi, 1962).

As mentioned above little lipid can be demonstrated in *Fasciola* in organs other than the excretory system. Some histochemical evidence has been presented showing that phospholipids occur in its Mehlis' gland (Rao, 1959). There is no indication that the vitellaria of this worm contain cholesterol esters, which have been found in abundance in those of *Gorgodera cygnoides* as well as in its eggs (Schmidt, 1930). Distinct lipid reactions have also been obtained in the vitelline cells of *Paragonimus ohirai* (Yokogawa and Yoshimura, 1957), the esophagus, and intestinal epithelium, as well as the parenchyma of *Clonorchis sinensis* (Takagi, 1962), the vitelline cells, and ova, and in the parenchyma of maturing males of *Schistosoma japonicum* (I-Hsun-Ho, 1963).

Among nematodes parasitic in vertebrates, *Ascaris lumbricoides* and *Parascaris equorum* have been investigated most often (von Kemnitz, 1912; Fauré-Fremiet, 1913a; Mueller, 1929; Hirsch and Bretschneider, 1937; Kessel *et al.,* 1961). The general aspects of fat deposition were similar in both species, the subcuticula, especially the chords, and the plasma bulbs of the body wall muscles being the most important storage places. Fat droplets were also found within the ganglion cells, the intestinal cells, and various structures of the reproductive tracts. As an example of invertebrate parasites the cockroach nematode *Thelastoma bulhoesi* may be mentioned. According to Lee (1960), the chief storage areas for fat are the chords, intestine, oocytes, oogonia, and ova. Fat globules were found occasionally within the lumen of the gut of this species, but much more often in that of the male *Hammerschmidtiella diesingi,* especially after a 24-hour starvation period. Lee (1960) considers it as possible that these lipid droplets have been shed into the lumen to be broken down by the lipase of the gut into compounds that are easily absorbed and transportable to other regions of the body.

Various other adult and larval nematodes have been studied in more or less detail by Payne (1922, 1923), Cort (1925), Giovannola (1935, 1936), Rogers (1939, 1940), Chitwood and Jacobs (1938), Chitwood and Chitwood (1938), Weinstein (1949), Elliott (1954), Nath *et al.* (1961), Münnich (1962, 1965), Engelbrecht (1963), and Engelbrecht and Palm (1964). Some observations on the larvae are of interest. Lipid accumulation, not only within the cells of the intestine, but within the lumen, is often pronounced. In some cases the fat content of the larvae is a good indicator of the physiological age, for example, in hookworms. Reduction in fat content and activity paralleled each other rather closely, but fat-free larvae (by morphological observation only, it is true, of some species at least, e.g., *Haemonchus placei*) are still infective, indicating that the presence of fat is not essential for infectivity (Durie, 1957). Remarkable differences between species exist in respect to the length of time fat reserves remain demonstrable. In embryonated *Ascaris* eggs, for instance, only a moderate diminution of fat reserves was discernible after 2 years' storage at room temperature (Münnich, 1962) and they were nearly exhausted only after 4 years (Münnich, 1965), while in *Ascaridia galli* (Elliott, 1954) most fat was lost within 10 months. Engelbrecht and Palm (1964) developed the theory that larval stages of helminths which live only a short time and are usually free-swimming, such as miracidia, cercariae, coracidia, or oncospheres, as well as larval *Enterobius vermicularis,* depend principally on stored glycogen, while others that stay alive a long time, such as the ascarid larvae, store and utilize lipids primarily.

The last group of helminths to be considered briefly are the Acanthocephala. A characteristic feature is that lipid droplets are found in the vessels of the lacunar system, although not in all species. Relevant data have been presented by Saefftigen (1885), Hamann (1891), Meyer (1931), von Brand (1939), and Bullock (1949b). The subcuticula contained relatively large amounts of lipids in all species studied, whereas specific differences occurred in respect to the muscles. Those of *Macracanthorhynchus* contained but little histochemically demonstrable fat, while those of *Echinorhynchus, Neoechinorhynchus,* and *Pomphorhynchus* showed marked accumulations. Some fat droplets were seen in the nervous and the male reproductive system. In the female reproductive system, the germ balls were especially rich in fat, as were some of the other structures, such as the vaginal glands. Histochemical tests showed that phospholipids, though not completely lacking in the other organs, were especially plentiful in the subcuticula, having a tendency to accumulate around the lacunae. Cholesterol and cholesterol esters, on the other hand, were found essentially limited to the inner layer of the subcuticula.

In contrast to what has been mentioned above for flatworms, quantitative determinations on certain organ systems of nematodes and Acanthocephala are feasible.

Some of the data available are shown in Table XXXVII. They indicate the percentage of lipid found in certain organs, but do not indicate what organs are quantitatively the most important storage areas, because they do not take into account the relative weight of the various organs. In the case of *Macracanthorhynchus,* for instance, the lipids of hypodermis plus muscles account for 61 % of the total body lipids and those of the female reproductive tract for 30 %, although the latter contains more lipid per unit weight than the former.

The only quantitative studies on lipids in isolated organs of parasitic arthropods have been done on the tracheal organ of *Gastrophilus intestinalis* larvae. It has been observed (Levenbook, 1951) that lipid accumulates in this organ throughout development, reaching a maximum of over 35 % of the dry tissue on the 7th to 10th day of pupation. Equally scarce are histochemical data. They are available only for *Peltogaster paguri* (Reinhard and von Brand, 1944). The root system of the parasite, which permeates the liver of the host, always contained some fat, but it was not seen in the bulbous tips of the roots which presumably are the main places of absorption. The external sacs of the parasites showed variable conditions, depending upon their age. The smallest, that is, the youngest, sacs were fat-free while the eggs and developing embryos of mature specimens were extremely rich in fat. Fully developed free-swimming nauplii, which do not feed, again showed a decrease in fat content.

IV. LIPID ABSORPTION AND DIGESTION

The mechanism of lipid absorption is still rather obscure. Wotton (1963) has listed the following processes as probably all involved in the actual uptake of fat into, or the release of fat from, cells: direct diffusion of molecules, ion pumping mechanisms, membrane flow with vesicle formation, direct porosities, and the rearrangement of protein molecules located on the outer surface of the cell membrane. Which one, if any, of the above mechanisms is involved in the uptake of particulate fat droplets by the blood-stream forms of *Trypanosoma lewisi* and *Trypanosoma equiperdum* (Wotton and Halsey, 1957; Wotton and Becker, 1963) is at present not known. Wotton and his co-workers assume that the process is largely a physical one, since such compounds as tryparsamide or

TABLE XXXVII

DISTRIBUTION OF LIPIDS IN VARIOUS ORGAN SYSTEMS OF HELMINTHS

| Species | Lipids in per cent of fresh substance occurring in | | | | References |
	Hemolymph	Cuticle	Muscle	Reproductive system	
Ascaris lumbricoides ♀	0.32–0.35	0.61	0.75	6.0	Fairbairn (1957); Cavier *et al.* (1958)
Ascaris lumbricoides ♂	0.33	0.98		3.2	Cavier *et al.* (1958)
Macracanthorhynchus hirudinaceus ♀	0.2	1.3		1.9	von Brand (1939)

acridine orange, when dissolved prior to the experiments in the food lipids, are absorbed together with the latter.

Whether analogous processes occur in other parasitic protozoa is unknown. Small amounts of microscopically demonstrable lipids became visible in *Endamoeba blattae* and *Nyctotherus ovalis* after their hosts had been kept for 6 to 8 weeks on a high fat diet, an observation possibly indicating a small-scale fat absorption (Armer, 1944), and metabolic studies indicate that probably fairly large amounts of lipids are absorbed by several species of rumen ciliates (Wright, 1959; Williams, *et al.*, 1963; Gutierrez *et al.*, 1962).

In other cases only indirect indications pointing toward fat absorption exist. It has thus been shown that stearic acid can fulfill an essential growth requirement of *Trypanosoma cruzi* (Boné and Parent, 1963) and that cholesterol plus Tween 80 (monooleate of polyethylene sorbitan) (Sanders, 1957), or a mixture of cholesterol and fatty acids can replace serum in the cultures of *Trichomonas foetus* (Wyss *et al.*, 1960a,b). The situation is complex, however, and far from clear in this last case. It appears that in the absence of cholesterol, stearic, elaidic, and oleic acids exerted a stimulatory influence on growth, while linoleic and linolenic acids did not. In the presence of cholesterol, on the other hand, stearic acid was inactive, while the doubly and triply unsaturated acids were active. The best combination was a mixture of cholesterol and elaidic acid which had a growth stimulatory activity almost equal to that shown by the ether-soluble fraction of serum.

A fairly clear indication for fat absorption is the observation reported by Shorb (1963) that the fatty acids occurring in *Trichomonas gallinae* grown in a medium containing, among other ingredients, trypticase, oleic, and palmitic acids, were identical with those found in the culture medium; oleic and palmitic acids predominated, but these acids were accompanied by the same complicated mixture of fatty acids characterizing the trypticase supplement.

It is unlikely that lipases secreted into the environment are of any importance in lipid absorption by parasitic protozoa that do not possess a cytostome, such as trypanosomes. Indeed, there is no indication that the blood-stream forms of African pathogenic trypanosomes contain this type of enzyme (Califano and Gritti, 1930; Krijgsman, 1936a,b). Protozoa that might engulf fat droplets via food vacuoles theoretically could use lipases to digest fat prior to absorption into the protoplasm, but no definite information is available. In *Opalina carolinensis* an intracellular mitochondria-bound lipase has been found that could hydrolyze oleate, but was inactive against stearate (Hunter, 1957). Its physiological role is obscure; it could serve to facilitate intracellular lipid movements.

Little is known about lipid absorption by multicellular parasites lacking an alimentary canal. The lipase activity of *Taenia taeniaeformis,* and *Taenia pisiformis* (but also of the gut-containing *Fasciola hepatica*) is low (Pennoit-DeCooman and van Grembergen, 1942), and Pflugfelder (1949) found that *Acanthocephalus ranae* does not liberate a lipase into the environment. He is of the opinion that these worms absorb the degradation products of the fat digested by the lipases of the host. He transplanted Acanthocephala that had been starved for 6 weeks *in vivo* and were devoid of microscopically demonstrable fat droplets to new hosts which were then fed with hog fat dyed with Scharlach R. First absorption of stained lipid could be demonstrated after 12 hours; after 4 days large amounts of fat were deposited within the tissues of the lemnisci, and in the following days even the latter's lacunae filled up with fat. Fat absorption apparently takes place only through lemnisci and the adjacent parts of the body wall, but the mechanism by which lipids are taken into the tissues is unknown.

Parasites possessing an alimentary tract can theoretically digest fats by means of lipases, that is, fat absorption could take place after hydrolysis and soap formation. Lipases occur in the intestinal canal of such nematodes as *Ascaris lumbricoides, Strongylus edentatus,* and *Leidynema appendiculata* (Rogers, 1941; Carpenter, 1952; Lee, 1958). Few details about these enzymes are known. The lipase of *Leidynema*, for instance, has a pH optimum of 7.0 and hydrolyzes glycerol tributyrate, but is inactive against olive oil or ethyl butyrate. However, the actual biological role of these lipases has not been established yet; lipid absorption has not been demonstrated unequivocally. In fact, only vague indications pointing toward utilization of any lipid exist. Thus, Rohrbacher (1957) found only slight beneficial influence of cholesterol during maintenance of bacteria-free *Fasciola hepatica* specimens *in vitro*.

Tissue lipases, that is, lipases presumably assisting in lipid movements within tissues rather than preparing lipids for absorption from the intestinal tract, may be fairly common in helminths. Lipase activity on tripalmitin at pH 8.0 has been found in extracts of the filariform larvae of *Strongyloides ratti* and *Nippostrongylus muris,* and less pronounced in cercariae of *Schistosoma mansoni* (Mandlowitz *et al.,* 1960). Due to the mode of extraction the exact localization of the enzyme is not known in these cases. Histochemical evidence indicated the presence of a lipase in ovary, testicle, and eggs advanced in development in the case of *Enterobius vermicularis* (Marzullo *et al.,* 1957) and in the subcuticula of the trunk as well as in the lemnisci of several acanthocephalan species (Bullock, 1949a). The perivisceral fluid of *Ascaris,* which is rich in many enzymes, does not show lipase activity (Monteoliva, 1960).

Insofar as endoparasitic arthropods are concerned, an enzyme capable of splitting tributyrin has been found in the mid-gut of *Gastrophilus* larvae and their hemolymph (Roy, 1937; Tatchell, 1958), as well as in *Cordylobia* larvae (Blacklock *et al.,* 1930). Furthermore, House (1954a,b) has shown that cholesterol is an essential constituent of the chemically defined medium on which he grew the larvae of the dipterous parasite *Pseudosarcophaga affinis* and that the addition of lard or domestic shortening to the medium improved growth. It has also been assumed that the abundant fat droplets in parasites like *Sacculina* essentially represent fat absorbed from the host's liver (Smith, 1911, 1913; Robson, 1911). This, of course, is quite possible, but has not yet been proved. Reinhard and von Brand (1944) pointed out that the bulbous root tips of the parasites are poor in fat, making a direct transition of lipid from host to parasite unlikely.

Related to lipases are various esterases described from numerous parasites. Nonspecific esterases have been found in the cuticle and various internal organs of *Ascaris lumbricoides* (Lee, 1961) and in *Diplostomum phoxini* (Lee, 1962). In tapeworms (Lee *et al.,* 1963) nonspecific esterases have been encountered in various organs, but of special interest is their occurrence in the walls of the main excretory canals, since this localization may indicate functional involvement in the excretion of lipids.

The best-known specific esterase is acetylcholinesterase. The older relevant experiments of Bacq and Oury (1937), Pennoit-DeCooman (1940), Artemov and Lure (1941), and Pennoit-DeCooman and van Grembergen (1942) had made the presence of the enzyme probable in cestodes, trematodes, and nematodes, but the methods used by these authors were not specific enough to prove strictly the presence of a specific acetylcholinesterase. The first definite identification was made by

Bueding (1952) in the case of *Schistosoma mansoni;* he established the following three facts: (1) In concentrations at which a high rate of hydrolysis of acetylcholine was observed, butyryl choline was not hydrolyzed; (2) reduction below or increase above optimal concentration of acetylcholine decreased enzymatic activity; and (3) triacetin was hydrolyzed at a slow rate. He points out that these three properties differentiate true acetylcholinesterase from other choline-splitting enzymes.

Bueding found the same enzyme also in *Litomosoides carinii* and, in low concentration, in *Ascaris lumbricoides.* Later workers, making use in part of histochemical methods, demonstrated cholinesterase in the miracidia of *Schistosoma mansoni* (Pepler, 1958), in *Diplostomum phoxini* (Lee, 1962), *Fasciola hepatica* (Chance and Mansour, 1953), *Dicrocoelium dendriticum* (Becejac *et al.,* 1964), *Diphyllobothrium latum,* and *Taenia saginata* (Pylkkö, 1956a,b), *Echinococcus granulosus* (Schwabe, 1959; Schwabe *et al.,* 1961), various ascarids (Lui *et al.,* 1964), and some plant-parasitizing nematodes (Rohde, 1960). The available histochemical evidence indicates that in some cases at least the acetylcholinesterase is localized within elements of the nervous system; a functional role in the nervous activity of the parasites appears therefore possible. It is in this connection of interest to note that the survey of Bacq (1941) shows the motor nerves of worms in general to be cholinergic.

Acetylcholine itself, or at any rate an acetylcholine-like substance, has been demonstrated in nematodes (Mellanby, 1955), in tapeworms (Artemov and Lure, 1941; Pylkkö, 1956a), and in *Fasciola* (Chance and Mansour, 1953). It occurs, however, not only in worms who have a more or less well-developed nervous system, but also in *Trypanosoma rhodesiense,* but not in *Plasmodium gallinaceum* (Bülbring *et al.,* 1949). These authors suggest that its occurrence in trypanosomes may be correlated with their vigorous motility as contrasted to the sluggish motion of the malarial parasites.

It should finally be kept in mind that acetylcholine-splitting enzymes, not specific enough to warrant identification with a true acetylcholinesterase, may also be present in parasites. While no pseudo-cholinesterase seems to occur in *Fasciola* (Chance and Mansour, 1953), a relevant enzyme has been observed in *Diphyllobothrium latum* and in *Taenia saginata* (Pylkkö, 1956b). It splits benzoylcholine which is not readily attacked by true acetylcholinesterase.

V. LIPID SYNTHESIS

The starting point for the synthesis of long-chain fatty acids is commonly acetyl-CoA which, by addition of CO_2, is transformed into malonyl-CoA and serves as a primer for the further synthetic steps. The other C_2 units are added as malonyl-CoA, with loss of one CO_2/malonyl unit. Whether a comparable sequence occurs in parasites has not yet been established. It has been found that acetate-1-C^{14} is incorporated into the lipid fraction, especially fatty acids of glycerides, and into phospholipids of various trypanosomids and *Trichomonas foetus* (Newton, 1956; Grant and Fulton, 1957; Halevy, 1962, 1963), but the details of the synthetic steps have not been elucidated.

It has been established that acetyl-CoA is not the only compound serving for synthesis of fatty acids. Korn and Greenblatt (1963) grew *Leishmania enrietti* in the presence of C^{14}-labeled stearic acid and recovered significant amounts of radioactivity from stearaldehyde, stearic, oleic, linoleic, and α-linolenic acids isolated from the flagellates, whereas no activity was found in any acid with less than 18 carbon atoms. They interpret this finding as indicating that the unsaturated 18-carbon acids and stearaldehyde were synthesized from stearic acid without previous degradation of the latter and without reutilization of 2-carbon units.

Later studies (Korn *et al.*, 1965), dealing with the synthetic capabilities of some trypanosomids, showed that *Leishmania tarentolae* and *Trypanosoma lewisi,* just as *Leishmania enrietti,* could synthesize oleic acid by direct desaturation of stearic acid. An interesting situation was observed in respect to octadecatrienoic acids. *Leishmania enrietti* is able to synthesize only one such acid, 18:3 (9,12,15), the numbers in brackets indicating the position of the double bonds counting from the carboxyl end of the molecule. *Leishmania tarentolae,* on the other hand, can form both 18:3 (9,12,15) and 18:3 (6,9,12) acids, while *Trypanosoma lewisi* produces only 18:3 (6,9,12) although also containing in its lipids some 18:3 (9,12,15). The extreme is represented by *Crithidia* sp. in which 18:3 (6,9,12) is found in abundance, while 18:3 (9,12,15) is completely absent. Further elongation of the 18-carbon acids appears to be achieved only slowly by trypanosomids. *Leishmania tarentolae,* grown on Trager's (1957) C medium, can use 18:3 (6,9,12) for the synthesis of 20:3 (8,11,14), 22:4 (7,10,13,16), and 22:5 (4,7,10,13,16); it can also use 18:3 (9,12,15) for the synthesis of 20:3 (11,14,17), 20:4 (8,11,14,17), 22:5 (7,10,13,16,19), and 22:6 (4,7,10,13,16,19). Some of these acids are formed in very small amounts only, others in larger ones, depending in part on the medium on which the organisms are grown. For instance, the 22:4 (7,10,13,16) acid comprises only 0.3 % of the total acids in the flagellates harvested from Trager's C medium. However, when the latter was supplemented with human serum albumin and arachidonate this figure rose to 18 %.

In rumen ciliates, on the other hand, hydrogenation rather than unsaturation occurs, although the latter process has also been found. *Iso-*

tricha intestinalis converts oleic acid into stearic, linoleic, and an unidentified acid, while stearic, linoleic, and palmitic acids gave rise only to
unidentified acids (Williams *et al.,* 1963). Hydrogenation of unsaturated
acids was especially pronounced in mixed material of holotrich and
oligotrich ciliates (Wright, 1959). When offered unsaturated C-18 acids,
they converted trienes to dienes and monoenes into stearic acid, but
curiously little conversion of dienes to monoenes occurred.

Nothing definite is known about the biosynthesis of sterols in parasites. Sterols, such as cholesterol or irradiated ergosterol, are often added
to media used in the cultivation of parasites, for example, the mosquito
phase of *Plasmodium relictum* (Ball and Chao, 1960), *Schistosoma
mansoni* (Senft and Senft, 1962), or *Pseudosarcophaga affinis* (House,
1954b), that is, protozoa, worms, or arthropods. It must be emphasized,
however, that the significance of these additions to culture media is
difficult to assess, even when it is shown that the sterol is required for
optimal growth, as in the case of *Pseudosarcophaga*. Evidently, it can
only be established by rather long series of experiments whether or not
the addition of the sterol as such is necessary, or whether it could be
synthesized from precursors, such as mevalonic acid and others.

Some definite information in this respect is available only for trichomonads. It was established early that such forms as *Eutrichomastix
colubrorum, Trichomonas foetus,* or *Trichomonas gallinae* require
cholesterol even when grown in a complex medium (Cailleau, 1936a,b,
1937, 1938), the last-named species being the one most thoroughly
studied. Cailleau (1936b, 1937) investigated 66 sterols and sterol derivatives and found that 18, among them dehydrocholesterol and ergosterol,
supported growth satisfactorily. These results have been confirmed in all
essentials by the newer experiments of Lund and Shorb (1962), who grew
Trichomonas gallinae in a synthetic medium. They came to the conclusion that the addition of a double bond in the ring structure at the 7–8
position, or the removal of the double bond in the 5–6 position does not
interfere with the activity of the compounds. On the contrary, such
changes as opening the ring structure at the 9–10 position, characteristic
for activation of D vitamins, or removal of the side chains destroy activity.
Steroid hormones are then inactive. Inactivity in respect to promotion
of growth does, however, not indicate that the compounds are metabolically completely inert. Indeed Sebek and Michaels (1957) found that
both *Trichomonas gallinae* and *Trichomonas foetus* contain a dehydrogenase which specifically interconverts 17-keto and 17-β-hydroxyl groups
of certain C_{18} and C_{19} steroids. The organisms are, for instance, capable
of reducing estrone to estradiol, or of oxidizing 17-β-hydroxy-4-estren-3-
one to 4-estren-3, 17-dione. The biological significance of such metabolic
activities is obscure.

While there can be no doubt that trichomonads can effect certain changes in the structure of sterols and related compounds, their ability to synthesize sterols appears to be minimal. Lund and Shorb (1962) found that typical precursors of cholesterol synthesis, such as acetate, mevalonic acid, or squalene, could not replace cholesterol in their medium.

A pronounced synthesis of phospholipids undoubtedly occurs in all rapidly growing or multiplying parasites. It has thus been found that in red cells parasitized by *Plasmodium knowlesi* the phospholipid-P is from 2 to 4 times higher than in normal erythrocytes. According to Ball *et al.* (1948) the increased synthesis is due to the parasites. A relatively high rate of phospholipid synthesis has also been demonstrated for *Trypanosoma equiperdum in vivo* (Moraczewski and Kelsey, 1948; Cantrell, 1953; Cantrell and Genazzani, 1955).

No details of phospholipid synthesis are known as yet. It is not evident to what extent the various components of the phospholipids can be formed by the parasites themselves or must be supplied by the environment. Choline, inositol, and serine are frequently components of media used in cultivating parasitic protozoa or worms (e.g., Trager, 1957; Taylor, 1963), but their essentiality has hardly been established. Indeed, Cowperthwaite *et al.* (1953) could eliminate choline and inositol from their synthetic medium used in the cultivation of *Herpetomonas culicidarum*. It did not contain serine at any time of development. Furthermore, the possibility should not be overlooked that the above compounds could serve other purposes than the synthesis of phospholipids. An interesting observation has been reported for *Leishmania tarentolae* by Trager (1957). In cultivating this organism he established an interchangeable requirement for either pyridoxine plus choline, for pyridoxal or pyridoxamine. Both of the former compounds could be eliminated from the medium without interference with growth of the flagellates induced by either pyridoxal or pyridoxamine. This finding was interpreted as meaning that either choline was required to form pyridoxine, or alternatively that pyridoxal has in this case a specific function in the biosynthesis of choline.

VI.   METABOLISM OF FATTY ACIDS AND THEIR GLYCERIDES

There is little experimental evidence indicating that parasitic protozoa are capable of utilizing lower volatile fatty acids for energy production. No stimulation of respiration with volatile fatty acids as substrate was observed with *Trypanosoma hippicum* (Harvey, 1949), *Trypanosoma lewisi* (Moulder, 1948), or trichomonads (Lindblom, 1961), and only a slight stimulation in the case of *Trypanosoma evansi* (Mannozzi-Torini,

1940), but the respiration of the culture form of *Leishmania brasiliensis* was double the endogenous rate when acetate was available (Medina *et al.,* 1955). Anaerobically, acetate and tributyrin increased significantly the gas production of *Isotricha intestinalis* and *Entodinium simplex* (Williams *et al.,* 1963), while that of *Isotricha prostoma* also increased when valeric or caproic acids were available (Gutierrez *et al.,* 1962)

Little is known in this respect for parasitic worms and arthropods. No utilization of acetate was demonstrable in the free-living third stage larvae of *Nippostrongylus muris* (Schwabe, 1957) or the larvae of *Gastrophilus intestinalis* (Van de Vijver, 1964), but a little acetate was used by *Litomosoides carinii* (Bueding, 1949). Definitive proof for large-scale utilization is available only for the eggs of ascarids. Szwejkowska (1929) found a diminution of volatile fatty acids from 0.46 to 0.34 % during the time elapsing from fertilization to the formation of the second polar body in the case of the *Parascaris* egg. More recently, Fairbairn (1955b) observed that during embryonation of the *Ascaris lumbricoides* eggs a large proportion of the volatile fatty acids is used up. He assumes that the acids found in the ovary are derived from fermentation acids produced in other tissues, which instead of being excreted are incorporated into ovarian glycerides and are thus being salvaged for subsequent oxidative energy production characteristic for the developing egg.

In the past, fatty acids were not considered as useful substrates for anaerobic energy production because their carbon atoms, with the exception of the carboxyl carbon, are largely reduced. It was thought that they would not lend themselves readily to the internal oxidation-reductions characteristic for anaerobic processes. However, theoretically, reactions characteristic of aerobic β-oxidation can proceed anaerobically if suitable mechanisms are at hand for regeneration of acceptors such as DPN or TPN (D. Fairbairn, personal communication, 1965). Some such mechanism may be realized in the case of rumen ciliates. It has been shown recently that these quite strictly anaerobic organisms seem to utilize certain higher fatty acids rather freely. The gas production (H_2 and CO_2) of *Isotricha intestinalis* was found markedly stimulated by oleate, in contrast to that of *Entodinium simplex* (Williams *et al.,* 1963), while *Isotricha prostoma* was intermediate (Gutierrez *et al.,* 1962). It was maximally stimulated by methyl myristate. The chemical processes involved have not yet been studied.

As explained in a previous section the large worms of the intestinal tract or the bile ducts elaborate fatty acids as an end product of their carbohydrate metabolism. When higher fatty acids are formed, as in *Fasciola* or *Moniezia,* they are either excreted or accumulate at least partially in the body. The question now arises whether under certain conditions this body fat can be utilized further. The eggs of these worms, in contrast to the adults, require oxygen, at least for full development, and it can be visualized, in parallel to the findings on lower fatty acids mentioned above, that fat could be metabolized once oxygen becomes available. This is indeed the case. Chemical analysis has shown that lipids disappeared from the *Parascaris* egg during aerobic development (Fauré-Fremiet, 1912, 1913a,b; Szwejkowska, 1929). In the case of *Ascaris* eggs, Passey and Fairbairn (1957) observed a pronounced decrease in fat during embryonation and a slower one in the infective embryo. They found indications (Fairbairn, 1960) that only part of the disappearing fat is completely oxidized, while part serves as substratum for carbohydrate resynthesis. A decrease in lipid has been reported also from anaerobically kept *Parascaris* eggs (Dyrdowska, 1931). This finding was based on histochemical evidence alone and is at present not supported by quantitative studies. Delayed oxidation of fat probably occurs also in *Gastrophilus*. There is no indication that the larva utilizes fats; its fat reserves are formed from carbohydrate, protein, or both (von Kemnitz, 1916). From analogy with other insects it is probable that this fat is largely utilized during pupal rest and during the adult life of the fly.

A different question is whether parasites living normally chiefly anaerobically can utilize fat when kept under aerobic conditions. Histochemical evidence on explanted fat-containing tissues of *Ascaris* (Mueller, 1929) or on the intestinal cells of aerobically kept ascarids (Hirsch and Bretschneider, 1937) seems to point in this direction, but there is no chemical proof. No significant fat decrease was found in starving ascarids during the first 24 hours of life *in vitro* (von Brand, 1934b). If starvation was continued for 5 days, a small decrease in body fat occurred, but it was accounted for by the fat recovered from the expelled eggs (von Brand, 1941). However, it can be expected that the glycogen stores of the worms were not completely exhausted after such limited periods of starvation and it is possible that a different result would have been obtained if longer starvation periods would have been feasible. Some decrease in petroleum ether extract was observed after 10 hours' starvation in the cases of *Paramphistomum explanatum* and *Fasciola gigantica* (Goil, 1958), but the decreases appear not to be statistically significant. Under comparable conditions an apparently significant lipid increase was found in *Gastrothylax crumenifer*.

Small intestinal parasites and tissue parasites probably have *in vivo* a greater opportunity to procure oxygen in significant amounts than the large intestinal worms like *Ascaris*. It is conceivable that they might be adapted to utilize lipids oxidatively more readily than the latter. Possibly suggestive in this direction is the observation of Pflugfelder (1949) that microscopically demonstrable fat droplets remain visible in *Acanthocephalus ranae* up to 4 months' starving *in vivo,* but it is not clear to what extent the original reserves were actually depleted. Definite proof for lipid disappearance during aerobic starvation has been presented for larval *Trichinella spiralis* (von Brand *et al.,* 1952) by quantitative determination; in contrast no lipid disappeared during comparable periods of anaerobic starvation.

A clearly aerobic life is led by the free-living stages of parasitic nematodes. A definite starvation-induced decrease in morphologically demonstrable fat droplets has been reported for various species (Payne, 1923; Rogers, 1939; Giovannola, 1936; Elliott, 1954; Durie, 1957; Münnich, 1965). Although no quantitative determinations have been done in these cases, and despite justification of cautious interpretation of histochemical evidence alone, it is probably justified to conclude that many larvae of parasitic nematodes are able to utilize lipid reserves aerobically.

VII. DISTURBANCES IN THE HOST'S LIPID METABOLISM DURING PARASITIC INFECTIONS

The blood levels of some lipids appear to be quite variable in protozoan diseases. In infections with trypanosomes and leishmanias the blood cholesterol level has been reported as normal (Linton, 1930a,b; Scheff, 1932), increased (Launoy and Lagodsky, 1937; Ada and Fulton, 1948), or decreased (Lippi and Sebastiani, 1958). Similar contradictions exist in respect to the phospholipid and fatty acid levels during trypanosome infections (Randall, 1934, and the authors quoted above).

In human malaria low cholesterol levels have often been observed (Crespin and Zaky, 1919; Fairley and Bromfield, 1933; McQuarrie and Stoesser, 1932; Kopp and Solomon, 1943), but approximately normal values have also been reported (Ross, 1932; Greig *et al.,* 1934). Similarly, both normal and subnormal values have been encountered in simian malaria (Krishnan *et al.,* 1936; Kehar, 1937). Variable findings have also been reported concerning the phospholipid content of the blood of malarious humans and monkeys with a preponderance of low values (Kopp and Solomon, 1943; Whitmore and Roe, 1929; Kehar, 1937).

The lipids of the liver frequently show abnormalities in protozoan infections. It has thus been known for years (Scheff and Horner, 1932; Scheff and Csillag, 1936) that the neutral fat of the liver, in contrast to phospholipids and cholesterol, was considerably increased in *Trypanosoma equiperdum* infections. Lipid infiltration in this and other trypanosome infections could also be demonstrated histochemically. The patterns shown by this infiltration were variable, however, in respect to the morphologically visible amount of fat and its localization, both centrilobular and periportal infiltrations occurring (Hara *et al.,* 1955; Mercado and von Brand, 1960). In contrast, cultured chicken macrophages infected with *Leishmania donovani* had lost almost all their stainable lipids (Read and Chang, 1955).

In *Babesia canis* (Maegraith *et al.,* 1957) and *Plasmodium berghei* infections (von Brand and Mercado, 1958) pronounced centrilobular lipid infiltrations have been observed. In contrast, a periportal fat deposition has been found in monkeys infected with *Plasmodium knowlesi* and the same type of lesion occurred in noninfected animals which had been injected with the plasma of heavily infected ones (Ray, 1958; Ray and Sharma, 1958). In rodent malaria, the amount of fat deposited in the liver was directly correlated to the severity of the infection. Fractionation of the liver lipids showed that phospholipids and unsaponifiable matter increased only to an extent corresponding to the liver hypertrophy, while the fatty acids, derived primarily from triglycerides, increased to a much higher degree (von Brand and Mercado, 1958). It is justifiable to assume that the morphologically visible lipid infiltration was due primarily to an increase in triglycerides.

The mechanism responsible for the changes mentioned has not been fully elucidated. Circulatory difficulties leading to tissue anoxia may be involved, but the participation of some physiologically active substance produced by the parasites cannot be ruled out and is even perhaps probable (Maegraith, 1948, 1956; von Brand, 1959).

Only isolated relevant observations are available for helminthic infections. Fat absorption appears reduced in patients infected with *Ancylostoma duodenale, Necator americanus, Taenia saginata,* or *Hymenolepis diminuta* (Sheehy *et al.,* 1962; Ciauri and Mastandrea, 1960). Blood lipids are variable, just as described above for protozoan infections. Normal cholesterol levels have been reported from humans infected with *Trichinella spiralis* (Pierce *et al.,* 1939; Hartman *et al.,* 1940). They have been found increased in animals infected with *Clonorchis sinensis* (Shigenobu, 1932), *Schistosoma japonicum* (Hiromoto, 1939), and humans infected with filarias (Boyd and Roy, 1930), but lowered values were obtained in several patients infected with *Schistosoma mansoni* (Coutinho and Loureiro, 1960). Contradictory evidence has been presented for ancylostomiasis. Donomae (1927) reported a decrease in the fatty acid, lecithin, and cholesterol content of the serum, but an increase in all these fractions in the blood cells. Villela and Teixeira (1929), on the contrary, found an increased blood cholesterol level in their patients.

Hardly anything is known that would relate organ lipids to helminthic infections. Uyeno (1935) showed that liver homogenates of rabbits infected with *Clonorchis sinensis* had a reduced hydrolyzing action on tributyrin. Sawada *et al.* (1956) observed a generalized lipid infiltration of the liver of mice infected with *Schistosoma japonicum,* while Münnich (1958, 1959) found no distinct lipid abnormalities of the liver attributable to migrating *Ascaris* larvae. The lipids of the adrenals have been found reduced in several helminthic infections, the damage to the gland being especially pronounced in infections with *Fasciola hepatica* (Takagi, 1956). In *Trichinella* infection the lipid depletion of the adrenals was rapid during the early development of the worms in the intestine, but it accumulated again during the migration phase (Ritterson and Mauer, 1957). Finally, it was observed that the jejunal mucosa of rats infected with *Nippostrongylus muris* contained, in per cent of dry weight, the same amount of total lipids as mucosa from noninfected rats, but the phospholipids constituted 40 % of the total lipids in the former as contrasted to 15 % in the latter. No such difference was found in the epithelial cell brush borders (Symons and Fairbairn, 1963).

The fat content of crustaceans infected by other crustaceans has been determined repeatedly with widely varying results (Table XXXVIII).

TABLE XXXVIII

INFLUENCE OF PARASITIC CRUSTACEA ON THE FAT CONTENT OF THEIR HOSTS

Parasite	Host	Lipid content of host	References
Gyge brachialis	*Upogebia* ♂	Increased	Hughes (1940)
Gyge brachialis	*Upogebia* ♀	Normal	Hughes (1940)
Peltogaster paguri	*Pagurus* ♂♀	Decreased	Reinhard and von Brand (1944)
Peltogasterella socialis	*Pagurus* ♂♀	Increased	Oguro (1958)
Sacculina carcini	*Carcinus* ♂	Increased	Frentz and Veillet (1953)
Sacculina carcini	*Carcinus* ♀	Decreased	Frentz and Veillet (1953)
Sacculina neglecta	*Carcinus, Inachus*	Increased	Smith (1911, 1913); Robson (1911)
Septosaccus cuenoti	*Diogenes*	Decreased	Pierre (1935)
Septosaccus cuenoti	*Diogenes* ♂♀	Increased	Rudloff and Veillet (1954)
Stegophryxus hyptius	*Pagurus* ♂♀	Normal	Reinhard *et al.* (1947)

The only conclusion possible at the present time is that various species of parasitic crustacea have a different influence on the fat content and presumably on the lipid metabolism of their hosts. The mechanism of this interference is rather obscure and its full eludication will have to wait for metabolic studies. Smith (1911, 1913) and Robson (1911) are of the opinion that an alleged fat consumption of the parasites is responsible for the changes they observed. Reinhard and von Brand (1944), on the other hand, are inclined to incriminate the toxic action of sacculinids, which has been demonstrated rather conclusively by Lêvy (1923, 1924).

Only one observation is available that indicates abnormalities in fat metabolism of parasitized insects. Male *Thelia bimaculata* parasitized by *Aphelopus theliae* contain, according to Kornhauser (1919), 47% more lipids than normal males.

REFERENCES

Ada, G., and Fulton, J. D. (1948). *Brit. J. Exptl. Pathol.* **29,** 524–529.

Agosin, M., Brand, T. von, Rivera, G. F., and McMahon, P. (1957). *Exptl. Parasitol.* **6,** 37–51.

Armer, J. M. (1944). *J. Parasitol.* **30,** 131–142.

Arndt, W. (1922). *Verhandl. Deut. Zool. Ges.* pp. 76–78.

Artemov, N. M., and Lure, R. N. (1941). *Bull. Acad. Sci. URSS* **2,** 278–282.

Bacq. Z. M. (1941). *Ann. Soc. Roy. Zool. Belg.* **72,** 181–203.

Bacq, Z. M., and Oury, A. (1937). *Bull. Cl. Sci. Acad. Roy Belg.* [5] **23,** 891–893.

Ball, E. G., McKee, R. W., Anfinsen, C. B., Cruz, W. O., and Geiman, Q. M. (1948). *J. Biol. Chem.* **175,** 547–571.

Ball, G. H., and Chao, J. (1960). *Exptl. Parasitol.* **9,** 47–55.

Beames, C. G. (1964). *Exptl. Parasitol.* **15,** 387–396.

Beames, C. G., and Fisher, F. M. (1964). *Comp. Biochem. Physiol.* **13,** 401–412.

Becejac, S., Lui, A., Krvavica, S., and Kralj, N. (1964). *Vet. Arhiv (Zagreb)* **34,** 87–89.

Blacklock, D. B., Gordon, R. M., and Fine, J. (1930). *Ann. Trop. Med. Parasitol.* **24,** 5–54.

Bondouy, T. (1910). Thesis, University of Paris.

Bonê, G. J., and Parent, G. (1963). *J. Gen. Microbiol.* **31,** 261–266.

Boyd, T. C., and Roy, A. C. (1930). *Indian J. Med. Res.* **17,** 949–951.

Brand, T. von (1928). *Z. Vergleich. Physiol.* **8,** 613–624.

Brand, T. von (1933). *Z. Vergleich. Physiol.* **18,** 562–596.

Brand, T. von (1934a). *Ergeb. Biol.* **10,** 37–100.

Brand, T. von (1934b). *Z. Vergleich. Physiol.* **21,** 220–235.

Brand, T. von (1938). *J. Parasitol.* **24,** 445–451.

Brand, T. von (1939). *J. Parasitol.* **25,** 329–342.

Brand, T. von (1940). *J. Parasitol.* **26,** 301–307.

Brand, T. von (1941). *Proc. Soc. Exptl. Biol. Med.* **46,** 417–418.

Brand, T. von (1952). "Chemical Physiology of Endoparasitic Animals." Academic Press, New York.

Brand, T. von (1957). *Z. Tropenmed. Parasitol.* **8,** 21–23.

Brand, T. von (1959). *Z. Tropenmed. Parasitol.* **10,** 135–146.

Brand, T. von (1962). *Rev. Inst. Med. Trop. Sao Paulo* **4**, 53–60.

Brand, T. von, and Bowman, I. B. R. (1961). *Exptl. Parasitol.* **11**, 276–297.

Brand, T. von, and Mercado, T. I. (1958). *Am. J. Hyg.* **67**, 311–320.

Brand, T. von, and Weinland, E. (1924). *Z. Vergleich. Physiol.* **2**, 209–214.

Brand, T. von, and Winkeljohn, M. I. (1945). *Proc. Helminthol. Soc. Wash., D. C.* **12**, 62–65.

Brand, T. von, Weinstein, P. P., Mehlman, B., and Weinbach, E. C. (1952). *Exptl. Parasitol.* **1**, 245–255.

Brand, T. von, McMahon, P., Tobie, E. J., Thompson, M. J., and Mosettig, E. (1959). *Exptl. Parasitol.* **8**, 171–181.

Brand, T. von, Mercado, T. I., Nylen, M. U., and Scott, D. B. (1960). *Exptl. Parasitol.* **9**, 205–214.

Brault, A., and Loeper, M. (1904). *J. Physiol. Pathol. Gen.* **6**, 503–512.

Bueding, E. (1949). *J. Exptl. Med.* **89**, 107–130.

Bueding, E. (1952). *Brit. J. Pharmacol.* **7**, 563–566.

Bülbring, E., Lourie, E. M., and Pardoe, U. (1949). *Brit. J. Pharmacol.* **4**, 290–294.

Bullock, W. L. (1949a). *J. Morphol.* **84**, 185–200.

Bullock, W. L. (1949b). *J. Morphol.* **84**, 201–226.

Cailleau, R. (1936a). *Compt. Rend. Soc. Biol.* **121**, 424–425.

Cailleau, R. (1936b). *Compt. Rend. Soc. Biol.* **122**, 1027–1028.

Cailleau, R. (1937). *Ann. Inst. Pasteur* **59**, 137–172 and 293–328.

Cailleau, R. (1938). *Compt. Rend. Soc. Biol.* **127**, 861–863.

Califano, L., and Gritti, P. (1930). *Riv. Patol. Sper.* **5**, 9–15.

Cantrell, W. (1953). *J. Infect. Diseases* **93**, 219–221.

Cantrell, W., and Genazzani, E. (1955). *Arch. Ital. Sci. Farmacol.* [3] **5**, 234–238.

Carpenter, M. F. P. (1952). Thesis, University of Michigan [not seen, quoted in Fairbairn (1960)].

Cavier, R., Savel, J., and Monteoliva, M. (1958). *Bull. Soc. Chim. Biol.* **40**, 177–187.

Chance, M. R. A., and Mansour, T. E. (1953). *Brit. J. Pharmacol.* **8**, 134–138.

Cheissin, E. (1930). *Arch. Protistenk.* **70**, 531–618.

Chitwood, B. G. (1938). *Proc. Helminthol. Soc. Wash., D.C.* **5**, 68–75.

Chitwood, B. G., and Chitwood, M. B. (1938). *Proc. Helminthol. Soc. Wash., D. C.* **5**, 16–18.

Chitwood, B. G., and Jacobs, L. (1938). *J. Wash. Acad. Sci.* **28**, 12–13.

Ciauri, G., and Mastandrea, G. (1960). *Parassitologia* **2**, 93–94.

Cmelik, S. (1952). *Z. Physiol. Chem.* **289**, 78–79.

Cmelik, S., and Bartl, Z. (1956). *Z. Physiol. Chem.* **305**, 170–176.

Cohn, L. (1896). *Zool. Jahrb. Abt. Anat.* **9**, 227–272.

Cort, W. W. (1925). *Am. J. Hyg.* **5**, 49–89.

Cosgrove, W. B. (1959). *Can. J. Microbiol.* **5**, 573–578.

Coutelen, F. R. (1931). *Ann. Parasitol. Humaine Comp.* **9**, 97–100.

Coutinho, A., and Loureiro, P. (1960). *Anales Fac. Med. Univ. Recife* **20**, 27–49.

Cowperthwaite, J., Weber, M. M., Packer, L., and Hutner, S. H. (1953). *Ann. N.Y. Acad. Sci.* **56**, 972–981.

Crespin, J., and Zaky, A. (1919). *Compt. Rend. Soc. Biol.* **82**, 216–218.

Crites, J. L. (1958). *Ohio J. Sci.* **58**, 343–346.

Daniels, M. I. (1938). *Quart. J. Microscop. Sci.* **80**, Part II, 293–320.

Das Gupta, B. (1960). *Parasitology* **50**, 501–508.

Doflein, F. (1898). *Zool. Jahrb., Abt. Anat.* **11**, 281–350.

Donomae, I. (1927). *Japan. J. Med. Sci., Part 8* **1**, 385–412.

Durie, P. H. (1957). *Australian Vet. J.* pp. 305–306.

Dutta, G. P. (1958a). *Quart. J. Microscop. Sci.* **99**, 517–521.

Dutta, G. P. (1958b). *Res. Bull. Panjab Univ., Zool.* **143,** 97–106.

Dutta, G. P. (1959). *Res. Bull. Panjab Univ.* [N.S.] **10,** Part I, 13–19.

Dyrdowska, M. (1931). *Compt. Rend. Soc. Biol.* **108,** 593–596.

Elliott, A. (1954). *Exptl. Parasitol.* **3,** 307–320.

Engelbrecht, H. (1963). *Z. Parasitenk.* **23,** 384–389.

Engelbrecht, H., and Palm, V. (1964). *Z. Parasitenk.* **24,** 88–104.

Erdmann, R. (1917). *Arch. Protistenk.* **37,** 276–326.

Fairbairn, D. (1955a). *Can. J. Biochem. Physiol.* **33,** 31–37.

Fairbairn, D. (1955b). *Can. J. Biochem. Physiol.* **33,** 122–129.

Fairbairn, D. (1956). *Can. J. Biochem. Physiol.* **34,** 39–45.

Fairbairn, D. (1957). *Exptl. Parasitol.* **6,** 491–554.

Fairbairn, D. (1958). *Nature* **181,** 1593–1594.

Fairbairn, D. (1960). *In* "Nematology" (J. N. Sasser and W. R. Jenkins, eds.), pp. 267–296. Univ. of North Carolina Press, Chapel Hill, North Carolina.

Fairbairn, D., and Jones, R. N. (1956). *Can. J. Chem.* **34,** 182–184.

Fairbairn, D., and Passey, B. I. (1955). *Can. J. Biochem. Physiol.* **33,** 130–134.

Fairbairn, D., Wertheim, G., Harper, R. P., and Schiller, E. L. (1961). *Exptl. Parasitol.* **11,** 248–263.

Fairly, N. H., and Bromfield, R. J. (1933). *Trans. Roy. Soc. Trop. Med. Hyg.* **27,** 289–314.

Fauré-Fremiet, E. (1912). *Bull. Soc. Zool. France* **37,** 233–234.

Fauré-Fremiet, E. (1913a). *Arch. Anat. Microscop. (Paris)* **15,** 435–757.

Fauré-Fremiet, E. (1913b). *Compt. Rend. Soc. Biol.* **75,** 90–92.

Faust, E. S., and Tallqvist, T. W. (1907). *Arch. Exptl. Pathol. Pharmakol.* **57,** 367–385.

Flury, F. (1912). *Arch. Exptl. Pathol. Pharmakol.* **67,** 275–392.

Flury, F., and Leeb, F. (1926). *Klin. Wochschr.* **5,** 2054–2055.

Fouquey, C. (1961). Thesis, University of Paris.

Fouquey, C., Polonsky, J., and Lederer, E. (1957). *Bull. Soc. Chim. Biol.* **39,** 101–132.

Fox, H. M. (1953). *Nature* **171,** 162–163.

Frentz, R., and Veillet, A. (1953). *Compt. Rend.* **236,** 2168–2170.

Gerzeli, G. (1954a). *Riv. Istochim.* **1,** 91–94.

Gerzeli, G. (1954b). *Riv. Istochim.* **1,** 205–210.

Gerzeli, G. (1955). *Riv. Parasitol.* **16,** 209–215.

Gerzeli, G. (1959). *Acta Histochim.* **8,** 191–198.

Giovannola, A. (1935). *Arch. Ital. Sci. Med. Coloniali* **16,** 430–436.

Giovannola, A. (1936). *J. Parasitol.* **22,** 207–218.

Goil, M. M. (1958). *Z. Parasitenk.* **18,** 320–323.

Goil, M. M. (1964). *Parasitology* **54,** 81–85.

Goodchild, C. G., and Vilar-Alvarez, C. M. (1962). *J. Parasitol.* **48,** 379–383.

Grant, P. T., and Fulton, J. D. (1957). *Biochem. J.* **66,** 242–250.

Greig, E. D. W., Hendry, E. B., and Rooyen, C. E. van (1934). *J. Trop. Med. Hyg.* **37,** 289–295.

Gurwitsch, B. M. (1927). *Arch. Protistenk.* **59,** 369–372.

Gutierrez, J., Williams, P. P., Davis, R. E., and Warwick, E. J. (1962). *Appl. Microbiol.* **10,** 548–551.

Hack, M. H., Gussin, A. E., and Lowe, M. E. (1962a). *Comp. Biochem. Physiol.* **5,** 217–221.

Hack, M. H., Yaeger, R. G., and McCaffery, T. D. (1962b). *Comp. Biochem. Physiol.* **6,** 247–252.

Halevy, S. (1962). *Bull Res. Council Israel* **10E,** 65–68.

Halevy, S. (1963). *Proc. Soc. Exptl. Biol. Med.* **113,** 47–48.

Halevy, S., and Girsy, O. (1964). *Proc. Soc. Exptl. Biol. Med.* **117,** 552–555.

Hamann, O. (1891). *Jena. Z. Naturw.* **25**, 113–231.

Hara, K., Oka, S., Takagi, K., Nagata, K., and Sawada, T. (1955). *Gunma J. Med. Sci.* **4**, 291–301.

Hartman, E., Foote, M., and Pierce, H. B. (1940). *Am. J. Hyg.* **31**, Sect. D, 74–75.

Harvey, S. C. (1949). *J. Biol. Chem.* **179**, 435–453.

Hedrick, R. M. (1958). *J. Parasitol.* **44**, 75–84.

Hiromoto, T. (1939). *Mitt. Med. Ges. Okayama* **51**, 1637 (German summary).

Hirsch, G. C., and Bretschneider, L. H. (1937). *Cytologia (Tokyo)* Fujii Jubilee Vol., 424–436.

House, H. L. (1954a). *Can. J. Zool.* **32**, 331–341.

House, H. L. (1954b). *Can. J. Zool.* **32**, 358–365.

Hughes, T. E. (1940). *J. Exptl. Biol.* **17**, 331–336.

Hunter, N. W. (1957). *Trans. Am. Microscop. Soc.* **76**, 36–45.

I-Hsun-Ho (1963). *Tung Wu Hsueh Pao* **15**, 363–370; *Chem Abstr.* **60**, 11101 (1964).

Ikejiani, O. (1947). *Am. J. Hyg.* **45**, 144–149.

Jacobs, L., and Jones, M. F. (1939). *Proc. Helminthol. Soc. Wash., D.C.* **6**, 57–60.

Joyet-Lavergne, P. (1926). *Arch. Anat. Microscop. (Paris)* **22**, 1–17.

Kedrowsky, B. (1931). *Z. Zellforsch. Mikroskop. Anat.* **12**, 666–714.

Kehar, N. D. (1937). *Records Malaria Survey India* **7**, 117–129.

Kemnitz, G. von (1912). *Arch. Zellforsch.* **7**, 463–603.

Kemnitz, G. von (1916). *Z. Biol.* **67**, 129–244.

Kent, N., Macheboeuf, M., and Neiadas, B. (1948). *Experientia* **4**, 193–194.

Kessel, R. G., Prestage, J. J., Sekhon, S. S., Smalley, R. L., and Beams, H. W. (1961). *Trans. Am. Microscop. Soc.* **80**, 103–118.

Kilejian, A., Sauer, K., and Schwabe, C. W. (1962). *Exptl. Parasitol.* **12**, 377–392.

Kligler, I. J., and Olitzki, L. (1936). *Ann. Trop. Med. Parasitol.* **30**, 287–291.

Kopp, I., and Solomon, H. C. (1943). *Am. J. Med. Sci.* **205**, 90–97.

Korn, E. D., and Greenblatt, C. L. (1963). *Science* **142**, 1301–1303.

Korn, E. D., Greenblatt, C. L., and Lees, A. M. (1965). *Lipid Res.* **6**, 43–50.

Kornhauser, S. I. (1919). *J. Morphol.* **32**, 531–636.

Krijgsman, B. J. (1936a). *Natuurw. Tijdschr. (Belg.)* **18**, 237–241.

Krijgsman, B. J. (1936b). *Z. Vergleich. Physiol.* **23**, 663–711.

Krishnan, K. V., Ghosh, B. M., and Bose, P. N. (1936). *Records Malaria Survey India* **6**, 1–12.

Kublickiene, O. (1963). *Lietuvos TSR Mokslu Akad. Darbai, Ser. C* pp. 79–84; *Chem. Abstr.* **61**, 1010. (1964)

Launoy, L. L., and Lagodsky, H. (1937). *Bull. Soc. Pathol. Exotique* **30**, 57–68.

Lavette, A. (1964). *Compt. Rend.* **258**, 1106–1108.

Lee, D. L. (1958). *Parasitology* **48**, 437–447.

Lee, D. L. (1960). *Parasitology* **50**, 247–259.

Lee, D. L. (1961). *Nature* **192**, 282–283.

Lee, D. L. (1962). *Parasitology* **52**, 103–112.

Lee, D. L., Rothman, A. H., and Senturia, J. B. (1963). *Exptl. Parasitol.* **14**, 285–295.

Lenel, R. (1954). *Compt. Rend.* **238**, 948–949.

Lesuk, A., and Anderson, R. J. (1941). *J. Biol. Chem.* **139**, 457–469.

Levenbook, L. (1951). *J. Exptl. Biol.* **28**, 173–180.

Lêvy, R. (1923). *Bull. Soc. Zool. France* **48**, 291–294.

Lêvy, R. (1924). *Bull. Soc. Zool. France* **49**, 333–336.

Lindblom, G. P. (1961). *J. Protozool.* **8**, 139–150.

Linton, R. W. (1930a). *J. Exptl. Med.* **52**, 103–111.

Linton, R. W. (1930b). *J. Exptl. Med.* **52**, 695–700.

Lippi, M., and Sebastiani, A. (1958). *Arch. Ital. Sci. Med. Trop. Parassitol.* **5**, 327–335.

Lui, A., Coric, D., and Krvavica, S. (1964). *Vet. Arhiv. (Zagreb)* **34**, 84–86.

Lund, P. G., and Shorb, M. S. (1962). *J. Protozool.* **9**, 151–154.

McMahon, P. (1961). *Exptl. Parasitol.* **11**, 156–160.

McQuarrie, I., and Stoesser, A. V. (1932). *Proc. Soc. Exptl. Biol. Med.* **29**, 1281–1283.

Maegraith, B. G. (1948). "Pathological Processes in Malaria and Blackwater Fever." Thomas, Springfield, Illinois.

Maegraith, B. G. (1956). *Ann. Soc. Belge Med. Trop.* **36**, 623–629.

Maegraith, B. G., Gilles, H. M., and Devakul, K. Z. (1957). *Z. Tropenmed. Parasitol.* **8**, 485–514.

Mandlowitz, S., Dusanic, D., and Lewert, R. M. (1960). *J. Parasitol.* **46**, 89–90.

Mannozzi-Torini, M. (1940). *Arch. Sci. Biol. (Italy)* **26**, 565–580.

Marzullo, F., Squadrini, F., and Taparelli, F. (1957). *Boll. Soc. Med.-Chir. Modena* **57**, 84–88.

Medina, H., Amaral, D., and Bacila, M. (1955). *Arquiv. Biol. Tecnol. Inst. Biol. Pesquisas Tecnol.* **10**, 103–119.

Mellanby, H. (1955). *Parasitology* **45**, 287–294.

Mercado, T. I., and Brand, T. von (1960). *J. Infect. Diseases* **106**, 95–105.

Meyer, A. (1931). *Z. Zellforsch. Mikroskop. Anat.* **14**, 255–265.

Monné, L. (1955). *Arkiv Zool.* [2] **9**, 93–113.

Monné, L., and Hönig, G. (1954a). *Arkiv Zool.* [2] **6**, 559–562.

Monné, L., and Hönig, G. (1954b). *Arkiv Zool.* [2] **7**, 261–272.

Monteoliva, M. (1960). *Rev. Iberica Parasitol.* **20**, 573–589.

Moraczewski, S. A., and Kelsey, F. E. (1948). *J. Infect. Diseases* **82**, 45–51.

Morrison, D. B., and Jeskey, H. A. (1947). *Federation Proc.* **6**, 279.

Moulder, J. W. (1948). *J. Infect. Diseases* **83**, 33–41.

Mueller, J. F. (1929). *Z. Zellforsch. Mikroskop. Anat.* **8**, 361–403.

Münnich, H. (1958). *Naturwiss.* **45**, 551–552.

Münnich, H. (1959). *Wiss. Z. Humboldt-Univ. Berlin, Math.-Naturw. Reihe* **9**, 389–403.

Münnich, H. (1962). *Naturwiss.* **49**, 66–67.

Münnich, H. (1965). *Z. Parasitenk.* **25**, 231–239.

Nadakal, A. M. (1960). *J. Parasitol.* **46**, 777–786.

Nath, V., Gupta, B. L., and Kochhar, D. M. (1961). *Quart. J. Microscop. Sci.* **102**, Part I, 39–50.

Newton, B. A. (1956). *Nature* **177**, 279–280.

Nomura, H. (1957). *J. Keio Med. Assoc.* **34**, 75–88.

Oesterlin, M., and Brand, T. von (1934). *Z. Vergleich. Physiol.* **20**, 251–254.

Ogimoto, S. (1956). *Fukuoka Acta Med.* **47**, 1077–1091.

Oguro, C. (1958). *J. Fac. Sci. Hokkaido Univ., Ser. VI* **14**, 64–68.

Palm. V. (1962). *Z. Parasitenk.* **22**, 261–266.

Pantelouris, E. M., and Threadgold, L. T. (1963). *Cellule* **64**, 63–67.

Panzer, T. (1913). *Z. Physiol. Chem.* **86**, 33–42.

Passey, R. F., and Fairbairn, D. (1957). *Can. J. Biochem. Physiol.* **35**, 511–525.

Patillo, W. H., and Becker, E. R. (1955). *J. Morphol.* **96**, 61–96.

Payne, F. K. (1922). *Am. J. Hyg.* **2**, 254–263.

Payne, F. K. (1923). *Am. J. Hyg.* **3**, 547–583.

Pennoit-DeCooman, E. (1940). *Ann. Soc. Roy. Zool. Belg.* **71**, 76–77.

Pennoit-DeCooman, E., and Grembergen, G. van (1942). *Verhandel. Koninkl. Vlaam. Acad. Wetenschap. Belg., Kl. Wetenschap.* **4**, No. 6, 7–77.

Pepler, W. J. (1958). *J. Histochem. Cytochem.* **6**, 139–141.

Petruschewsky, G. K. (1932). *Arch. Protistenk.* **78**, 542–556.

Pflugfelder, O. (1949). *Z. Parasitenk.* **14**, 274–280.

Pierce, H. B., Hartman, E., Simcox, W. J., Aitken, T., Meservey, A. B., and Farnham, W. B. (1939). *Am. J. Hyg.* **29**, Sect. D, 75–81.

Pierre, M. (1935). *Trav. Sta. Biol. Roscoff* **13**, 179–208.

Pintner, T. (1922). *Sitzber. Akad. Wiss. Wien, Math.-Naturw. Kl., Abt. I* **131**, 129–138.

Polonsky, J., Fouquey, C., Ferreol, G., and Lederer, E. (1955). *Compt. Rend.* **240**, 2265–2267.

Prenant, M. (1922). *Arch. Morphol. Gen. Exptl.* **5**, 1–474.

Pylkkö, O. O. (1956a). *Ann. Med. Exptl. Biol. Fenniae (Helsinki)* **34**, Suppl. 8, 1–81.

Pylkkö, O. O. (1956b). *Ann. Med. Exptl. Biol. Fenniae (Helsinki)* **34**, 328–334.

Randall, R. (1934). *Philippine J. Sci.* **53**, 97–105.

Rao, K. H. (1959). *Experientia* **15**, 464.

Rao, K. H. (1960). *Parasitology* **50**, 349–350.

Ray, A. P. (1958). *Indian J. Med. Res.* **46**, 359–367.

Ray, A. P., and Sharma, G. K. (1958). *Indian J. Med. Res.* **46**, 367–376.

Read, C. P., and Chang, P. (1955). *J. Parasitol.* **41**, Suppl., 21.

Reid, W. M. (1942). *J. Parasitol.* **28**, 319–340.

Reinhard, E. G., and Brand, T. von (1944). *Physiol. Zool.* **17**, 31–41.

Reinhard, E. G., Brand, T. von, and McDuffie, S. F. (1947). *Proc. Helminthol. Soc. Wash., D.C.* **14**, 69–73.

Reznik, G. K. (1963). *Trudy Vses. Inst. Gel'mintol.* **10**, 245–250.

Ritterson, A. L., and Mauer, S. I. (1957). *Science* **126**, 1293–1294.

Roberts, L. S. (1961). *Exptl. Parasitol.* **11**, 332–371.

Robson, G. C. (1911). *Quart J. Microscop. Sci.* **57**, 267–278.

Rogers, W. P. (1939). *J. Helminthol.* **17**, 195–202.

Rogers, W. P. (1940). *J. Helminthol.* **18**, 183–192.

Rogers, W. P. (1941). *J. Helminthol.* **19**, 35–46.

Rogers, W. P., and Lazarus, M. (1949). *Parasitology* **39**, 302–314.

Rohde, R. A. (1960). *Proc. Helminthol. Soc. Wash., D.C.* **27**, 121–123.

Rohrbacher, G. H. (1957). *J. Parasitol.* **43**, 9–18.

Ross, G. R. (1932). *Mem. London Sch. Trop. Med.* **6**, 1–262.

Roy, D. N. (1937). *Parasitology* **29**, 150–162.

Rudloff, O., and Veillet, A. (1954). *Compt. Rend. Soc. Biol.* **148**, 1464–1467.

Saefftigen, A. (1885). *Morphol. Jahrb.* **10**, 120–171.

Salisbury, L. F., and Anderson, R. J. (1939). *J. Biol. Chem.* **129**, 505–517.

Sanders, M. (1957). *J. Protozool.* **4**, 118–119.

Sassuchin, D. N. (1928). *Arch. Protistenk.* **64**, 71–92.

Sawada, T., Hara, K., Takagi, K., Nagazawa, Y., and Oka, S. (1956). *Am. J. Trop. Med. Hyg.* **5**, 847–859.

Scheff, G. (1932). *Biochem. Z.* **248**, 168–180.

Scheff, G., and Csillag, Z. (1936). *Arch. Exptl. Pathol. Pharmakol.* **183**, 467–477.

Scheff, G., and Horner, E. (1932). *Biochem. Z.* **248**, 181–188.

Schiefferdecker, P. (1874). *Jena. Z. Naturw.* **8**, 458–487.

Schimmelpfennig, G. (1903). *Arch. Wiss. Prakt. Tierheilk.* **29**, 332–376.

Schmidt, W. J. (1930). *Zool. Jahrb., Abt. Allgem. Zool. Physiol.* **47**, 249–258.

Schulte, H. (1917). *Arch. Ges. Physiol.* **166**, 1–44.

Schulz, F. N., and Becker, M. (1933). *Biochem. Z.* **276**, 253–259.

Schwabe, C. W. (1957). *Am. J. Hyg.* **65**, 325–337.

Schwabe, C. W. (1959). *J. Trop. Med. Hyg.* **8**, 20–28.

Schwabe, C. W., Koussa, M., and Acra, A. N. (1961). *Comp. Biochem. Physiol.* **2**, 161–172.

Sebek, O. K., and Michaels, R. M. (1957). *Nature* **179,** 210–211.

Senft, A. W., and Senft, D. G. (1962). *J. Parasitol.* **48,** 551–554.

Sheehy, T. W., Meroney, W. H., Cox, R. S., and Soler, J. E. (1962). *Gastroenterology* **42,** 148–156.

Shigenobu, T. (1932). *Mitt. Med. Ges. Okayama* **44,** 1099–1112.

Shorb, M. S. (1963). *In* "Progress in Protozoology" (J. Ludvik *et al.,* eds.), pp. 153–158. Czech. Acad. Sci. Prague.

Smith, G. (1911). *Quart. J. Microscop. Sci.* **57,** 251–265.

Smith, G. (1913). *Quart. J. Microscop. Sci.* **59,** 267–295.

Smorodincev, I. A., and Bebesin, K. W. (1935). *Biochem. Z.* **276,** 271–273.

Smorodincev, I. A., and Bebesin, K. W. (1936a). *J. Biochem. (Tokyo)* **23,** 19–20.

Smorodincev, I. A., and Bebesin, K. W. (1936b). *J. Biochem. (Tokyo)* **23,** 21–22.

Smorodincev, I. A., and Bebesin, K. W. (1936c). *J. Biochem. (Tokyo)* **23,** 23–25.

Smorodincev, I. A., and Bebesin, K. W. (1936d). *Compt. Rend. Acad. Sci. URSS* [N.S.] **2,** 189–191.

Smorodincev, I. A., and Bebesin, K. W. (1939). *Bull. Soc. Chim. Biol.* **21,** 478–482.

Smorodincev, I. A., Bebesin, K. W., and Pawlowa, P. I. (1933). *Biochem. Z.* **261,** 176–178.

Smyth, J. D. (1947). *Biol. Rev. Cambridge Phil. Soc.* **22,** 214–238.

Smyth, J. D. (1949). *J. Exptl. Biol.* **26,** 1–14.

Stein, G. A. (1963). *In* "Progress in Protozoology" (J. Ludvik *et al.,* eds.), pp. 294–295. Czech. Acad. Sci. Prague.

Stephenson, W. (1947). *Parasitology* **38,** 140–144.

Sukhanova, K. M. (1963). *In* "Progress in Protozoology" (J. Ludvik *et al.,* eds.), p. 296. Czech. Acad. Sci., Prague.

Symons, L. E. A., and Fairbairn, D. (1963). *Exptl. Parasitol.* **13,** 284–304.

Szwejkowska, G. (1929). *Bull. Intern. Acad. Polon. Sci., Cl. Sci. Math. Nat.* **B1928,** 489–519.

Takagi, K. (1956). *Gunma J. Med. Sci.* **5,** 190–208.

Takagi, K. (1962). *Tukushima J. Exptl. Med.* **9,** 60–66.

Tatchell, R. J. (1958). *Parasitology* **48,** 448–458.

Taylor, A. E. R. (1963). *Exptl. Parasitol.* **14,** 304–310.

Thompson, M. J., Mosettig, E., and Brand, T. von (1960). *Exptl. Parasitol.* **9,** 127–130.

Tötterman, G., and Kirk, E. (1939). *Nord. Med.* **3,** 2715–2716.

Trager, W. (1957). *J. Protozool.* **4,** 269–276.

Uyeno, H. (1935). *Mitt. Med. Ges. Okayama* **47,** 1094–1108.

Van Cleave, H. J., and Rausch, R. L. (1950). *J. Parasitol.* **36,** 278–283.

Van de Vijver, G. (1964). *Exptl. Parasitol.* **15,** 97–105.

Villela, G. G., and Teixeira, J. C. (1929). *Mem. Inst. Oswaldo Cruz* Suppl. 6, 62–68.

Vogel, H., and Brand, T. von (1933). *Z. Parasitenk.* **5,** 425–431.

von Brand, T., *see* Brand, T. von

von Kemnitz, G., *see* Kemnitz, G. von

Waitz, J. A. (1963). *J. Parasitol.* **49,** 73–80.

Wantland, W. W., Wantland, E. M., and Weidman, T. A. (1962). *J. Parasitol.* **48,** 305.

Warren, Mc., and Daugherty, J. (1957). *J. Parasitol.* **43,** 521–526.

Weinland, E. (1901). *Z. Biol.* **42,** 55–90.

Weinland, E., and Brand, T. von (1926). *Z. Vergleich. Physiol.* **4,** 212–285.

Weinstein, P. P. (1949). *J. Parasitol.* **35,** Suppl., 14.

Whitmore, E. R., and Roe, J. H. (1929). *Rept. Med. Dept. United Fruit Co. (Boston)* **18,** 59 (not seen).

Williams, P. P., Gutierrez, J., and Davis, R. E. (1963). *Appl. Microbiol.* **11,** 260–264.

Williamson, J. (1963). *Proc. 16th Intern. Congr. Zool., Washington, D. C., 1963* Vol. 4, pp. 189–195.

Wilson, P. A. G., and Fairbairn, D. (1961). *J. Protozool.* **8,** 410–416.
Wottge, K. (1937). *Protoplasma* **29,** 31–59.
Wotton, R. M. (1963). *Intern. Rev. Cytol.* **15,** 399–420.
Wotton, R. M., and Becker, D. A. (1963). *Parasitology* **53,** 163–167.
Wotton, R. M., and Halsey, H. R. (1957). *Parasitology* **47,** 427–431.
Wright, D. E. (1959). *Nature* **184,** 875–876.
Wyss, W., Kradolfer, F., and Meier, R. (1960a). *Experientia* **16,** 141–142.
Wyss, W., Kradolfer, F., and Meier, R. (1960b). *Exptl. Parasitol.* **10,** 66–71.
Yokogawa, M., and Yoshimura, H. (1957). *Kiseichugaku Zasshi* **6,** 546–554.
Zawadowsky, M. (1928). *Trans. Lab. Exptl. Biol., Zoopark, Moscow* **4,** 201–206.

Chapter 6

PROTEINS

I. TOTAL PROTEIN CONTENT AND PROTEIN FRACTIONS

The protein content of parasites (Table XXXIX) often has been calculated, as is customary for free-living organisms, by multiplying the experimentally determined N content by 6.25, or one of the other conventional factors. While this procedure undoubtedly gives fairly accurate values in many instances, its validity is open to question (Reid, 1942; J. W. Campbell, 1960) when an organism contains an abnormally large amount of nonprotein N. In this connection cestodes, in which Eisenbrandt (1938), Salisbury and Anderson (1939), and J. W. Campbell (1960) found 10 to 16% of the total N to consist of nonprotein N, must be mentioned. Campbell's (1960) figures for protein (Table XXXIX) are derived from his determinations of the protein carboxyl nitrogen and are characteristically lower than those obtained by other authors. There are clear indications, however, that in some cestodes the conventional procedure is acceptable (von Brand and Bowman, 1961). In evaluating the data of Table XXXIX it should be kept in mind that the percentage of protein depends largely on the amounts of nonprotein reserve substances present at any one time in a given parasite. Interesting in this connection is Goodchild's (1961) finding that *Hymenolepis diminuta* isolated from adequately fed rats contained 32% protein, while the corresponding figure for worms taken from starved rats was 59.5%.

The soluble proteins of some parasites have been fractionated in a few instances by physical methods, largely in attempts to localize antigens of protein nature. Desowitz (1959) and Williamson and Desowitz (1961) subjected particle-free supernatants of homogenates prepared from several trypanosome species to electrophoretic analysis and usually obtained four fractions, one of which, however, did not occur regularly. Subsequent centrifugal fractionation of *Trypanosoma rhodesiense*

231

TABLE XXXIX

PROTEIN CONTENT[a] OF SOME PARASITES[b]

Species	Protein in per cent of dry substance	References
Flagellates		
Trypanosoma cruzi, culture form	43–53	von Brand *et al.* (1959)
Sporozoa		
Eimeria acervulina, oocysts	41	Wilson and Fairbairn (1961)
Ciliates		
Entodinium caudatum	25	Abou Akkada and Howard (1960)
Trematodes		
Fasciola hepatica	58	Weinland and von Brand (1926)
Fasciola gigantica	67	Goil (1958)
Gastrothylax crumenifer	49	Goil (1958)
Paramphistomum explanatum	53	Goil (1958)
Cestodes		
Cittotaenia perplexa	21	J. W. Campbell (1960)
Echinococcus granulosus, scoleces	61	Agosin *et al.* (1957)
Hymenolepis diminuta	32–33	Goodchild (1961); Goodchild and Vilar-Alvarez (1962)
Moniezia expansa	22	J. W. Campbell (1960)
Raillietina cesticillus	36	Reid (1942)
Schistocephalus solidus, plerocercoids	36	Hopkins (1950)
Taenia taeniaeformis, larval	27–29	von Brand and Bowman (1961)
Taenia taeniaeformis, adult	45	von Brand and Bowman (1961)
Thysanosoma actinioides	29	J. W. Campbell (1960)
Nematodes		
Ascaris lumbricoides	48–57	Weinland (1901); Flury (1912); Smorodincev and Bebesin (1936c); Savel (1954)
Acanthocephala		
Macracanthorhynchus hirudinaceus	70	von Brand (1939)
Arthropods		
Gastrophilus intestinalis, larval	43	von Kemnitz (1916)

[a] $N \times 6.25$

[b] Data on additional species of helminths, or additional data on species listed above, will be found in the following papers: von Brand (1933); Smorodincev and Bebesin (1936a,b); Smorodincev *et al.* (1933); Wardle (1937); Salisbury and Anderson (1939).

homogenates (K. N. Brown and Williamson, 1964) demonstrated highest antigen concentration in the cell sap fraction. Further analysis by the Ouchterlony immunodiffusion test and other methods revealed that the antigens are manifold, but no details will be given here, since the chemical nature of the antigens has not yet been clarified. It may be mentioned that according to Williamson and Brown (1964) the variant-specific antigens of *Trypanosoma rhodesiense* consist of two groups of unconjugated proteins. The major group has a molecular weight of $5-16 \times 10^4$ and its antigenicity apparently depends on tertiary hydrogen-bonded structures, probably involving tyrosine. The minor group has a molecular weight of $1-2 \times 10^4$, is diffusible through cellophane, and only incompletely precipitated by trichloracetic acid.

While there is no indication that the above antigens have polysaccharide or lipopolysaccharide components (Williamson and Brown, 1964), it should be recalled (see Chapter 2) that in *Trypanosoma cruzi* (Gonçalves and Yamaha, 1959) and *Trichomonas foetus* (Feinberg and Morgan, 1953) antigenic fractions have been found which are conjugates of proteins and polysaccharides. Similarly, in helminths conjugated proteins are potent antigens. N. H. Kent (1963) has pointed out that the relevant heteroproteins are often complexed with carbohydrates, usually glycogen. From *Ascaris lumbricoides,* for instance, he isolated five protein fractions. One was carbohydrate-free and was only weakly antigenic, the others were more strongly antigenic and contained from 14 to 76.5 % carbohydrate. Similarly, aqueous extracts of *Trichinella spiralis* larvae contained large amounts of protein-bound carbohydrate (N. H. Kent, 1963). The complexity of the antigens is illustrated by the observation of Tanner and Gregory (1961) that the larvae contain at least eleven electrophoretically distinct saline-soluble antigens. Four moved like human γ-globulin, one each like β_1- and β_2-globulins and albumin, while two each moved like α_1- and α_2-globulins. In the case of *Echinococcus granulosus,* fractionation of the hydatid fluid yielded three protein fractions and that of the cyst eight fractions (N. H. Kent, 1963). The major fraction of both preparations had the electrophoretic mobility of serum albumin (Del Bono, 1955; Kagan and Norman, 1961; Goodchild and Kagan, 1961; N. H. Kent, 1963). As a final example the antigenic fractions of *Schistosoma mansoni* may be mentioned. Biguet *et al.* (1962) isolated by electrophoresis five proteins, five glycoproteins, and one lipoprotein fraction.

Data on electrophoretic separation of proteins are also available for the perivisceral fluid of *Ascaris,* but in these cases no attempts were made to identify the various fractions with antigens. Savel (1954) and Benedictov (1962) both found that the albumin fraction corresponded to more than 50% of the total proteins. The former author reported in addition small amounts of α- and β-globulin, as well as the surprisingly high value of 31.7% γ-globulin, a figure in approximate agreement with that reported by Yasuo (1961). The occurrence of phospholipoproteins, glucoproteins, and acetal lipoprotein in three to four fractions of the *Ascaris* perivisceral fluid has been observed by Giraldo Cardona (1960).

Older data on fractionation of proteins of cestodes and roundworms will be found in the papers by E. S. Faust and Tallqvist (1907); Smorodincev and Pawlowa (1936); F. N. Kent (1947); Bondouy (1910); and Flury (1912).

Insoluble proteins, the scleroproteins or albuminoids, have essentially a supporting or protective function and hence are widely distributed among both parasites and free-living organisms. The cyst walls of such protozoa as *Entamoeba histolytica, Endolimax nana,* and *Giardia lamblia* (Kofoid *et al.,* 1931), or the spore wall of *Goussia gadi* (Panzer, 1911, 1913) have been thought to consist of a keratin- or elastin-like albuminoid. However, more recent investigators (Monné and Hönig, 1954a; Ratnayake, 1960) identified the main component of the coccidian or gregarine oocyst walls as a quinone-tanned protein, that is, a tanned collagen.

True keratin, a protein with molecules cross-linked by cystine bridges, probably occurs only in vertebrates (C. H. Brown, 1949), but keratin-like proteins have been described from the external cortical layer of the *Ascaris* cuticle (Chitwood, 1936), as well as from the cortical layer of the cuticle, the esophageal, and cloacal linings of several other nematode species (Chitwood, 1938b). A similar protein perhaps occurs also in the cuticle of Acanthocephala; suggestive in this connection is Mueller's (1929) finding that the cuticle of *Macracanthorhynchus* contains 14.78% N and 0.564% S. The best evidence, however, for a keratin-like protein in helminths has been provided by Gallagher's (1964) investigation of the hooks of *Echinococcus granulosus;* his findings fully support the earlier experiments of Dollfus (1942) and Crusz (1947, 1948). Gallagher (1964) bases his identification on elemental analysis (15.6% N, 5.6% S), the amino acid composition of hydrolyzates (Table XL), and the fact that the hooks were resistant to digestion with ficin, papain, and trypsin. The substance found in the hooks differs from typical vertebrate keratin by its higher aspartic acid, tyrosine, and histidine, and its lower glutamic acid content. Histochemical evidence for keratin-like proteins, finally, is available for the fibrillar coat of the embryonic envelopes of some Acanthocephala (Monné and Hönig, 1954b; Monné, 1955a) and the primary eggshell of *Contracoecum osculatum* (Monné, 1963).

Excellent evidence has been presented for the occurrence of collagen

TABLE XL

AMINO ACIDS ISOLATED FROM SOME PARASITES[a,b]

Amino acid	Trypanosomidae (8 species) (1) Protein and free acids	Trichomonas foetus (2) Free acids	E. granulosus (3–6a) Cyst fluid, free acids	Cyst fluid, protein acids	Membrane proteins	Hooks	Moniezia expansa (7)	Posthodiplostomum minimum (8) Body	Cyst	Anuran lung flukes (9)	Ascaris lumbricoides (10–15) Body	Ovary, free acids	Ovary, protein acids	Perienteric fluid	Larvae	Egg, protein coat	Egg, middle coat	Egg, vitelline membrane	Adult, cuticle	Gastrophilus intestinalis (16) Larval hemolymph
Alanine	X	X	X	X	X		X	X	X	X	X	X	X	X	X				X	X
Glycine	X	X	X	X	X		X			X	X	X	X	X	X	X	X		X	X
Valine	X	X	X	X	X	X		X	X	X	X	X	X	X	X	X			X	X
Leucine	X	X	X	X	X	X	X	X	X	X	X	X	X	X	X	X		X	X	X
Isoleucine	X	X	X	X	X	X	X	X	X		X						X	X	X	X
Proline	X	X	X	X	X	X	X				X	X	X	X	X	X	X	X	X	X
Phenylalanine	X	X	X	X	X	X		X	X		X	X	X	X	X	X		X	X	X
Tyrosine	X	X	X	X	X	X		X	X		X	X	X	X	X	X	X	X	X	X
Serine	X	X	X	X				X	X		X	X	X	X	X	X	X		X	X
Threonine	X	X	X	X	X	X		X	X	X	X	X	X	X	X				X	
Cystine	X		X	X	X											X	X	X	X	X
Cysteine	X	X								X	X	X								
Methionine		X	X		X											X	X	X	X	
Arginine	X	X	X	X	X	X	X	X	X		X						X	X	X	X
Lysine	X	X	X	X	X			X	X		X	X	X	X	X	X			X	X
Histidine	X	X	X				X	X			X	X	X	X	X	X			X	X
Aspartic acid	X	X	X	X	X		X	X	X		X	X	X	X	X	X	X	X	X	X
Glutamic acid	X	X	X	X	X	X		X	X		X	X	X	X	X	X			X	X
Hydroxyproline			X																X	
Tryptophane			X	X			X				X	X	X	X	X	X				
Ornithine		X	X																	
Asparagine			X								X									
Glutamine											X	X								

[a] Further data on additional species or additional data for some of the species mentioned above will be found in the following papers: protozoa: Becker and Geiman (1954); Mehra et al. (1960); helminths: Aldrich et al. (1954); Savel (1954); Bird (1954); Ogimoto (1956); Goodchild and Wells (1957); J. W. Campbell (1960, 1963a); Monteoliva et al. (1962).

[b] KEY: (1) Williamson and Desowitz (1961); (2) Johnson (1962); (3) Sanz Perez (1956); (4) Mastandrea et al. (1962); (5) Popov and Sorokin (1962); (6) Pozzi and Pirosky (1953); (6a) Gallagher (1964); (7) F. N. Kent (1947); (8) Lynch and Bogitsh (1962); (9) Goodchild and Vilar-Alvarez (1955); (10) Flury (1912); (11) Yoshimura (1930); (12) Pollak and Fairbairn (1955a); (13) Salmenkova (1962); (14) Jaskoski (1962); (15) Watson and Silvester (1958); (16) Levenbook (1950).

in the cuticle and other structures of nematodes, especially *Ascaris*. Characteristic X-ray diffraction patterns have been reported (Fauré-Fremiet and Garrault, 1944; Picken *et al.*, 1947), but some differences to vertebrate collagens have been found (Watson and Silvester, 1958). Chemical analysis of the cuticle (Table XL) revealed all the common amino acids; especially characteristic for collagen is hydroxyproline, which repeatedly has been found in abundance (Bird, 1956, 1957; Bird and Rogers, 1956; Simmonds, 1958: Watson and Silvester, 1958). Furthermore, the cuticle of *Ascaris* (with the exception of the cortical layer), the basal lamella of the intestine, and the sheaths surrounding the muscle cells disappear upon incubation with collagenase (Dawson, 1960).

The chemical constitution of the external cortex of *Ascaris* cuticle is somewhat obscure. It is high in sulfur-containing amino acids (4.42% S), does not appear to contain hydroxyproline, but does contain a fairly high percentage of tyrosine, features not usually associated with collagen (Savel, 1954). The ratio histidine:lysine:arginine of 1:5:13 is considered by Savel (1954) to be within the range of keratins. On the other hand, the cortex contains polyphenols and polyphenol oxidase (C. H. Brown, 1950; Monné, 1955b; Bird, 1957), which are usually found when tanning of collagen occurs. D. Fairbairn (1960) has pointed out that if any tanning occurs, it cannot be pronounced since a well-known by-product of tanning, color development, is essentially missing in the nematode cuticle. Furthermore, well-tanned proteins resist the action of papain, while the enzyme attacks the cuticle, at least of adult nematodes (Berger and Asenjo, 1940). Chemical differences seem to exist between the cuticles of adult and larval nematodes; in contrast to the adult cuticle, the cuticle of some larval roundworms is not attacked by papain (Monné, 1955b) and no evidence for tanning was found in some larval species (Bird and Rogers, 1956). The cuticle of *Fasciola* also appears to consist largely of protein; although containing some polyphenols (Monné, 1959) there is no indication for pronounced tanning. Björkman *et al.* (1963) found that the cuticle of this worm is readily attacked by various proteolytic enzymes, amongst them papain and ficin.

Typical quinone-tanned proteins are the main component of the egg shells of trematodes and pseudophyllidean cestodes (Stephenson, 1947b; Smyth, 1954; Smyth and Clegg, 1959; Johri and Smyth, 1956; Monné and Borg, 1954; Monné, 1955b, 1960). The often-described refringent spheres in the vitellarian cells of these parasites contain large amounts of polyphenols and polyphenol oxidase. Both are incorporated into the eggshells and are responsible for the latter turning brown on exposure to air. Furthermore, it could be shown that *Schistocephalus solidus* upon being matured anaerobically *in vitro* produced normal eggs that tanned after exposure to air. If the worms, however, were cultured aerobically, the vitellaria themselves turned brown, indicating abnormal pretanning of eggshell material within the vitellarian cells. No such pretanning occurs in trematodes such as *Haematoloechus* which normally live under aerobic conditions. Evidently, they must possess an inhibitory mechanism preventing tanning within the vitellaria (Smyth, 1954). It is probable that the dark metacercarial cyst of *Fascioloides magna* contains quinone-tanned proteins, since a phenolase was found in the cystogenous granules occurring in the body of the cercariae (W. C. Campbell, 1960b).

The eggshells of numerous parasitic nematodes, for instance, *Syngamus, Passalurus, Trichuris,* and others, also probably contain quinone-tanned proteins which are derived from refringent protein granules rich in phenolic groups occurring in their oocytes (Monné and Borg, 1954; Monné and Hönig, 1954c,d). Whether they are identical with the refringent protein granules (Fauré-Fremiet *et al.,* 1954) of the *Parascaris* oocytes is open to question. The latter contain 14 amino acids, among them proline as quantitatively the most important one (Ebel and Colas, 1954) and are also incorporated into the hard shell (Yanagisawa, 1955; Yanagisawa and Ishii, 1954). The hard shell of the *Ascaris* egg seems not to give reactions characteristic of quinone tanning (Monné and Borg, 1954). However, the jelly coat of ascarid eggs does contain polyphenols bound to proteins which are responsible for the vigorous tanning of this layer (Monné, 1960). A word of caution may be indicated; the so-called tanning of this layer appears to take place in the O_2-poor intestine, while the usual tanning process is a clearly aerobic process.

Another unusual protein constitutes the basis of the conspicuous refringent bodies of the ascarid sperm cells. The compound, first isolated by Fauré-Fremiet (1913a) and called ascaridine, is an albuminoid protein containing 17.5% nitrogen, but neither sulfur nor phosphorus. The compound is insoluble in cold distilled water, but dissolves suddenly at 50°–51°C. This temperature of dispersion, however, is not a fixed point. It can be altered both ways by salts (Fauré-Fremiet and Filhol, 1937). Champétier and Fauré-Fremiet's (1937) X-ray studies have shown ascaridine to be a semicrystalline substance when precipitated from solution. It is, however, amorphous when the globules are centrifuged and desiccated. The function of ascaridine is not precisely known; it is possible that it is in some way connected with the synthesis of ribonucleoproteins in the egg after fertilization (Panijel, 1947).

The amino acids participating in the constitution of parasites either as free acids or protein amino acids have been determined repeatedly, especially in recent years. Examples are shown in Table XL. It is evident that, on the whole, few qualitative differences have been uncovered. The majority of the common amino acids are encountered in practically all animals studied. The apparent absence of some amino acid in one or the other case should not be taken too seriously, since various authors have used different techniques of separation and identification which have not all the same sensitivity. Some puzzling facts, however, remain. Thus, according to Pollak and Fairbairn (1955a), the ovaries of *Ascaris* from American pigs contain no arginine, although ascarids from Australian origin studied by the same methods have it. Less surprising is the fact that specialized structures, such as the vitelline membrane of the *Ascaris* egg, contain a smaller variety of amino acids than the body proteins (Table XL). Of interest also is that a purified antigen isolated from *Fasciola hepatica* contains fifteen amino acids (Maekawa and Kushibe, 1956).

Free and protein amino acids are usually qualitatively quite similar, while their relative abundance may vary considerably. Thus, in *Ascaris* ovaries leucine represents 1.5% of the total α-amino N of the free amino acids, but 12.7% of the protein N, while on the contrary the corresponding figures for proline are 0.5 and 8.2%, respectively (Pollak and Fairbairn, 1955a). Similarly, parasites belonging to the same group, even if not very closely related, show considerable similarities in amino acid composition, even in quantitative respects. Characteristic is, for instance, that Williamson and Desowitz (1961) found no significant quantitative differences between Group A and Group B trypanosomes, although the members of the two groups differ considerably in many other biochemical respects. Curiously, they found the greatest difference, and the only one of probable statistical significance, between two members of Group A: 19.1 and 7.4% alanine in *Trypanosoma cruzi* and *Trypanosoma lewisi*, respectively.

II. HEME COMPOUNDS

Hemoglobin has not yet been reported from parasitic protozoa, cestodes, or Acanthocephala. It has been found in trematodes, nematodes, and endoparasitic arthropods, as follows: Trematodes: *Allassostoma* and *Telorchis* (Wharton, 1938, 1941); *Dicrocoelium* and *Fasciola hepatica* (van Grembergen, 1949); *Fasciola gigantica, Cotylophoron,* and *Gastrothylax* (Goil, 1959, 1961); *Paramphistomum* (Lazarus, 1950), and *Proctoeces* (Freeman, 1962, 1963); Nematodes: *Ascaris* (Flury, 1912; Davey, 1938; Krueger, 1936; Davenport, 1949a; Treibs *et al.,* 1950; Smith, 1962, 1963; Smith and Lee, 1963; Smith and Morrison, 1963; Hamada *et al.,* 1962, 1963a,b); *Camallanus* (Wharton, 1938, 1941); *Cooperia* (Davey, 1938); *Dioctophyme* (Aducco, 1889); *Eu-*

strongylides, larval (von Brand, 1937; von Brand and Simpson, 1945); *Haemonchus* (Rogers, 1949); *Heterakis* (van Grembergen, 1954); *Ostertagia* (Davey, 1938); *Parascaris* (Faure-Fremiet, 1913b; Hurlaux, 1947); *Nematodirus* (Davey, 1938; Rogers, 1949); *Nippostrongylus* (Davenport, 1949b); *Spirocerca* (Hsü, 1938); *Tetrameres* (Villela and Ribeiro, 1955a,b; Ribeiro and Villela, 1956); *Toxocara* (Davey, 1938); *Trichinella,* larval (Stannard *et al.,* 1938; Goldberg, 1957); Arthropods: *Gastrophilus,* larval (von Kemnitz, 1916; Dinulescu, 1932; Keilin and Wang, 1946); *Peltogaster* (Fox, 1953); *Septosaccus* (Perez and Bloch-Raphael, 1946); and several ectoparasitic crustacea (literature in Nadakal, 1963).

Hemoglobin appears in parasites partly as tissue hemoglobin, or, in nematodes, also dissolved in the perienteric fluid. Occasionally, the pigment is especially concentrated in certain organs. Thus, in *Fasciola* (Stephenson, 1947b) it is found primarily in the vitellaria and the vicinity of the anterior uterine coils, or in *Gastrophilus* larvae within the cells of the red organ. In some nematodes, such as *Ascaris,* at least two types of hemoglobin occur. One is localized in the body wall, the other in the perienteric fluid. Both are clearly differentiated by spectral characteristics, oxygen affinity, reaction velocities (Keilin, 1925; Davenport, 1949a), the Q_{10} of deoxygenation velocity (Smith, 1963), isoelectric points, and molecular weights (Smith and Morrison, 1963). While the perienteric hemoglobin of *Ascaris* appears to be a uniform compound, some doubts exist whether this is true in respect to the body wall pigment. Hamada *et al.* (1963a,b) separated it by column chromatography into two components, but Smith and Morrison (1963) are of the opinion that their products had undergone partial denaturation. Contrary to the situation existing in *Ascaris,* it was the hemocele hemoglobin of *Tetrameres* that separated upon electrophoretic analysis into three components, all giving positive benzidine tests (Ribeiro and Villela, 1956).

All parasite hemoglobins studied in some detail differ from the hemoglobins of their hosts in one or several of the above characteristics. Since the color of the worms, even when maintained *in vitro* in hemoglobin-free solutions, remains unchanged (e.g., in the case of larval *Eustrongylides* up to 4 years according to von Brand and Simpson, 1945), a direct connection between parasite and host hemoglobin is very unlikely. Evidently, it cannot exist in the case of *Proctoeces* whose lamellibranch host has no hemoglobin (Freeman, 1963). However, in some cases at least indirect connections between parasite and host hemoglobin seem to exist. Smith and Lee (1963) observed an increase in perienteric hemoglobin of *Ascaris* upon *in vitro* incubation in presence of horse hemoglobin. Further analysis showed that the worms depend for hemoglobin synthesis on the availability of porphyrins or metalloporphyrins containing at least one vinyl group among their side chains. Positive results were thus obtained with protohematin, protoporphyrin, or chlorophyll as substrates. Smith and Lee (1963) developed the idea that *Ascaris* can, in its intestinal cells, degrade ingested hematin to bile pigments which would then be used as substrate for hemoglobin synthesis, i.e., the relationships between hemoglobin and bile pigments would be just the opposite from what is usually assumed. Substances giving reactions like bile pigments, but not really identified as such, may be fairly widespread in parasites. Such substances have, for instance, been found in the hemoglobin-containing *Septosaccus*. In this case, Perez and Bloch-Raphael (1946) take the orthodox view that the pigments are derived from hemoglobin destruction rather than considering them as substrate for synthesis. However, bile pigments absorbed from the environments and definitely not used for hemoglobin synthesis occur in other parasites, for instance, opalinids (Kedrowsky, 1931). They are reduced to stercobilin and may stay in the body for a long time as crystals (Brookes and Mohr, 1963).

Of considerable interest are the oxygen relationships of parasite hemoglobins. They all show an unusually high affinity to oxygen, e.g., the body wall hemoglobin of *Nippostrongylus* is half saturated with oxygen at 0.1 mm partial pressure (Davenport, 1949b; Rogers, 1949). The oxygen dissociation curves of the hemoglobins of this and other small nematodes are then unusually steep (Fig. 9), steeper than those of the host (Wharton, 1941; Davenport, 1949b; Rogers, 1949). This implies that the worms will be able to extract oxygen from very oxygen-poor surroundings. Conversely, the oxygen tension of their own tissues will have to be extremely low before the oxygen bound to the pigment will be released. It has been shown several times, however, (von Brand, 1937; Wharton, 1941; Rogers, 1949) that the respiratory activities of small nematodes, such as *Heterakis* (van Grembergen, 1954), are sufficient to deoxygenate their hemoglobins when the oxygen of the surroundings is depleted. The same has been found for the body wall hemoglobin of *Ascaris* (Davenport, 1949a). It is likely, therefore, that in these cases the biological significance of the hemoglobins must be sought in their oxygen-carrying capacity.

It is unlikely, on the other hand, that the same assumption should be made for the hemocele hemoglobins of such worms as *Dioctophyme, Ascaris,* or *Strongylus,* or the tissue hemoglobin of *Proctoeces.* They are extremely resistant to deoxygenation; it is almost impossible to dissociate the oxygen by evacuation. Even chemical deoxygenation is difficult (Aducco, 1889; Davenport, 1949a,b). A variety of views as to the significance of these hemoglobins has been expressed. They have

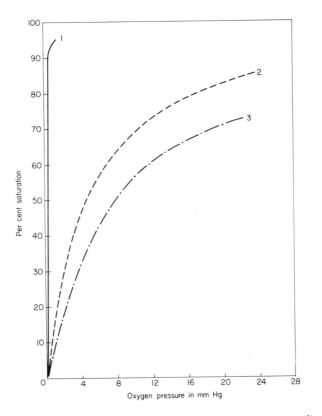

Fig. 9. Oxygen dissociation curves of parasite hemoglobins: *Nematodirus* spp. (1) (after Rogers, 1949); *Gastrophilus intestinalis* (2) (after Keilin and Wang, 1946); *Camallanus trispinosus* (3) (after Wharton, 1941).

been regarded as "functionless by-products of the nutrition of the worms" (Davenport, 1949b) or as important by eliminating peroxides via the peroxidase activity of methemoglobin (Laser, 1944). More recently other possibilities have been discussed. Freeman (1963) thinks their function might be to facilitate oxygen diffusion, a possibility demonstrated by Scholander (1960) in model systems. Smith and Lee (1963), on the other hand, look upon the hemocele hemoglobin of *Ascaris* as a metabolic pool of hematin from which other hemoproteins can be synthesized. They point out that this might be the mechanism enabling maintenance of maximal egg production. Evidently, then, experimental work is needed to elucidate this problem.

Other important heme pigments are the cytochromes. They are universally distributed in free-living organisms where they constitute an integral part of the respiratory chain. They are found also in many parasites, both protozoa and helminths (Table XLI), while parasites belonging to other phyla have not yet been studied in this respect. In some forms, such as *Trichuris,* cytochrome activity is high enough to account for the entire oxygen consumption (Bueding *et al.,* 1960). In schistosomes, on the other hand, the system is so weakly developed as to mediate only a small fraction (Bueding and Charms, 1952). In a last group, finally, no functional cytochrome system can be detected. It is curious that this group contains both parasites that evidently lead primarily aerobic lives, such as the blood-stream forms of the African pathogenic trypanosomes (Harvey, 1949; Ryley, 1956; Fulton and Spooner, 1959), or *Litomosoides* (Bueding and Charms, 1952) and parasites normally leading a primarily anaerobic existence. To this latter group belong *Trichomonas foetus* (Ryley, 1955b) and *Ascaris* (Bueding and Charms, 1952; Rathbone, 1955). The case of this latter worm is of interest from several standpoints. Even though it does not appear to have a functional cytochrome system, spectral lines characteristic for cytochromes have been observed in its tissues (Keilin, 1925). Furthermore, it is a good example for the fact that various stages in the life cycle of a parasite may differ in respect to their electron transport mechanisms. It has been shown conclusively (Table XLI) that the eggs of *Ascaris,* especially the embryonated ones, have, in contrast to the tissues of the adult worms, a functional cytochrome system. A similar situation prevails also in some protozoa. It has thus been found that only the culture forms, but not the blood-stream form, of *Trypanosoma rhodesiense* contain a functional cytochrome system (Ryley, 1962).

Other iron porphyrin compounds of biological significance are the catalases and peroxidases which have been reported repeatedly from parasites. Catalase activity is quite weak in the blood-stream forms of pathogenic African trypanosomes (Strangeways, 1937; Harvey, 1949), or may even be absent (Fulton and Spooner, 1956). It is more pronounced in *Trypanosoma lewisi,* bird and amphibian trypanosomes (Tasaka, 1935), insect trypanosomids (Wertlieb and Guttman, 1963), and *Trichomonas* spp. (Asami, 1956; Doran, 1957, 1958). The catalase activity of parasitic helminths seems to be low. This has been observed in *Fasciola hepatica,* larval and adult *Taenia pisiformis* (Pennoit-DeCooman and van Grembergen, 1942), *Heterakis gallinae* (Glocklin and Fairbairn, 1952), and *Ascaris lumbricoides* (Lesser, 1906). It has been assumed that the well-established toxicity of high oxygen tensions to this worm is due to its low catalase content (Laser, 1944) which would be insufficient to decompose the toxic hydrogen peroxide accumulating under the influence of surplus oxygen. Monteoliva (1961) recently re-

TABLE XLI
CYTOCHROMES IN PARASITES

Species	Cytochrome[a] a/a$_3$	b	c	Cytochrome oxidase	References
Protozoa					
Strigomonas fasciculata		x	x		A. Lwoff (1934)
Strigomonas oncopelti	x	x	x	x	Ryley (1955a)
Trypanosoma cruzi	x	x	—	x[b]	Baernstein and Tobie (1951); Ryley (1956); Fulton and Spooner (1959)
Trypanosoma gambiense, culture form	x	x			Fulton and Spooner (1959)
Trypanosoma lewisi	x	x	x	x	Ryley (1951, 1956)
Trypanosoma rhodesiense, culture form	x	x	—		Ryley (1962)
Trichomonas foetus		x			Suzuoki and Suzuoki (1951)
Trichomonas foetus	—	—	—	—	Ryley (1955b)
Trichomonas vaginalis	—	—	—	—	Wellerson et al. (1959)
Opalina carolinesis				x	Hunter (1957)
Trematodes					
Allassostoma magnum			x		Wharton (1941)
Fasciola hepatica		x	x		van Grembergen (1949)
Schistosoma mansoni			x	x	Bueding and Charms (1951, 1952)
Schistosoma japonicum				x	Huang and Chu (1962)
Cestodes					
Diphyllobothrium latum			x		Friedheim and Baer (1933)
Hymenolepis diminuta				x	Read (1952)
Moniezia benedeni		x	x		van Grembergen (1944)
Triaenophorus lucii			x		Friedheim and Baer (1933)
Nematodes					
Ascaris lumbricoides, adult	x	x	x	—[c]	Keilin (1925); Bueding and Charms (1951, 1952); Rathbone (1955)
Ascaris lumbricoides, eggs				x	Costello et al. (1963); Oya et al. (1963); Kmetec et al. (1963)
Camallanus trispinosus			x		Wharton (1941)
Ditylenchus triformis	x	x		x	Krusberg (1960)
Litomosoides carinii		—		—	Bueding and Charms (1952)
Trichinella spiralis, larval	x	x	x	x	Agosin (1956); Goldberg (1957)
Trichuris vulpis		x		x	Bueding et al. (1960)

[a] Not all authors quoted in this table differentiate between cytochromes a and a$_3$. Although the identity of these cytochromes with cytochrome oxidase is generally assumed, a special column for cytochrome oxidase has been retained in this table because in some cases the identification of cytochromes a or a + a$_3$ rests only on spectroscopic evidence without an oxidase activity having been demonstrated. According to Bueding (1949), absorption spectra simulating those of cytochromes could also be given by some other hematin-like pigment.

[b] No cytochrome c oxidase.

[c] In contrast to the authors quoted, Kikuchi et al. (1959) reported evidence for the presence of cytochrome oxidase in adult *Ascaris*.

ported both catalase and peroxidase activity from the perivisceral fluid of *Ascaris*. His paper electrophoretic analysis showed peroxidase activity in three of the four fractions obtained from female specimens, while only two fractions isolated from males showed corresponding activity. Catalase was localized in both sexes in a single fraction.

Little is known about the ability of parasites to synthesize their essential heme compounds other than the previously mentioned hemoglobin. Quite evidently considerable differences exist in this respect even between closely related species. It is thus well known that some trypanosomids require hematin or related compounds in culture, while others do not (literature in M. Lwoff, 1951). Of interest is that in such cultures hematin could be replaced successfully by iron porphyrin compounds having protohemin as prosthetic group; for example, veal liver catalase in cultures of *Leptomonas pyrrhocoris* (Zotta, 1923), or peroxidases of plant origin in those of *Strigomonas fasciculata* (M. Lwoff, 1933). A. Lwoff (1934) studied a series of porphyrin compounds as to their ability to support growth and stimulate respiration of this flagellate. He found that only blood, hematin, protohemin, and protoporphyrin will do so. This last finding is of special interest because protoporphyrin is iron-free. If A. Lwoff's (1934) assumption is correct that the above compounds serve primarily to build the flagellate's iron-catalyzed respiratory enzyme system, it follows that it must be able to incorporate iron into the protoporphyrin molecule.

The heme compounds discussed so far play a role in dynamic metabolic phases while those to be mentioned now represent end products of hemoglobin utilization. The best known is malaria pigment, usually designated as hemozoin. Although known for more than 200 years, chemical studies with modern methods of analysis go back only to Sinton and Ghosh (1934a,b), Ghosh and Sinton (1934), and Ghosh and Nath (1934). They concluded that the pigment isolated from *Plasmodium knowlesi* was hematin. Later investigators (Devine and Fulton, 1941, 1942; Morrison and Anderson, 1942; Rimington *et al.,* 1947), using successively more sophisticated techniques of extraction and analysis, reached essentially the same conclusion for the pigments of *Plasmodium knowlesi* and *Plasmodium gallinaceum*. More recently Deegan (1956) and Deegan and Maegraith (1956a,b) extracted the pigment from several species of mammalian malaria parasites or the organs of their hosts with borate and observed that the absorption spectra differed definitely from that of hematin. Treatment of the pigment (chiefly that isolated from *Plasmodium knowlesi*) with dithionite had little effect on the spectrum, indicating that no rapid production of hemochrome took place. The latter was formed slowly only upon treatment with pyridine or NaOH, suggesting presence of the intact iron porphyrin bound to another compound, possibly a denatured polypeptide or protein. Similarly, Sherman and Hull (1960) could not identify the pigment of *Plasmodium lophurae* with hematin. They also assume combination of hematin with a proteinaceous moiety, the nature of which remains, however, obscure.

Hematin, or occasionally hemin, derived from digested hemoglobin has been found repeatedly in the intestine of helminths, or their cyst fluids. Such pigments have been described from schistosomes (Rogers, 1940); *Fasciola* (Stephenson, 1947a), *Paragonimus* (Ogimoto, 1956), and several species of monogenetic trematodes (Llewellyn, 1954; Jennings, 1959). The pigments found in the Kupffer cells of the liver or in mononuclear leucocytes of other organs during schistosomiasis (Fairley, 1920), or in various organs of sheep infected with *Fascioloides magna* (W. C. Campbell, 1960a) are also probably heme pigments, but their exact chemical constitution has not yet been elucidated. Still less proof is available for the assumption made by Porter (1935) that the pigment occurring in the larvae of *Nippostrongylus muris* and in the lungs of infected animals belongs into the same group.

III. PROTEASES

Proteases can be discharged by parasites into the environment, either to prepare food material for ingestion (extracorporeal digestion), for penetration into the tissues of the host, or for migration through the latter. As D. Fairbairn (1960) has pointed out, it is frequently difficult to separate these functions, since tissue destruction due to penetration or migration will lead to the production of substances potentially useful for the alimentation of the parasites.

There can, however, be no doubt that tissue penetration or migration involves enzymatic activity originating in parasites. Tissue-penetrating protozoa and helminths frequently contain enzymes capable of producing changes in the acellular components of the dermal connective tissues (Table XLII). The relevant enzymes have often, especially in the older literature, been called hyaluronidase. However, hyaluronidase proper is a mucopolysaccharidase (Lee and Lewert, 1957) which does not occur in typical form in such skin penetrators as cercariae of *Schistosoma mansoni* or larval *Strongyloides ratti*. These worms contain a collagenase-like enzyme or enzyme complex which is active against skin glycoproteins, but differs in some aspects from true collagenase (Milleman and Thonard, 1959, for cercariae). They are furthermore capable of decapsulating streptococci, that is, they bring about alterations and dissolution of compounds having hyaluronic acid as major component (Evans, 1953) and

TABLE XLII

DISTRIBUTION OF HYALURONIDASE- OR COLLAGENASE-LIKE ENZYMES IN PARASITES

Species	References
Protozoa	
Entamoeba histolytica[a]	Lincicome (1953); Bradin (1953)
Balantidium coli	Tempelis and Lysenko (1957)
Ichthyophthirius multifiliis	Uspenskaya (1963)
Trichomonas vaginalis	Boni and Orsi (1958)
Trematodes	
Schistosoma bovis, cercariae	Deiana (1954)
Schistosoma mansoni, cercariae	Stirewalt and Evans (1952); Lewert and Lee (1956, 1957)
Nematodes	
Ancylostoma duodenale	Bruni (1939); Bruni and Passalaqua (1954)
Ancylostoma caninum, filariform larvae	Lincicome (1953)
Strongyloides ratti, larvae	Lewert and Lee (1956, 1957)
Strongylus edentatus	Deiana (1955)
Strongylus equinus	Deiana (1955)
Arthropods	
Hypodermis bovis, larvae	Lienert and Thorsell (1955)

[a] Neal (1960) found neither hyaluronidase nor collagenase in *Entamoeba histolytica.*

they have a factor similar to the "spreading factor." Recently, the elastolytic properties of the cercarial protease complex have been emphasized (Gazzinelli and Pellegrino, 1964).

The properties of helminthic collagenase-like enzymes vary according to species and they differ from those of bacterial collagenase or trypsin. Thus, SH-binding substances interfere effectively with the schistosome enzyme, but they show little activity against that of the *Strongyloides* larvae. The latter is more sensitive to chelating agents and SH-containing substances. Other differences exist in respect to such factors as sensitivity to metal ions or pH optimum (Lewert and Lee, 1956, 1957).

A naturally occurring inhibitor of the schistosome collagenase-like enzyme has been described from the blood of infected hosts (Lewert *et al.,* 1959). It has the same electrophoretic mobility as α-globulin and is apparently a protein. It is probably not an antibody, but a nonspecific substance occurring at low level in noninfected individuals which is increased sharply during active infection. It is of special interest that such inhibitory substances are not limited to infected vertebrates, but occur even in plants. Myuge (1960) thus observed in plants infected with *Heterodera* spp. substances inhibiting the proteolytic activity of the nematodes.

While it is reasonable to assume that the main, though possibly not the only, function of the enzymes discussed so far is facilitation of entry into the host or of migration through its tissues, other cases exist where the main function of proteases secreted into the environment is probably extracorporeal digestion in the narrow sense of the word, i.e., preparation of food material for ingestion. There is thus good histological evidence that several species of intestinal nematodes produce lesions in the host by extracorporeal digestion of the latter's intestinal mucosa (von Linstow, 1907; Hoeppli, 1927; Hoeppli and Feng, 1931; Wetzel, 1927, 1931; Schuurmans-Stekhoven and Botman, 1932). Thorson (1956a) found pronounced proteolytic activity in extracts of the esophagus of *Ancylostoma caninum* which probably can be considered to play a role during extracorporeal digestion. Interestingly, the enzymatic activity was largely inhibited by the serum of previously infected dogs, but not by that of noninfected ones. Whether a similar protease occurring in the esophagus of *Ascaris lumbricoides* (Chitwood, 1938a) has a similar biological role is problematical, since the worm is not usually considered as a tissue feeder.

Proteolytic digestive enzymes functionally comparable to those secreted into the intestinal lumen of free-living organisms occurs in many gut-possessing parasites, that is, essentially, trematodes, nematodes, and arthropods. Thus, to quote some of the older observations first, a polypeptide-splitting enzyme was found in the intestine of *Toxocara* by Abderhalden and Heise (1909), an enzyme splitting egg albumin rapidly and fibrin more slowly was found in *Ascaris* by Flury (1912), and trypsin-like enzymes have been reported from the gut of *Cordylobia* larvae (Blacklock *et al.*, 1930) and *Gastrophilus* larvae (Roy, 1937). More detailed are the observations of Rogers (1941a), who studied the ability of intestinal extracts of *Ascaris lumbricoides* and *Strongylus edentatus* to digest gelatin, blood albumin, and casein. Quantitative estimation showed that the proteolytic enzymes of *Strongylus* were considerably more active than those of *Ascaris*. The pH optimum of the enzymes of both worms was 6.2, that is, it was on the alkaline side of the isoelectric points of the digested proteins. A similar value (pH 6.0) has more recently been found optimal for the protease of the gut of *Leidynema appendiculata* (Lee, 1958), but a higher one (pH 8.3) has been observed in the case of the mid-gut protease of *Gastrophilus intestinalis* larvae (Tatchell, 1958). There is no indication that any of the above worms has an intestinal proteolytic enzyme active at a pH characteristic for mammalian pepsin. All enzymes studied so far are rather more trypsin-like, but failing purification they should not be identified with mammalian trypsin as yet.

Besides the enzymes mentioned so far, most of which can be classified as endopeptidases, enzymes have been reported which belong to the exopeptidases, that is, enzymes splitting off successively terminal amino groups of polypeptides and dipeptides. Four different peptidases have been found with the help of microchemical procedures in the intestine of *Ascaris* (Carpenter, 1952). Histochemical evidence (Lee, 1962) indicates that one of them at least, leucine aminopeptidase, is not limited to the intestinal tract, but occurs also in the walls of the anterior parts of the excretory canals and in the hypodermis. Similarly, Savel (1954) found peptidase (and protease) activity in the intestine, the perivisceral fluid (see also Ichii *et al.,* 1959) and the muscle layer of *Ascaris.* Peptidases are evidently widely distributed in parasites with intestinal tract. Relevant enzymes, among them a prolidase splitting glycyl-L-proline, have been found in *Leidynema appendiculata* (Lee, 1958). In the mid-gut of *Gastrophilus intestinalis* larvae a peptidase with a double pH optimum (7.5 and 8.7) has been found when glycyl-glycine was the substrate tested while a single peak (pH 7.5) was observed when DL-leucyl-glycyl-glycine was split (Tatchell, 1958).

There is no indication that metazoan parasites lacking an intestinal tract secrete proteolytic enzymes into the environment to prepare food for absorption. They nevertheless have such enzymes which then probably serve as tissue enzymes used in the movements of the parasite's own proteins. Specifically, such enzymes with apparently fairly high rates of activity have been reported from *Diphyllobothrium latum, Taenia saginata,* and *Taenia solium* (Tallqvist, 1907; Smorodincev and Bebesin, 1936d). Pennoit-DeCooman and van Grembergen (1942), on the other hand, found only a very low proteolytic activity in several species of cestodes. These investigators also reported the absence of polypeptidases but the presence of a strong dipeptidase in the same worms. The biological significance of the proteolytic enzymes encountered by Lemaire and Ribêre (1935) in the *Echinococcus* cystic fluid requires further clarification.

Corresponding enzymes found in *Fasciola hepatica* (Abderhalden and Heise, 1909; Flury and Leeb, 1926; Pennoit-DeCooman and van Grembergen, 1942) and in the cercariae of *Schistosoma mansoni* (Mandlowitz *et al.,* 1960) cannot be properly assessed as yet; for obvious anatomical reasons no distinction between tissue and truly digestive enzymes can be made in these cases.

Insofar as protozoa are concerned, it is often difficult to differentiate between enzymes used for the dissolution of host tissues, those possibly digesting proteins within food vacuoles, and finally true tissue enzymes. This uncertainty exists especially in the case of *Entamoeba histolytica.*

It has been found that trophozoites as well as freeze-dried extracts were able to hydrolyze a wide spectrum of protein substrates, among them guinea pig caecal epithelial cells, by means of a trypsin-like enzyme (Jarumilinta and Maegraith, 1961a). Enzymatic activity was not inhibited by iodoacetate or stimulated by cysteine (Neal, 1956). Serum did inhibit proteolysis, but typical trypsin inhibitors, such as crystalline soy bean inhibitor, did not (Harinasuta and Maegraith, 1958; Neal, 1960). Besides this trypsin-like enzyme the amoebas also contained a pepsin-like enzyme, with a pH optimum of 4.1. Three types of peptidases were found in non-pathogenic strains, while, interestingly, pathogenic strains lacked one of them, carboxypeptidase (Jarumilinta and Maegraith, 1961b). Other proteolytic enzymes described from *Entamoeba histolytica* are a gelatinase (Nakamura and Edwards, 1959a), a casease (Nakamura and Edwards, 1959b), and a glutaminase (Nakamura and Goldstein, 1957). The latter enzyme was activated by phosphate like the corresponding mammalian enzyme, but not by NaCl, which activates the enzyme of *Clostridium perfringens.*

A Ca^{++}- and cysteine-activated protease has been reported from *Entodinium caudatum;* the same ciliate also possessed a peptidase active against 10 different peptides. The peptidase could be separated from the protease by paper electrophoresis at pH 8.6 (Abou Akkada and Howard, 1962).

Clearly, purely intracellular proteolytic enzymes occur in the blood-stream form of trypanosomes. Evidently all enzymes occurring in a parasite whirled constantly around in the blood stream can only have a significance if they act on substrates present within the cell. In *Trypanosoma evansi,* cathepsin, carboxypolypeptidase, aminopolypeptidase, and dipeptidase have been found by Krijgsman (1936).

The digestion of one naturally occurring substrate, blood, requires special discussion. It is of course well known that malaria parasites destroy hemoglobin at a rapid rate. Groman (1951) has estimated that the rate of decomposition amounts to 0.27% of the total hemoglobin/hour in a *Plasmodium gallinaceum* infection of average parasitemia, while *Plasmodium knowlesi* is about 4 to 5 times as destructive (Ball *et al.,* 1948; Morrison and Jeskey, 1948). Moulder and Evans (1946) and Groman (1951) observed rapid production of amino nitrogen by erythrocytes parasitized by *Plasmodium gallinaceum,* indicating the probability that hemoglobin was the substrate utilized. However, cell-free extracts of the parasites hydrolyzed hemoglobin only slowly, but they did, on the other hand, rapidly utilize denatured globin. Moulder and Evans (1946) assume that in intact parasites an enzyme system occurs which splits hemoglobin into heme and globin, the latter then being readily available for the action retained by the lysed parasites. The relevant enzymes of two species have recently been studied by Cook *et al.* (1961). Cell-free preparations of *Plasmodium berghei* showed proteinase activity against mouse globin, the two pH maxima (pH 4 and 8) found indicating that two proteases may have been present. The relative activity was low against crystalline hemoglobin, but high against the globin derived from it, the cytoplasmic protein of mouse reticulocytes and especially the cytoplasmic protein remaining after removal of crystalline hemoglobin. *Plasmodium knowlesi* also gave evidence of possessing two proteases with pH maxima of 5 and 8. The latter enzyme was partly purified and some of its properties determined. It was not inhibited by cyanide or SH-inhibitors, but its activity was markedly reduced by diisopropyl phosphorofluoridate and to a lesser degree by chelating agents, the inhibitory action of the latter not being reversible by a variety of divalent ions. The partly purified enzyme released free phenylalanine from the oxidized β-chain of bovine insulin and it liberated ammonia from the chymotrypsin substrate, acetyl-L-tyrosinamide, indicating that the enzyme could hydrolyze a peptide bond to which an aromatic amino acid contributes a carbonyl group.

Malaria parasites live in the closest possible connection with hemoglobin, while many metazoan parasites must gain access to the blood in order to ingest it, in other words, they suck blood out of blood vessels. Since blood removed from the vascular system usually clots very rapidly, it is not surprising that many bloodsucking organisms secrete anticoagulants in order to assure a flow of blood through the punctured blood vessel and to prevent an obstruction of their own alimentary passages. This is well known about free-living organisms such as leeches or mosquitoes, but relatively little information is available about helminths and endoparasitic arthropods.

Anticoagulants have been reported from the following nematodes: *Ancylostoma caninum* (Loeb and Smith, 1904; Loeb and Fleisher, 1910), various members of the family Strongylidae (Schwartz, 1921), and *Bunostomum trigonocephalum* (Hoeppli and Feng, 1933). The exact mode of action of these anticoagulants has not yet been established. Thorson (1956b) states that extracts of esophagus, amphidial glands, or excretory glands of *Ancylostoma caninum* either do not contain the anticoagulant described by Loeb and associates, or the activity is not directed at the thrombin-fibrinogen stage of coagulation. Thorson (1956b) observed that extracts of amphidial glands did prolong the prothrombin time; the activity of these glands seems to be directed against the formation of thrombin from prothrombin, but it is not yet known whether the action is directed directly against the latter compound or against thrombo-plastin. The prothrombin time of the blood of *Rana pipiens* and *Bufo americanus* infected respectively with *Pneumoneces* sp. and uniden-tified lung flukes was longer than that of uninfected specimens, pointing toward the release of anticoagulating factors by the worms (Dent and Schuellein, 1950). Finally, an anticoagulant has been found in the salivary gland of larval *Gastrophilus* (Dinulescu, 1932; Tatchell, 1958), this being apparently the only recorded instance for endoparasitic arthropods.

As to the fate of the ingested blood, Rogers (1941a) found in *Ascaris* first a reduction of oxyhemoglobin to hemoglobin, the latter substance then being split into globin and hematin. The same process probably took place in *Strongylus,* and the hematological observations of Rogers (1940) on the gut content of other species of nematodes and of schisto-somes made it probable that an identical sequence occurred also in such forms as *Syngamus trachea, Schistosoma mattheei,* and *Schistosoma mansoni.* Furthermore, Timms and Bueding (1959) found that an amino acid mixture containing the amino acids of globin prolonged the *in vitro* life of this last worm. This can be considered as rather clear indication that globin can provide some of the animal's nutritional requirements and that the required amino acids are liberated in the worm's intestine by digestion of ingested erythrocytes. It is very likely that this digestion is due to a remarkably substrate-specific proteolytic enzyme found by Timms and Bueding (1959) in homogenates of whole worms. The enzyme had a sharp peak of activity at pH 3.9. It could be purified 20-fold by ultracentrifugation. It proved to be quite specific for hemoglobin and globin and did not attack serum proteins, with the possible exception of bovine serum mercaptalbumin, at pH 7.7. There is a possibility that the schistosomes have a second enzyme capable of degrading hemoglobin, since the crude preparation digested hemoglobin not only at pH 3.9, but also at pH 6.0.

A different type of enzyme evidently occurs in the gut of *Fasciola hepatica.* Rijavec *et al.* (1962) found that liver flukes incubated in radio-iodine-tagged blood serum did digest the albumins of the blood to amino acids, the latter apparently being readily absorbed.

Gastrophilus larvae, though probably not constant bloodsuckers (Roy, 1937) seem at least intermittently to ingest blood. Dinulescu (1932) relates that the blood clots in the gut, that it is then hemolyzed and split into globin and hematin. Part of the globin is supposedly used for the synthesis of fat reserves of the larvae while the pigmented prosthetic group is decomposed to a hemochromogen-like substance and iron. Dur-ing pupation the hemoglobin of the red organ and other body tissues is transformed into biliverdin, a process occasionally also observed in third-stage larvae where the pigment originates from ingested blood (Beaumont, 1948).

IV. ANTIENZYMES

Antienzymes, that is, enzymes inhibiting the activity of the digestive enzymes of the host, are widespread in intestinal worms. They have been reported primarily from ascarids and tapeworms (Weinland, 1902; Dastre and Stassano, 1903; Hamill, 1906, Fetterolf, 1907; Tallqvist, 1907; Mendel and Blood, 1910; Harned and Nash, 1932; Sang, 1938; von Bonsdorff, 1939, 1948) but have also been found in smaller nematode species (Stewart, 1933b; Bushnell and Erwin, 1949). Shearer and Stewart (1933) assumed that the antienzymatic activity of stomach worms of sheep was pronounced enough to explain the nutritional disorders evidenced by parasitized sheep, a view which has not been substantiated subsequently, however (Andrews, 1938). Generalizations are not possible; it thus seems probable that *Nippostrongylus* does not produce antienzymes (Symons and Fairbairn, 1963).

The antienzymes extracted from helminths are usually either antitryptic, or antitryptic and antipeptic. However, relatively little is known about their chemical constitution and specificity. Collier (1941) isolated from *Ascaris* a polypeptide which was fairly similar to a trypsin inhibitor occurring in beef pancreas. Green (1957) reached the conclusion that the body wall of female *Ascaris* contains two antienzymes, a trypsin and a chymotrypsin inhibitor. Although both enzymes were not separated it was shown that the antichymotrypsin activity was inactivated by heat (80°C) and trichloracetic acid, while the antitrypsin activity was not. It was furthermore possible to determine the rate constant of the combination between enzyme and inhibitor: reaction with trypsin 2.1×10^6 1/mole/sec (ionic strength 0.007), with chymotrypsin 1.5×10^6 1/mole/sec (ionic strength 0.016). Subsequently, Peanasky and Laskowski (1960) isolated and purified the chymotrypsin inhibitor which in the end yielded a crystalline product. During this process specific activity against α-chymotrypsin increased 100-fold. Chymotrypsin B was also inhibited, but not trypsin.

The most recent investigators of the problem, Rhodes *et al.* (1963), found trypsin and chymotrypsin inhibitors not only in the body wall of *Ascaris,* but also in its intestine, ovaries, uteri, and perienteric fluid. Extracts of body wall and perienteric fluid were fractionated and purified on carboxymethylcellulose and it was found that both contained a trypsin inhibitor and two distinct chymotrypsin inhibitors. One of the latter apparently corresponded to the crystalline product isolated by Peanasky and Laskowski (1960). All inhibitors isolated were proteins of low molecular weight, varying from 4650 (trypsin inhibitor from body wall) to 12,400 (chymotrypsin inhibitor No. 2 from perienteric fluid).

It has been assumed that the antienzymes play a role in protecting parasites from being digested by the digestive juices of the host. It has been shown that both intestinal nematodes and cestodes withstand trypsin digestion *in vitro* (Fredericq, 1878; Burge and Burge, 1915; DeWaele, 1933) as long as they are living and intact, but that they are digested when dead or when their cuticle is injured. This resistance is, however, not confined to helminths. It is a property which they have in common with the mucosa of the intestinal tract itself and many free-living organisms (Fermi, 1910; Northrop, 1926). It is hence difficult to ascribe to the antienzymes the primary role in protecting helminths from digestion, although they may be of some significance in this respect. It is probable that at least two more factors are involved: the impermeability of living cells and the impermeability of the external cuticle. The peculiar chemical constitution of the cuticle may also be of importance, at least in some cases. Bird (1955) stated that pepsin rapidly attacks proteins which have a high content of aromatic amino acids, and he explains the resistance of the cuticle of larval *Haemonchus contortus* against pepsin with its lack of the aromatic amino acids lysine and arginine. An exact assessment of the importance of these various factors as protective mechanisms is hardly possible at present (Bueding, 1949).

Insofar as intestinal protozoa are concerned, it is difficult to see how they could secrete sufficient antienzymes to protect themselves if this were the only important mechanism. In general, they do not have a thick cuticle. It is possible, therefore, that here the impermeability of living membranes may be of prime importance.

V. ABSORPTION OF AMINO ACIDS

Protozoa can take up amino acids either through the surface, as all forms lacking a cytostome must be assumed to do, from food vacuoles, or possibly in some forms from both these routes. However, no information on the relative importance of the various potential ways of entry is available, nor have the mechanisms of absorption been studied.

At least four different types of experiments described in the literature throw some light on the amino acids that are being absorbed by protozoa. They have commonly been used to elucidate some special question and do not represent systematic studies dealing specifically with the question as to which amino acids are absorbed and which ones may not be. One method consists in incubating the organisms in solutions containing labeled acids and to study the latter's incorporation into various constituents of the body. In two other procedures use is made of the power of the organisms to degrade amino acids. In one, the rates of decarboxylation are measured, that is, the rates of ammonia production. In the other, a stimulation of the oxygen consumption over the endogenous rate serves as measure of utilization. A final method is to investigate which amino acids have to be present in the medium to allow growth of the protozoa in culture, that is, which amino acids belong to the groups of acids commonly termed essential for a given organism. It is reasonable to assume that all amino acids which cannot be synthesized by the body must be absorbed from the environment. Clearly, however, such a study does not clear up the question whether or not nonessential amino acids are also absorbed. As the data assembled in Table XLIII indicate, our knowledge in this field is very limited and spotty.

Essentially the same criteria for amino acid utilization used for protozoa can be employed in the case of helminths. It has thus been found by Hankes and Stoner (1956, 1958) and Stoner and Hankes (1955, 1958) that labeled alanine, glycine, tryptophane, and tyrosine were absorbed rather readily by *Trichinella spiralis* larvae both *in vivo* and *in vitro*. There is no information available whether in this instance the amino acids were absorbed from the intestinal tract or via the cuticle, but more recently Weatherly *et al.* (1963) found the cuticle of *Ascaridia galli* permeable to labeled alanine and glucose, a finding in contrast to the evidence presented or discussed by previous workers (Rogers and Lazarus, 1949; Cavier and Savel, 1952; D. Fairbairn, 1960; Rogers, 1962). It would seem desirable to reinvestigate *Ascaridia galli* with methods differing from that (comparison of celloidin-coated and non-coated worms) employed by Weatherly *et al.* (1963). It should furthermore be realized that from a quantitative standpoint the rates of cuticular absorption reported by Weatherly *et al.* (1963) are almost negligible.

Little of interest in the present connection can be deduced from the amino acids constituting ingredients of the media used in the cultivation or the *in vitro* maintenance of parasitic worms, since, in general, a complex mixture of amino acids is added to an already complicated medium. So far, very few attempts have been made to study the question which amino acids are actually absorbed or at least can be assumed to have been absorbed by proving essential. However, Jackson (1962) has reported indications that *Neoaplectana glaseri* apparently requires in axenic cultures arginine, histidine, isoleucine, leucine, and lysine; Senft (1963) provided evidence, by quantitative analysis, that *Schistosoma mansoni* absorbs *in vitro* out of a complex mixture only aspartic and probably glutamic acid, as well as histidine, tryptophane, and arginine.

No information is available as to whether amino acids are absorbed by

TABLE XLIII

AMINO ACIDS ABSORBED BY SOME PARASITIC PROTOZOA[a]

Species	Alanine	Arginine	Asparagine	Aspartic acid	Cysteine	Glutamic acid	Glutamine	Glycine	Histidine	Isoleucine	Leucine	Lysine	Methionine	Phenylalanine	Proline	Serine	Threonine	Tryptophane	Tyrosine	Valine	Method	References
Flagellates																						
Crithidia fasciculata		x							x	x	x	x	x	x			x	x	x	x	E	Cowperthwaite *et al.* (1953); Kidder and Dutta (1958)
Leishmania donovani				x																	O	Chatterjee and Ghosh (1959)
Leishmania tarentolae		x		x		x		x	x	x	x	x		x	x	x	x	x	x	x	E	Trager (1957)
Strigomonas oncopelti		x		x		x	x		x	x	x	x		x	x	x	x	x	x	x	O	Ryley (1955a)
Strigomonas oncopelti	x																				L	Gill and Vogel (1962)
Strigomonas oncopelti													x								E	Newton (1956, 1957)
Trichomonas foetus						x															O	Ryley (1955b)
Trichomonas foetus		x						x	x	x	x	x		x	x	x	x			x	E	Weiss and Ball (1947)
Trichomonas vaginalis		x			x				x				x								D	Iyori (1959)
Trypanosoma lewisi, B			x	x		x	x														O	Ryley (1951); Moulder (1948)
Trypanosoma lewisi, B			x	x		x	x														D	Thurston (1958)
Trypanosoma rhodesiense, C						x	x														O	Ryley (1962)
Sporozoa																						
Plasmodium knowlesi					x								x								L	Fulton and Grant (1956)
Plasmodium knowlesi													x								E	McKee *et al.* (1947)
Ciliates																						
Epidinium ecaudatum	x										x								x	x	L	Gutierrez and Davis (1962)
Ophryoscolex caudatus	x										x								x	x	L	Williams *et al.* (1961)

[a] KEY: E = essential in culture; O = stimulated O_2 consumption; L = incorporated labeled compound; D = deaminated compound; B = blood-stream form; C = culture form.

active transport mechanisms or by simple diffusion in the intestine of the above nematodes. Pertinent evidence has been presented for cestodes which of course absorb amino acids through their external surface. Daugherty (1957a,b) studied the uptake of labeled cystine and methionine by *Hymenolepis diminuta*. Because the Q_{10}, in the temperature range 4° to 38°C, was considerably higher than expected for simple diffusion and because certain amino acids, such as alanine or glycine, interfered with the absorption of cystine or methionine, the conclusion was drawn that the absorption involved active transport mechanisms. Similar experiments done with *Raillietina cesticillus* gave analogous results, but showed considerably higher absorption rates (Daugherty and Foster, 1958). Although the above experiments suggest strongly the participation of active transport mechanisms, they are not sufficiently clear-cut to prove them definitely, as Read *et al.* (1960b) have emphasized.

More sophisticated experiments were then carried out by Read *et al.* (1960a,b) with *Calliobothrium verticillatum*. They showed that at low external concentrations the absorption of L-valine and L-leucine followed first-order kinetics, while at concentrations above those yielding maximum penetration rates zero-order reaction kinetics prevailed. The amino acids in question accumulated against a concentration gradient and there was competitive inhibition between valine and leucine in respect to absorption. Metabolic inhibitors, such as iodoacetate or dinitrophenol, inhibited permeation at least of leucine. These experiments were sufficiently detailed to prove definitely that amino acids are taken up by active transport. It is of interest to note that no such assumption can be made for the permeation of urea. This compound apparently enters and leaks out of *Calliobothrium* and *Onchobothrium* by simple diffusion (Simmons *et al.*, 1960).

In further experiments Read *et al.* (1963) examined in detail the absorption of amino acids, especially methionine, by *Hymenolepis diminuta*. Accumulation against a concentration gradient, and noncompetitive inhibition of uptake by iodoacetate were proved, but dinitrophenol did not interfere with methionine uptake. Changing the Na/K ratio of the external medium, or addition of G-strophanthin were without effect, indicating, but not proving definitely, that a "sodium pump" may not be involved in the absorptive processes. Next, the influence of a large number of amino acids, tested in pairs, blocks of four, or in complex mixtures, was investigated in respect to influence on the uptake of methionine or other amino acids such as L-glutamic acid (cf. also Read and Simmons, 1962, for comparable experiments on *Calliobothrium*). Furthermore, similar studies were conducted with a series of analogs. The most significant result of this approach was the recognition of at least four qualitatively different absorption loci for amino acids: One for arginine-lysine, one for phenylalanine-tyrosine, one for dicarboxylic amino acids, and one for glutamic acid. Some of these loci, which, incidentally, do not necessarily represent fixed places in space, but may just as well involve some types of mobile carrier, appear to have overlapping affinities. Thus, evidence was adduced that methionine can enter the worms by more than one locus. Read *et al.* (1963) finally developed an equation that allows predictions concerning the rate at which a single component of an amino acid mixture is absorbed, as well as concerning the effects of altering individual components of the mixture. The equation reads as follows:

$$ v = \frac{V}{\frac{(K_t)}{(S)} + 1 + \frac{(K_t)\ (S^1)}{(K_{t1})\ (S)} + \frac{(K_t)\ (S^2)}{(K_{t2})(S)} \cdots\cdots + \frac{(K_t)\ (S^n)}{(K_{tn})\ (S)}} $$

In this equation v stands for the velocity of transport, V for the maximum velocity of transport when the transport loci are saturated, K_t for a transport constant and S for the substrate concentration. Since the S values will be known, and V as well as the K values can be determined independently, the equation can be tested by varying (S^1), (S^2) ... (S^n) and comparing v observed with v calculated for any (S).

Experiments essentially similar to those described above have also been done with the acanthocephalans *Moniliformis* and *Macracanthorhynchus* (Rothman and Fisher, 1964) yielding comparable results: concentration of methionine, and competitive inhibition of L-methionine uptake by a mixture of leucine, isoleucine, serine, alanine, and others.

The absorption of amino acids by endoparasitic arthropods seems not yet to have been studied. The only indirect evidence is due to House (1954). He found the following amino acids essential for *in vitro* growth of *Pseudosarcophaga affinis:* L-arginine, *l*-histidine, *dl*-isoleucine, *l*-leucine, *l*-lysine, *dl*-methionine, *dl*-phenylalanine, *dl*-threonine, *dl*-tryptophane, and *dl*-valine, and possibly glycine. It can be presumed that these compounds were actually taken up.

VI.   SYNTHETIC PROCESSES

Although no exact data are available it follows from differences in growth patterns that the extent of protein synthesis varies in different parasite species and often also at different periods in the life cycle of one species.

Large-scale protein synthesis takes place, for example, during the infection of small rodents with pathogenic trypanosomes. Hoppe and Chapman (1947) observed that *Trypanosoma equiperdum* increased in sugar-fed rats from about 20 million/ml blood to about 4 billion/ml within 100 hours. Other examples of pronounced protoplasm synthesis are the malarial parasites. Morrison and Jeskey (1948) estimated that about half the amino acids liberated from the breakdown of the erythrocytes are used by *Plasmodium knowlesi* for the synthesis of the parasites' body substance. Gregarines, on the other hand, only need to replace what nitrogenous compounds are being used up once the trophozoites are fully grown until they encyst and a new growth cycle sets in.

Similar differences occur also in parasitic worms. Tapeworms often grow very rapidly and they produce proglottids over long periods of time. *Hymenolepis diminuta* thus reached an average length of 35 cm in 14 days (Addis and Chandler, 1946), *Diphyllobothrium latum* specimens in dogs increased 61.5 mm in length daily from the fifteenth to thirtieth day after infection (Wardle and Green, 1941), and *Raillietina kashiwarensis* increased in weight from 0.10 mg to 142.5 mg in the interval from the third to the thirteenth day after infection (Sawada, 1959).

Rapid growth is also common in larval trematodes where 10,000 cercariae may be derived from a single miracidium of *Schistosoma japonicum* and more than 200,000 from one miracidium of *Schistosoma mansoni* (E. C. Faust and Hoffman, 1934).

Trematodes, nematodes, and Acanthocephala cease growing once they have reached adulthood. They must nevertheless possess marked powers of protein synthesis as evidenced by the fact that most parasitic helminths produce much greater numbers of reproductive cells than their free-living relatives. One *Haemonchus contortus* produces 5000 eggs daily on an average (Martin and Ross, 1934), one *Ancylostoma duodenale* 24,000 eggs (Augustine *et al.,* 1928), one *Ascaris lumbricoides* 200,000 eggs (H. W. Brown and Cort, 1927), and one *Fasciolopsis buski* 25,000 eggs (Stoll *et al.,* 1927). A graphic illustration of the protein synthesis necessarily involved is provided by the estimation of D. Fairbairn (1957) that the weight of the eggs and accompanying secretions produced by one *Ascaris* female in 24 hours corresponds to about 10% of the worm's total body weight. The actual nitrogen content of the eggs of human ascarids is 4.24 mg/million (Venkatachalam and Patwardhan, 1953).

Many phytoflagellates can satisfy their nitrogenous requirements from inorganic compounds such as nitrite or nitrate. Utilization of these latter compounds has never been demonstrated in parasites. It would, perhaps, be of interest to study in this respect forms like *Euglenomorpha hegneri* or *Hegneria leptodactyli,* which appear to be true parasites of amphibians (Kirby, 1941) and which are close relatives of free-living phytoflagellates.

The simplest nitrogenous compound utilized by some parasites is ammonia. The process has not been described so far from protozoa, but only from some helminths. Reductive amination of keto acids was first observed by Daugherty (1954) in *Hymenolepis diminuta*. He incubated worms in a medium containing ammonium carbonate and a keto acid (pyruvic, α-ketoglutaric, or oxalacetic acid) and observed after 90 minutes a rather considerable synthesis of amino nitrogen, the major amino acid formed in all cases being identified as alanine. Glucose also could serve as substrate, the keto acids produced during its utilization evidently being involved.

Reductive amination occurs also in *Ascaris lumbricoides*. Pollak and Fairbairn (1955b) found that ovary homogenates synthesized in the presence of pyruvate and ammonium chloride both alanine and aspartic acid, quantitative considerations leading to the conclusion that amination of both pyruvate and oxalacetate had taken place. The rates observed indicated that the process may be of biological significance for the protein synthesis of the ovaries. Pollak (1957a) showed subsequently that worms kept *in vitro* maintained the normal, relatively high levels of free ammonia and nonprotein amino acids in the ovaries only when the incubation medium contained ammonia, both levels decreasing rapidly and sharply in its absence. Pollak (1957b) then showed that alanine synthesis by ovary homogenates was greatly enhanced by the addition of chloramphenicol and ascorbic acid and that in the presence of the former compound ATP and DPNH increased alanine formation. Methylene blue could not substitute effectively for DPNH, indicating that the reductive amination of pyruvate by the worm tissues depended on a hydrogen donor such as a reduced coenzyme and thus on anaerobiosis. The continuity of the reaction requires effective removal of the newly formed alanine. It seems to be achieved by transamination, both a nonspecific alanine-α-ketotransaminase and a more specific alanine-glutamic acid transaminase occurring in the ovaries.

Incubation of parasites in solutions containing labeled glucose or acetate proves that carbon atoms derived from these substances can rather readily be incorporated into proteins. Relevant observations are available for *Entamoeba histolytica* where only radioactive aspartic acid, glutamic acid, and alanine were recovered (Becker and Geiman, 1955), while in the case of the blood-stream form of *Trypanosoma rhodesiense* labeling was confined to aspartic acid, glycine, serine, and alanine, with little activity in glutamic acid. Less incorporation of isotopes from C^{14}-glucose into proteins has been reported from the blood-stream forms of *Trypanosoma equiperdum* and *Trypanosoma cruzi* (Pizzi and Taliaferro, 1960). Ready use of labeled acetate for protein synthesis has been found in *Strigomonas oncopelti;* 13 labeled amino acids were recovered in this instance (Newton, 1957).

Alimentary amino acids can also be used rather freely for protein synthesis, a fact which evidently is not surprising. Pizzi and Taliaferro (1960) incubated trypanosomes in solutions containing S^{35}-amino acids and found rapid incorporation into proteins. The relative rates of synthesis by the various forms used were: "released" adults of *Trypanosoma lewisi* (i.e., washed adults injected into fresh rats before the beginning of multiplication) and dividing *Trypanosoma equiperdum* > dividing *Trypanosoma lewisi* > blood-stream form of *Trypanosoma cruzi* > adults of *Trypanosoma lewisi. Strigomonas oncopelti* is another trypanosomid capable of incorporating labeled amino acids into its protoplasm (Newton, 1957). It can also interconvert certain amino acids, e.g., C^{14}-labeled glutamic acid was utilized for the synthesis of 12 amino acids, especially arginine and proline. On the other hand, when labeled arginine was given the radioactivity was confined almost exclusively to the arginine of the protein fraction, indicating that no large-scale conversion to other amino acids had taken place. Glycine and serine readily interconverted and also gave rise to cysteine (Newton, 1957). There is some question whether all the synthetic capabilities of *Strigomonas oncopelti* are due to the organism itself. Gill and Vogel (1962, 1963) studied the incorporation of labeled C atoms of aspartate and alanine into lysine and found in *Strigomonas* a labeling pattern similar to that characteristic for bacteria. They are of the opinion that lysine is formed via α, ϵ, -diaminopimelic acid and they found a diaminopimelic decarboxylase localized in the so-called bipolar bodies of the flagellates, which in reality may be endosymbionts and in part responsible for the synthetic processes found.

Malaria parasites also can interconvert certain amino acids. Fulton and Grant (1956) showed that S^{35}-methionine is rapidly incorporated into the proteins of *Plasmodium knowlesi,* but it is in part also converted to cystine. It was furthermore shown by these investigators that the parasites can hydrolyze globin and utilize the degradation products for protein synthesis, but that free amino acids of the blood plasma also can probably be utilized for this purpose.

Little relevant information is available for helminths. Hankes and Stoner (1956) showed that labeled glycine and alanine are incorporated into the proteins of *Trichinella spiralis* larvae during incubation *in vitro.*

As indicated in a previous section, certain amino acids must be present in the food to allow growth of parasites. These are the essential amino acids (Table XLIII) which cannot be synthesized by the body. All the other amino acids participating in the structure of proteins which do not have to be provided in the diet evidently can be synthesized by the organisms themselves. However, hardly anything is known about the mechanisms involved. One possibility is the reductive amination mentioned above, another transamination, that is, the transfer of an amino group from one amino acid to a keto acid by means of an enzymatic reaction, a process giving rise to a new amino acid. Often studied systems, and frequently the most potent ones, are the α-ketoglutaric ⟶ glutamic acid and the pyruvic acid ⟶ alanine systems. In both, many amino acids, and much less readily such substances as some purines or pyrimidines, can serve as amino group donors (Tables XLIV and XLV). In general, it would seem that protozoa have in this respect a wider range of activity than helminths, although data on so few species are available that this conclusion can be considered only as tentative. It is evident, however, that the helminths studied so far have only a quite restricted range of amino acids that can be used as substrates in the two above systems.

Keto acids other than α-ketoglutaric or pyruvic acid, can also serve as substrates of transamination. Oxalacetate is an example; it has been found active in *Hymenolepis diminuta* (Aldrich *et al.,* 1954) and in the ovaries of *Ascaris lumbricoides* (Pollak and Fairbairn, 1955b).

The question as to whether the various transaminase systems are mediated by a common enzyme or by specific enzymes has been elucidated only for *Ascaris*. It appears very probable (Pollak and Fairbairn, 1955b) that at least two major systems (alanine ⟶ glutamic acid, and aspartic acid ⟶ glutamic acid) involve two separate enzymes which differ slightly in pH optima (7.8 and 7.4, respectively).

VII. METABOLIC END PRODUCTS AND SOME METABOLIC PATHWAYS

To what extent either aerobically or anaerobically living parasites utilize proteins for energy production is difficult to state at present. Especially scanty is our knowledge about the extent, nature, and significance of the anaerobic processes involving proteins. Indeed, we cannot state categorically whether they are primarily anabolic or catabolic in nature.

Moulder and Evans (1946) showed that anaerobiosis inhibited the liberation of amino nitrogen by erythrocytes parasitized by *Plasmodium gallinaceum* from 40 to 80%. They point out that such an inhibition does not usually occur during simple enzymatic protein hydrolysis and they assume that the production of amino nitrogen is in this case somehow linked to oxidative processes. Groman (1951) reinvestigated the problem with the same organism. On the basis of inhibition studies with cyanide and malonate as well as observations on the relations between oxygen uptake, substrates, and amino acid production, he concluded that only a

TABLE XLIV

AMINO GROUP DONORS FOR THE α-KETOGLUTARIC ACID ⟶ GLUTAMIC ACID TRANSAMINATION SYSTEM[a,b]

Species	Alanine	Arginine	Asparagine	Aspartic acid	Cysteine	Cystine	Glutamine	Glycine	Histidine	Isoleucine	Leucine	Lysine	Methionine	Phenylalanine	Serine	Tryptophane	Tyrosine	Valine	References
Flagellates																			
Endotrypanum schaudinni	×	—	×	×	—		—		×		—	—	×	×		×	×	×	Zeledon (1960)
Leishmania donovani	×	(×)	—	×	×		—		×		×	×	×	×		×	×	×	Chatterjee and Ghosh (1957)
Leishmania enrietti	×	—	—	×	—	—	—		—		×	×	×	×		×	×	(×)	Zeledon (1960)
Trypanosoma cruzi	×	×	×	×	×	×	×		×		×	—	×	×		×	×	×	Zeledon (1960); Bash-Lewinson and Grossowicz (1957)
Trypanosoma vespertilionis	×	×	×	×	×	—	×		×		×	—	×	×		×	×	×	Zeledon (1960)
Cestodes																			
Hymenolepis citelli	×	+	×	×	—	—	—		—		—	—	—	—		—	—	—	Wertheim et al. (1960)
Hymenolepis diminuta	×	×	×	×	—	—	—		—		—	—	—	—		—	—	—	Aldrich et al. (1954); Wertheim et al. (1960)
Hymenolepis nana	—	—	×	×	—	—	—		—		—	—	—	—		—	—	—	Wertheim et al. (1960)
Nematodes																			
Ascaris lumbricoides	×	×	—	×	—	—	—		—		—	—	×	×	—	—	—	—	Cavier and Savel (1954a)
Ascaris lumbricoides	×	—	—	×	—	—	—		—		—	—	—	—	×	—	—	—	Pollak and Fairbairn (1955b)

[a] With the exception of *Ascaris*, whole animals or extracts therefrom were used as enzyme source; in the case of *Ascaris* preparations of intestinal tissues, testicle, muscle, and especially ovaries were employed.

[b] KEY: × = positive reaction; (×) = very weak reaction; — = no reaction.

TABLE XLV

Amino Group Donors for the Pyruvic Acid ⟶ Alanine Transamination System[a,b,c]

Species	Arginine	Asparagine	Aspartic acid	Cysteine	Cystine	Glutamine	Glutamic acid	Glycine	Histidine	Isoleucine	Leucine	Lysine	Methionine	Ornithine	Phenylalanine	Serine	Tryptophane	Tyrosine	Valine	References
Flagellates																				
Endotrypanum schaudinni	x	x	–	–		x	x	x	x	x	x	x	x	x	x	x	x	–	–	Zeledon (1960)
Leishmania donovani	x	x	(x)	(x)		–	x	x	x	x	x	x	x	x	x	x	x	–		Chatterjee and Ghosh (1957)
Leishmania enrietti	–	–	–	–		x	x	x	–	x	–	x	x	x	x	x	–	–	–	Zeledon (1960)
Trypanosoma cruzi	x	x	x	x	x	x	x	x	x	x	x	x	x	x	x	x	x	–	x	Bash-Lewinson and Grossowicz (1957); Zeledon (1960)
Trypanosoma vespertilionis	x	x	x	x	x	x	x	x	x	x	x	x	x	x	x	x	x	–	x	Zeledon (1960)
Cestodes																				
Hymenolepis citelli	–	–	–	–	–	–	x	–	–	–	–	–	–	–	–	–	–	–	–	Wertheim *et al.* (1960)
Hymenolepis diminuta	–	x	x	–	–	–	x	–	–	–	–	–	–	–	–	–	–	–	–	Aldrich *et al.* (1954); Wertheim *et al.* (1960)
Hymenolepis nana	–	–	–	–	–	–	x	–	–	–	–	–	–	–	–	–	–	–	–	Wertheim *et al.* (1960)
Nematodes																				
Ascaris lumbricoides	–	–	x	–	–	–	x	x	–	–	–	–	–	–	–	x	–	–	–	Pollak and Fairbairn (1955b)

a With the exception of *Ascaris* whole animals or extracts therefrom were used as enzyme source; in the case of *Ascaris* homogenates of ovaries were used primarily.

b Data on some additional compounds tested in respect of their ability of serving as amino group donors will be found in some of the papers quoted in this and the foregoing table.

c KEY: x = positive reaction; (x) = very weak reaction; – = no reaction.

secondary relationship exists between aerobic oxidations and protein hydrolysis. He could, however, not exclude the participation of anaerobic degradations.

A different situation seems to prevail in *Ascaris lumbricoides*. It was found to excrete identical amounts of nitrogenous material under anaerobic and aerobic conditions (von Brand, 1934; Savel, 1954), but it is unknown whether the waste products were derived from anabolic or catabolic processes.

Fairly good indications exist that several species of parasitic protozoa can utilize proteins, or at least some amino acids, as energy source under aerobic conditions. Thus, ammonia production, either recognizable only in sugar-free media or increased over that produced in the presence of sugar, has been reported for the culture forms of *Leishmania tropica* (Salle and Schmidt, 1928), *Trypanosoma cruzi* (von Brand *et al.*, 1949; Tobie *et al.*, 1950), for *Trichomonas vaginalis* (Iyori, 1957), and *Plasmodium gallinaceum* (Moulder and Evans, 1946; Groman, 1951). It has furthermore been shown that the oxygen uptake of several protozoan species is significantly increased when certain amino acids are available (Table XLIII). It must be stressed, however, that the mere demonstration of oxidative utilization of amino acids does not necessarily indicate that an organism can fill all its energy requirements by this mechanism. Thus, Mannozzi-Torini (1940) reported significant increases in oxygen consumption of *Trypanosoma evansi* in the presence of several amino acids, especially marked ones in the presence of histidine, asparagine, valine, and cysteine. Doubtless, however, the blood-stream form of *Trypanosoma evansi,* just like those of related species, dies very rapidly in the complete absence of an available carbohydrate. In the case of *Trypanosoma equiperdum* only very low respiratory rates were observed with yeast extract, casein hydrolyzate, or Bactopeptone as substrates (Thurston, 1958).

Some relevant data have also been obtained from studies of the endogenous metabolism of protozoa, the most convincing example being *Entodinium caudatum*. Abou Akkada and Howard (1962) showed that this ciliate lost large amounts of nitrogen during maintenance in non-fortified buffer solutions, 50 to 70% of the excreted nonprotein N appearing in the form of ammonia and about 20% in the form of free amino acids. Probable endogenous utilization of proteins has also been shown for *Crithidia fasciculata* by Cosgrove (1959). He observed a respiratory quotient of 0.85 and a distinct increase in ammonia nitrogen during periods of inanition. Less clear is the case of *Plasmodium lophurae*. Hellerman *et al.* (1946) observed a rather stable rate of respiration in the absence of an exogenous energy source. Since malaria parasites store but little polysaccharides, the possibility that proteins or lipids may serve as energy source offers itself.

Little corresponding information is available for helminths. Schulte (1917) determined the heat of combustion of fresh and starved *Ascaris* and concluded that carbohydrate metabolism accounted only for 80% of the total loss of calories. Since this species does not consume fat during short-term starvation experiments, it would seem possible that the remaining 20% is derived from protein utilization. There is no indication that protein is metabolized during the development of the eggs of ascarids. Szwejkowska (1929) did not find changes in their nitrogen content during maturation; 1.78% nitrogen was found by Kosmin (1928) both in undeveloped and developed eggs. This investigator points out that the apparent constancy in nitrogen content does not necessarily exclude an active protein metabolism since it could be related to an impermeability of the egg membranes preventing the excretion of nitrogenous end products. However, Passey and Fairbairn (1957) found the concentrations of protein and nonprotein nitrogen unchanged during embryonation of the *Ascaris* egg, that is, they found no indication that proteins participate in the energy production of the eggs.

Insofar as endoparasitic arthropods are concerned, von Kemnitz (1916) relates that protein in the medium exerts a glycogen-sparing action in the case of *Gastrophilus* larvae kept *in vitro,* an observation possibly indicating the utilization of protein.

A great variety of nitrogenous compounds is excreted by parasites (Tables XLVI and XLVII), but their significance varies. It must be emphasized that nitrogenous substances recovered from the medium after incubation of organisms having an intestinal tract often do not represent end products of actual intracellular protein utilization. They are usually a composite between such end products, fecal material, and regurgitated half-digested food. It is thus very likely that the peptones found among the excreta of *Ascaris* by Flury (1912), or the hemoglobin, coagulated proteins, albumoses, and peptones encountered in the dejections of *Fasciola* by Flury and Leeb (1926) stem from the latter sources. It is furthermore possible that some of the compounds listed in Tables XLVI and XLVII are lost through the orifices of the sex organs (Rogers, 1955), or represent glandular secretions (Haskins and Weinstein, 1957b).

Especially difficult to assess is the significance of amino acid excretion. The liberation of amino acids during the metabolism of malarial parasites (Moulder and Evans, 1946; Groman, 1951) can perhaps best be understood on the assumption that only a part of the degraded hemoglobin is actually absorbed and utilized by the parasites while the rest diffuses through the parasites' bodies. A similar assumption would hardly

TABLE XLVI

NITROGENOUS METABOLIC END PRODUCTS OF SOME PARASITES

Species	Material	Ammonia	Urea	Uric acid	Methylamine	Ethylamine	Propylamine	Butylamine	Amylamine	Heptylamine	Ethylenediamine	Cadaverine	Ethanolamine	1-Amino-2-propanol	References
Protozoa															
Leishmania tropica	Culture	x													Salle and Schmidt (1928)
Plasmodium gallinaceum	Incubates	x													Moulder and Evans (1946); Groman (1951)
Trichomonas vaginalis	Culture	x													Iyori (1959)
Trypanosoma cruzi	Culture	x													Tobie et al. (1950)
Trypanosoma lewisi	Blood form	x													Thurston (1958)
Trematodes															
Fasciola gigantica	Excreta	x		x											Goil (1958)
Fasciola hepatica	Excreta, body	x	x												Flury and Leeb (1926); van Grembergen and Pennoit-DeCooman (1944); Ehrlich et al. (1963)
Gastrothylax crumenifer	Excreta	x		x											Goil (1958)
Paramphistomum explanatum	Excreta	x		x											Goil (1958)
Schistosoma mansoni	Excreta	x	x												Senft (1963)

Cestodes

Organism	Source		References
Echinococcus granulosus[a]	Cyst fluid	x x	Mazzocco (1923); Flössner (1925); Lemaire and Ribère (1935); Codounis and Polydorides (1936)
Cysticercus tenuicollis[b]	Cyst fluid	x x	Schopfer (1932)
Hymenolepis diminuta	Excreta	x x x	D. Fairbairn *et al.* (1961); J. W. Campbell (1963a)
Lacistorhynchus tenuis	Excreta	x	Simmons (1961)
Moniezia benedeni	Body	x	van Grembergen and Pennoit-De-Cooman (1944)
Taenia taeniaeformis, larval	Excreta, body	x x x x x x x x	Salisbury and Anderson (1939); Haskins and Olivier (1958)

Nematodes

Organism	Source		References
Ascaridia galli	Excreta	x x	Rogers (1952)
Ascaris lumbricoides	Excreta, body fluid	x x	Weinland (1901); Flury (1912); Chitwood (1938a); Savel (1954); Guevara *et al.* (1961)
Ascaris lumbricoides larval	Excreta	x x x x	Haskins and Weinstein (1957a)
Ascaris lumbricoides,[c] eggs	Egg fluid	x x x x x	Haskins and Weinstein (1957a)
Nematodirus spp.		x	Rogers (1952)
Nippostrongylus muris, filariform larvae	Excreta	x x x	Weinstein and Haskins (1955)
Trichinella spiralis, larval	Excreta	x x x x x x x x x	Haskins and Weinstein (1957a,b)

[a] Also excretes creatinine and betaine.
[b] Also excretes creatinine.
[c] Also excretes 2 unidentified hydroxyamines, and possibly allylamine.

TABLE XLVII

EXCRETION OF AMINO ACIDS, PEPTIDES, AND PEPTONES BY SOME HELMINTHS

Species	Alanine	Aspartic acid	Glutamic acid	Glycine	Isoleucine	Leucine	Methionine	Ornithine	Phenylalanine	Proline	Serine	Tyrosine	Valine	α-Amino nitrogen	Peptides	Peptones	References
Trematodes																	
Fasciola hepatica																x	Flury and Leeb (1926)
Schistosoma mansoni	x				x			x		x							Senft (1963)
Cestodes																	
Hymenolepis diminuta														x			D. Fairbairn *et al.* (1961)
Nematodes																	
Ascaridia galli	x	(x)	(x)			x			x	x		(x)	x		x		Rogers (1955)
Ascaris lumbricoides	x	(x)	(x)			x			x	x			x		x		Flury (1912); Savel (1954); Rogers (1955)
Nematodirus spathiger,																	
Nematodirus filicollis	x	(x)	(x)			x			x				x		x		Rogers (1955)
Trichinella spiralis,																	
larval	x	x	x			x			x	x	x	x	x		x		Haskins and Weinstein (1957b,c)

be justified in the case of *Entodinium caudatum* which apparently releases during starvation large amounts of amino acids into the medium (Abou Akkada and Howard, 1962), nor in that of amino acid leakage by helminths (Table XLVII). It should be realized in this connection that amino acids are found also in the excreta of some free-living invertebrates; the significance of the process in the latter is just as obscure as in parasites.

While thus the exact nature of the compounds listed in Table XLVII is far from clear, it is reasonable to assume that those listed in Table XLVI are true metabolic end products, that is, it can be assumed that they are derived from compounds utilized intracellularly. Especially widespread is ammonia production. It is common among protozoa and occurs, although apparently not as regularly, also in helminths. Quantitatively, ammonia is the most important identified nitrogenous end product in such forms as *Leishmania, Trypanosoma cruzi, Fasciola,* and others. Especially interesting is the case of the adult *Ascaris.* If the worm is kept in large amounts of medium, ammonia accounts for about 70% of the excreted nitrogen and urea for about 7%. However, if it is confined to a narrow glass tube, the ammonia excretion is reduced by more than 50% and the urea excretion increases sharply, accounting now for 51% of the excreted nitrogen (Savel, 1954; Cavier and Savel, 1954b). Biologically, the significance of this shift lies in the reduction of potentially toxic ammonia concentrations in the immediate vicinity of the worms and substitution of the less toxic urea. Most parasites live normally in more or less fluid and constantly changing environments which will rather rapidly dilute any excreted material. In this respect they resemble aquatic animals rather than terrestrial ones. Characteristically, ammonia excretion is common only among the former.

Ammonia can be formed by several different enzymes. One well-known group of enzymes are the L- and D-amino acid oxidases, of which only the former appear to be of biological significance, since animal tissues do not commonly contain D-amino acids. Daugherty (1955) reported that *Hymenolepis diminuta* showed amino acid oxidase activity only against L-glutamic acid. A somewhat wider spectrum of activity, but always at rather low levels, has been found in the muscles and the intestine of *Ascaris,* arginine, aspartic acid, and glutamic acid being most readily attacked (Cavier and Savel, 1954a). Homogenates or minces of *Ascaris* ovaries, on the other hand, seem to contain neither L- or D-amino acid oxidases. They do, however, contain glutamic acid dehydrogenase, which also leads to ammonia formation (Pollak and Fairbairn, 1955b). A third way of ammonia production, observed in some helminths, is by means of urease. The enzyme does not occur in *Fasciola hepatica, Moniezia benedeni,* or *Taenia pisiformis* (van Grembergen and Pennoit-DeCooman, 1944), or in tetraphyllidean tapeworms (Simmons, 1961). It has, however, been found in some trypanorhynchid cestodes, especially *Lacistorhynchus tenuis* and *Pterobothrium lintoni,* but not in *Grillotia erinaceus.* The urease of *Lacistorhynchus* has been studied in some detail by Simmons (1961). Its activity shows a sharp maximum at pH 7.0 in phosphate buffer. Main activity occurred at substrate concentrations of 250 and 350 m*M,* an observation of special interest, because the urea concentrations in the blood and the gut contents of the host are approximately 330 m*M.* It is furthermore noteworthy that urea utilization could be shown not only in homogenates, but also when whole worms were employed. The latter produced ammonia and C^{14}-CO_2 from C^{14}-urea. Both compounds can conceivably be reutilized in synthetic processes. Some urease activity has also been described from nematodes: minces of *Nematodirus* spp., *Ascaridia galli,* and least pronounced *Haemonchus contortus* (Rogers, 1952). It has also been found in the intestine of *Ascaris lumbricoides,* but was hardly detectable in ovaries and muscle (Rogers, 1952; Savel, 1954), while the perivisceral fluid was intermediate.

Urea excretion has not yet been reported from parasitic protozoa, but is fairly common in helminths (Table XLVI). In vertebrates, urea is produced by the Krebs-Henseleit ornithine cycle. As the data summarized below indicate, the occurrence of this sequence in parasites has not yet been demonstrated conclusively, but there are indications that it, or an approximation of it, may be functional.

The first definite information to this effect was reported by Rogers (1952) for *Ascaridia galli, Nematodirus* spp., and *Ascaris lumbricoides.* He found that urea production was increased in the presence of arginine, the arginase being activated by Co^{++}, and in the presence of ornithine and citrulline. These findings were fully confirmed by Savel (1954), who observed a stronger arginase activity in the intestine of *Ascaris* than in its hemolymph or muscle layer.

It has furthermore been known for a long time (van Grembergen and Pennoit-DeCooman, 1944) that arginase occurs in parasitic flatworms, such as *Cysticercus pisiformis, Moniezia benedeni, Taenia pisiformis,* and *Fasciola hepatica.* However, only in recent years has more complete information come to light. J. W. Campbell (1963a) studied urea formation in *Hymenolepis diminuta,* establishing that it was increased by arginine and that it involved incorporation of CO_2. This latter observation indicates that an initial CO_2-activating step was involved prior to the actual reactions of the ornithine cycle. However, all attempts to demonstrate synthesis of one of the key compounds, carbamyl phosphate, failed. J. W. Campbell (1963a) could demonstrate and partially characterize two important enzymes of the cycle, ornithine transcarbamylase and arginase. The former was localized in the particulate fraction of the homogenates, the latter essentially in the soluble one. Arginase had a sharp pH optimum at pH 9.5 and was dependent on the presence of Mn^{++} or Co^{++} in the system. The pH optimum of the ornithine transcarbamylase was 7.8–8.0, differentiating it from the corresponding bacterial and vertebrate enzymes. J. W. Campbell and Lee (1963) encountered the same two enzymes in some other tapeworms and the trematodes *Fasciola hepatica* and *Fascioloides magna,* although in some species, such as the ectoparasite *Entobdella bumpusi* or the endoparasite *Phyllobothrium foliatum,* no ornithine transcarbamylase was found. Of all species tested, *Lacistorhynchus tenuis* had by far the most active transcarbamylase and it was the only species in which the activity of this enzyme surpassed that of arginase.

Şome further relevant data for *Fasciola hepatica* have been provided by Ehrlich *et al.* (1963). They showed C^{14}-CO_2 fixation into urea, proved the occurrence of the essential amino acids of the ornithine cycle (ornithine, citrulline, arginine, aspartic, and glutamic acid) as free amino acids within the tissues of the worms, and finally showed an increase in urea formation under the influence of ornithine.

It has been mentioned above that urea formation has not yet been reported for parasitic protozoa. This does not imply that the compound is inert for them. In at least one case a very curious physiological action of urea has been reported. Steinert (1958) found that urea provides the stimulus for the transformation of the crithidia of *Trypanosoma mega* into the blood-stream form. This seems to be a unique case. In the few other instances in which transformation of similar nature was achieved *in vitro* (*Trypanosoma vivax,* according to Trager, 1959; *Trypanosoma theileri,* according to Ristic and Trager, 1958; and *Trypanosoma conorhini,* according to Deane and Deane, 1961), elevation of the temperature proved to be the decisive factor.

Of considerable interest is the excretion of a great variety of amines, a process described so far only for nematodes (Table XLVI). These compounds undoubtedly originate from amino acids through decarboxylation. Pronounced decarboxylation activity has been reported from *Ascaris* with histidine, lysine, and ornithine leading respectively to histamine, cadaverine, and putrescin. There was less activity with arginine, phenylalanine, tryptophane, and tyrosine, and none with alanine, glycine, leucine, and valine (Savel, 1954; Cavier and Savel, 1954a). Mettrick and Telford (1963) found histidine decarboxylase activity in *Mesocoelium monodi,* which contained also considerably more histamine in its tissues (58.3 μg/gm) than *Fasciola hepatica* (5.2 μg/gm) and

Oochoristica ameivae (13.0 μg/gm). The latter two worms showed no measurable histidine decarboxylase activity. Little is known about the actual occurrence of histamine in roundworms. The only observation available seems to be that of Deschiens (1948), who reported 2 μg histamine/ml perienteric fluid of *Ascaris lumbricoides*.

The occurrence of histamine in, or its excretion by, helminths requires special comment, because the compound may be involved in the production of toxic phenomena due to parasitization. The question concerning production of true toxins by helminths is controversial (review of older literature in von Brand, 1952; newer data concerning *Ascaris* in Nakajima, 1954, and concerning *Setaria* in Taniguchi *et al.*, 1961). It is, however, generally conceded that many symptoms observed after injection of flatworm or roundworm extracts into experimental animals can best be explained by assuming that they had histamine-like action (e.g., Deschiens and Poirier, 1947a,b, 1949, 1953; Rocha e Silva *et al.*, 1946; Gurtner, 1948). This does evidently not necessarily prove that the histamine present in the worms, or excreted by them, is directly responsible. Indeed, the amount of histamine found by Deschiens (1948) in 1 ml perienteric fluid of *Ascaris* was only 1.2% of a dose lethal to guinea pigs, despite the fact that the injection of 1 ml perienteric fluid will kill them. It is probable that in this and similar cases anaphylactic reactions were involved which involve the release of histamine from the tissues of the host (Rocha e Silva and Grana, 1946a,b, Rocha e Silva *et al.*, 1946). This latter aspect has been proven for *Ascaris*. Högberg *et al.* (1957a, b), Uvnäs *et al.* (1960), and Diamant (1961) prepared potent histamine-releasing extracts from this worm. The effectiveness of these extracts is attested to by the observation of Diamant (1961) that fully 50% of the releasable histamine is liberated within 1 minute of adding the extract. He found some indication that the process is dependent on enzymatic reactions yielding high-energy compounds.

Serotonin (5-hydroxytryptamine) is another amine that deserves to be discussed briefly. It, or at any rate a compound resembling it, has been found in *Fasciola hepatica* (Mansour *et al.*, 1957). Serotonin significantly stimulated motility, glucose uptake, and lactate production of the liver fluke, inducing a certain shift from fatty acid to lactic acid fermentation (Mansour, 1959). It was also found that the compound activated the worm's phosphofructokinase and the suggestion has been advanced that it may have a regulatory role on its carbohydrate metabolism (Mansour and Mansour, 1962).

The last end product of protein metabolism to be considered is a group of brownish to black pigments, the melanins. They are usually derived from tyrosine, tryptophan, or phenylalanine and their formation is mediated through a phenolase, such as tyrosinase. Convincing evidence for the presence of such a system in parasites has been presented by Blacklock *et al.* (1930) and Dinulescu (1932) for the larvae of *Cordylobia anthropophaga* and *Gastrophilus intestinalis,* respectively; the findings in both cases were essentially similar. Tyrosinase was found in greatest concentration in the hemocele fluid, while various organs contained but little, if any, of the enzyme. Tyrosinase was most concentrated in the last prepupal instar and only then, in *Cordylobia,* could tyrosine be demonstrated. The presence of the complete melanin-forming system at this point of the development is understandable since large amounts of the pigment are used during the blackening of the pupal case. It can be presumed that the system is functional also in the earlier instars, since the spines of the second instar *Cordylobia* are black.

Little definite information concerning the possible occurrence of melanin in other groups of parasites is available. Nadakal (1960) considers the dark pigment of the body and the eye spot of the cercaria *Euhaplorchis californiensis* and an unidentified schistosome cercaria to consist of melanin. He found indications for the presence of tyrosine, but attempts to demonstrate a tyrosinase were inconclusive. Whether the conspicuous black or dark-brown color of many trematode eggs is due to melanin is so far an open question. It has been demonstrated that polyphenols which could serve as mother substance participate in the formation of the eggshell of *Fasciola* (Stephenson, 1947b), and Mansour (1958) found in this helminth a phenol oxidase.

VIII. DISTURBANCES IN THE HOST'S PROTEIN METABOLISM DURING PARASITIC INFECTIONS

Interference with protein digestion or absorption seems not to be very pronounced in most parasitic infections studied in this respect. Thus, even heavy infections with hookworms reduced nitrogen absorption only slightly in humans (Holmes and Darke, 1958; Darke, 1959), while a somewhat more significant depression of protein digestion and absorption has been observed during *Ascaris* infections of children (Venkatachalam and Patwardhan, 1953). A certain depression of protein digestion coupled with a slight reduction in absorption has been demonstrated by Symons (1960b) with the help of radioiodine-tagged albumin in the case of rats infected with *Nippostrongylus muris.* However, malabsorption, studied with L-histidine and D-glucose as substrates, is not an important factor in the disease. Absorption was decreased in the jejunum of infected rats (Symons, 1960a), but increased in the distal ileum (Symons, 1960c); in effect the over-all absorption rate of histidine proved essentially unchanged. Trypsin secretion was normal, but leucine-aminopeptidase, an enzyme confined to the cell surface, was distinctly reduced in the jejunum (Symons and Fairbairn, 1962, 1963). Some contradictory information is available in respect to digestion and utilization of food material by sheep infected with nematodes of various species. Stewart (1933a) and Shearer and Stewart (1933) observed a lowered digestion coefficient of crude protein and crude fiber in heavily infected lambs, findings not fully confirmed by Andrews (1938) and Andrews et al. (1944). These investigators studied the effects of pure infections with Cooperia curticei and Trichostrongylus colubriformis. They found in the majority of their lambs approximately normal digestibility coefficients but did observe that the infected lambs were less efficient than controls in transforming food into body substance. Andrews (1938) ascribed this primarily to a nervous excitation due to irritation and inflammation of the intestinal mucosa. Franklin et al. (1946) confirmed essentially the work of Andrews et al. (1944) and described a depression in crude fiber digestibility.

The observations quoted so far were all derived from studies conducted with heavily infected animals. Spedding (1954) on the contrary investigated the influence of subclinical infections with Trichostrongylus axei and Strongyloides papillosus on the digestive efficiency of sheep. Infected specimens had somewhat less appetite than noninfected ones, and showed a distinctly lowered digestion of crude protein, but not of crude fiber. Spedding (1954) considers these two factors the main reasons why infected sheep gained less weight than worm-free controls.

Little attention seems to have been given so far to the question whether comparable changes occur in parasitized invertebrates. Only Degkwitz (1958) has considered the question for sacculinized Carcinus maenas. He found decreased digestion of casein and edestin, and he is of the opinion that the well-known changes in metabolism of infected crabs are due in part to a disturbance in protein digestion resulting from changed production of proteolytic digestive enzymes.

One of the most characteristic abnormal symptoms involving proteins concerns changes in the blood proteins. The literature covering these alterations is so voluminous that no attempt at complete coverage was undertaken; some representative newer data are summarized in Tables XLVIII and XLIX. The most characteristic symptom, almost invariably present, is a more or less marked decline in the albumin fraction, while one or more of the globulin fractions usually are increased. As a consequence, the over-all changes in total protein are sometimes not marked, even though the relative proportions of albumin and globulin have changed considerably. Evidently, a further consequence of these changes

TABLE XLVIII

Plasma Proteins During Infections with Parasitic Protozoa[a,b]

Parasite	Host	Total protein	Albumin	Globulin α	Globulin β	Globulin γ	References
Flagellates							
Leishmania donovani	Man	±	−	−	±	−	Pitzus (1957); Kumar et al. (1958)
Leishmania donovani	Hamster, mouse		−	±	±	+	Rossan (1960)
Trypanosoma brucei	Guinea pig	±	−	± or +	±	± or +	Olberg (1955); Lippi and Benedetto (1958)
Trypanosoma gambiense	Man		−	±	±	+	Gall (1956)
Trypanosoma evansi	Guinea pig		−	+	±	−	Bellelli and Caraffa (1956)
Rhizopods							
Entamoeba histolytica	Man			+	−	± or +	Powell (1959); Fuhrmann (1962)
Entamoeba histolytica	Guinea pig		−	+	+	±.	Atchley et al. (1961)
Sporozoa							
Eimeria bovis	Calf	−	−	+	± or +	± or −	Fitzgerald (1964)
Eimeria tenella	Chicken		−	+	−	±	Martynowicz and Seniow (1956)
Plasmodium berghei	Mouse, rat		− or ±	± or −	± or +	+	Corradetti et al. (1955); Briggs et al. (1960)
Plasmodium falciparum	Man	−	−	±	±	+	Van Sande (1956)
Plasmodium vivax	Man	−	−	±	±	+	Van Sande (1956); Schneider (1958)
Toxoplasma gondii	Rat		−	±	±	+	Alosi and Andrini (1957); Wildführ et al. (1958)

[a] Numerous older references concerning infections with the above parasites, and some additional parasites in Stauber (1954); see also Angeloff et al. (1958); Arnaki et al. (1957); Dunlap et al. (1959); Gionta and Marioni (1957); Hara et al. (1955); Schinazi (1957); Seneca et al. (1958); Shumard (1957); Woodruff (1957); Mazzetti and Mele (1961); Desowitz (1960b).

[b] KEY: + = increase; ± = normal, or minor deviations from normal; − = decrease.

TABLE XLIX

PLASMA PROTEINS DURING INFECTIONS WITH PARASITIC HELMINTHS[a,b]

Parasite	Host	Total protein	Albumin	Globulin			References
				α	β	γ	
Trematodes							
Clonorchis sinensis	Rabbit		−	+	+	+	Kuwamura (1958)
Fasciola gigantica	Zebu cattle	±	−	−	±	+	Weinbren and Coyle (1960)
Schistosoma bovis	Cattle	±	−	+	−	−	Arru and Parriciatu (1960)
Schistosoma japonicum	Man, monkey	+	−	+	+	+	Sadun and Walton (1958); Smithers and Walker (1961)
Schistosoma mansoni	Man	±	−	±	±	+	Coutinho and Loureiro (1960); Ramirez et al. (1961)
Nematodes							
Ancylostoma caninum	Dog	−	−	±	+	+ or −	Hara (1956)
Gnathostoma spinigerum	Rabbit		−	+	+	+	Kitsuki (1958)
Trichinella spiralis	Guinea pig, rabbit	−	−	+	± or −	+	Seniow (1956, 1961)
Trichostrongylus axei	Calve	−	−	+	−	−	Leland et al. (1959)
Trichostrongylus axei	Lamb	−	−	±	±	+	Leland et al. (1960)
Wuchereria bancrofti	Man	−	−	+	±	+	Bénex and Deschiens (1960)

[a] Some additional data for infections with the above and other helminths in von Brand (1952) and Stauber (1954). See also Baba *et al.* (1956); Bersohn and Lurie (1953); Congiu and Pirlo (1956); Kona (1957a,b); Kuttler and Marble (1960); Marco Ahuir and Bellod Garcia (1958); Turner (1959); Turner and Wilson (1962); Varleta *et al.* (1961); Weimer *et al.* (1955, 1958); DeWitt (1957a); Bremner (1961).

[b] KEY: + = increased, ± = normal or minor deviations from normal; − = decreased.

is an altered albumin/globulin ratio, which quite generally is changed in favor of globulin.

The mechanisms responsible for the alterations in blood proteins are probably not uniform and difficult to evaluate for the individual case at the present state of our knowledge. The decrease in albumin can be due, and probably is due not rarely, to leakage into the lumen of the injured intestine, as has been assumed, for instance, in the case of coccidian infections (Fitzgerald, 1964). Reduction in albumin, but also of other protein fractions, entails a lowering of the osmotic pressure of the blood. A consequence may be a loss of fluid from the capillaries leading to edema, a symptom not rarely observed in malaria, ankylostomiasis, or schistosomiasis. Attempts to explain this symptom on the basis of changed blood protein concentration have, in the case of malaria, not been entirely successful (Boyd and Proske, 1941; Kopp and Solomon, 1941). The latter authors assume that the anemia developing during the disease is a contributing factor, a plausible explanation, since the effects of anoxia on capillary permeability are well established (Maegraith, 1948). Similarly, the anemic condition developing during schistosomiasis or ankylostomiasis may be a contributing factor toward the origin of edema (Salah, 1938), although in these diseases the lowered albumin content of the blood plasma has been incriminated with greater emphasis than in malaria (Villela and Teixeira, 1937; Salah, 1938). Certainly, however, the above concept cannot be applied indiscriminately to all edemas of verminous origin. Filarial elephantiasis, for example, is due largely to an obstruction of the lymphatic vessels. Drinker et al. (1934) could produce marked edemas in dogs by blocking the lymphatics.

Changes in blood proteins can be caused by liver damage. More or less severe signs of disturbed liver function, accompanied by changes in blood proteins, have thus been reported for gnathostomiasis (Kitsuki, 1958), clonorchiasis (Kuwamura, 1958), or fasciolodiasis (Weinbren and Coyle, 1960). However, no generalizations are possible. In chronic human schistosomiasis, for example, no overt signs of liver involvement have been observed, despite changes in blood proteins (Ramirez et al., 1961). In this and similar cases probably immunological mechanisms are involved. The presence of antibodies has thus been demonstrated, or at least made likely, in the β- and γ-globulin fractions during strongyloidiasis (Turner, 1959), and in rat malaria (Causse-Vaills et al., 1961), to give only two examples.

It is possible that the appearance of antibodies is also responsible for the relatively rare cases of qualitative changes in serum proteins described so far, as contrasted to the numerous quantitative ones reviewed above. Qualitative changes have been deduced from changes in electro-

phoretic mobility which lead either to the appearance of a new component, or to a divided peak of a known component. In human infect-
tions with *Leishmania donovani* Benhamou (1947) and Benhamou *et al.*
(1949) found a protein fraction with a mobility faster than albumin;
according to these authors and to Cooper *et al.* (1946), the γ-globulin
fraction contains an abnormally slow moving component. It seems that
various host species react in a different way to infections with *Leishmania donovani.* A slow moving γ-globulin develops, according to
Rossan (1960), during infections of cotton rats, golden and Chinese
hamsters, but not of chinchillas, mice, or gerbils. In pigeons infected
with *Plasmodium relictum* Schinazi (1957) observed a component moving faster than albumin which may have been a lipoprotein, while in
chicken infected with *Plasmodium lophurae* the electrophoretic mobility
of γ-globulin increased with the rise of the infection (Sherman and Hull,
1960). Some qualitative changes have also been reported for trypanosomiasis. In human infections with *Trypanosoma gambiense* an extra component appeared as a shoulder on the peak, between β- and γ-globulin
(Gall, 1956), and in rabbits infected with *Trypanosoma equiperdum* the
α- and β-globulin peaks, which appeared as single peaks in controls,
divided into distinct α_1 and α_2, and β_1 and β_2 peaks, respectively (Angeloff
et al., 1958). A similar double peak for α-globulin has been described
from guinea pigs infected with *Entamoeba histolytica* (Atchley *et al.*,
1961). D'Alesandro (1959) studied *Trypanosoma lewisi* infections and
found that ablastin and the two trypanocidal antibodies migrated between β- and γ-globulin, but he nevertheless is of the opinion that no
new protein component was associated with the antibody activities.

Changes in proteins, similar in principle to those described above for
blood proteins, occur in the cerebrospinal fluid during the later stages
of human sleeping sickness. The protein content is usually increased, but
the data are difficult to evaluate properly because, as Hill (1948) pointed
out, various methods give different results and different authors report
differing results from normal persons upon applying the same method. It
does, however, seem fairly certain that any increase is due to an increase
in γ-globulin (Sicé, 1930; Zschucke, 1932; H. Fairbairn, 1934). More recently, Janssens *et al.* (1961) studied the proteins of the cerebrospinal
fluid by agar electrophoresis. They found all γ-globulin fractions, but
especially the γ_2 and γ_3 fractions, increased, but they could not detect
any qualitative deviations from normal protein composition. Corresponding changes, increase in total protein due largely to increase in γ-globulin,
have also been found during infections of the human central nervous system with *Cysticercus cellulosae* (Varleta *et al.*, 1961).

While the literature on protein changes during parasitic infections is extremely extensive, only few data are available concerning changes in blood amino acids. Matsumoto (1960) found an increase in total amino acids in the blood of *Toxoplasma*-infected mice; Rama Rao and Sirsi (1958) reported that the free amino acids, with the exception of cystine and histidine, increased in erythrocytes, but decreased in blood plasma during *Plasmodium gallinaceum* infections of chickens. Rama Rao and Giri (1952) had previously observed a 5-fold increase in free glutamic acid of the whole blood and the erythrocytes, surmising that this may have been due to an increase in transamination activity. However, only a transitory increase in transaminase activity has been found during human infections with *Plasmodium falciparum* (Fuhrmann, 1962) and a moderate increase in glutamic-oxalacetic transaminase in human infections with *Schistosoma mansoni* (Coutinho and Loureiro, 1960).

Still less is known about the amino acids of tissues. Rama Rao and Sirsi (1958) described a steady decline of all amino acids studied in liver and brain of chicken infected with *Plasmodium gallinaceum,* the only exception being cystine, which increased in the liver. Ramaswamy (1956) investigating the same infection, found an increased proline content of infected livers. What is more curious, however, he observed in the spleen of infected chickens allohydroxy-L-proline which he could not find in the spleens of control animals. The latter contained only γ-hydroxyproline.

The nonprotein nitrogen and the urea content of the blood usually appear approximately normal in the hitherto studied parasitic diseases. In the terminal stages of trypanosomiasis, where many vital functions fail, an increase in nonprotein nitrogen and urea occurs, while usually normal values are found during earlier stages (Scheff, 1928; Linton, 1930; Jones, 1933; Randall, 1934; Launoy and Lagodsky, 1936, 1937; French, 1938a,b). In malaria, these blood constituents frequently show a sharp increase in cases of partial or complete anuria, a natural consequence of nitrogen retention which is especially frequent in blackwater fever (Lahille, 1915; Patrick, 1922; Owen and Murgatroyd, 1928). Cases of increased blood urea have, however, also been reported from malarial patients who showed no obvious signs of renal involvement; this has been interpreted as being due to an increased tissue catabolism (Driver *et al.,* 1926). Similarly, Ohta and Nishizaki (1936) found an increased urinary excretion of ammonia, amino acids, and purine compounds in rabbits infected with *Schistosoma japonicum,* which they explained by assuming a faulty liver function. Some evidence to this effect is the observation that minced livers from infected animals formed markedly less allantoin than normal ones when incubated with uric acid (Nishizaki, 1938). The same author (Nishizaki, 1940) correlated an increase of urinary amino nitrogen with disturbed deamination in the liver of rabbits infected with *Clonorchis sinensis.*

Increased catabolism during infection has also been reported in respect to the turnover of albumin. It was observed only prior to death in some calves infected with *Ostertagia* and *Trichostrongylus.* In parasitized calves the total exchangeable albumin was significantly smaller than in noninfected controls, apparently because the synthesis was reduced in the former (Cornelius *et al.,* 1962). In rhesus monkeys infected with *Schistosoma mansoni* studies conducted with I^{131}-labeled albumin indicated that concomitant with serum protein changes a transient fall of total body and intravascular albumin occurred. Apparently at that time an increase in albumin catabolism took place which was not sufficiently compensated by anabolic processes (Smithers and Walker, 1961).

Finally, interesting observations are available on the nitrogen metabolism during trichinosis. Flury and Groll (1913) found a nitrogen retention during the period of development of the larvae in the muscles, but an increased nitrogen excretion began with formation of the capsules, probably resulting from the elimination of waste products originating from destroyed muscle fibers. Detailed studies were then done by Rogers (1941b, 1942). He found that the protein digestion of infected rats fell to a low point 8 to 12 days after infection. The urinary nitrogen and urea output rose immediately after infection, fell off then, to rise again sharply beginning about 13 days after infection. These changes were attributed to a toxic action of the parasites, since they occurred before a large-scale invasion of the muscle fibers took place. Urinary creatine and creatinine were markedly increased only after about 13 days, while the excretion of these compounds was abnormally low during the first 4 to 12 days. This finding somewhat parallels the observation of Markowicz and Bock (1931), who reported a similar decrease in infected humans during the acute febrile stage, while in all fatal cases a sharp increase in output occurred before death. As in other conditions leading to extended lysis of necrotic tissues, guanidine or guanidine derivatives are at abnormally high levels in the blood of animals dying of trichinosis and it has been suggested that guanidinemia may be an important factor in producing many of the symptoms described for this infection (Harwood *et al.,* 1937).

Hardly any data are available concerning changes in proteins of animals infected by parasitic arthropods, the only papers shedding some light on this question dealing with sacculinized crabs. Both Damboviceanu (1928) and Drilhon (1936) found the total proteins of their hemolymph abnormally high and the former investigator stated that this increase was due to a rise in the pseudoglobulin fraction.

IX. HOST DIETARY PROTEINS AND PARASITES

Most investigators of the question agree that a high protein diet of the host creates unfavorable conditions for intestinal protozoa. These can become so extreme as to lead to a severe reduction in the number of parasites maintaining themselves in the intestinal tract, or even to complete extinction of the infections. This has been shown for intestinal amoebas and flagellates of rats, monkeys, human beings, and hamsters (Hegner, 1923; Hegner and Eskridge, 1937; Ratcliffe, 1930; Kessel, 1929; Kessel and Huang, 1926; and Wantland and Johansen, 1954). Corresponding observations have also been reported for *Endamoeba blattae* and intestinal flagellates of cockroaches by Sassuchin (1931) and Armer (1944). In this instance, however, no unanimity of opinion exists. Morris (1936) indicates that in his experience better infections with *Endamoeba blattae* can be maintained in roaches kept on a high protein diet than in insects getting but little protein.

The mechanisms responsible for creation of conditions unfavorable to intestinal protozoa by dietary proteins are rather obscure. Diets high in protein are by their nature often deficient in carbohydrates and a lack of available carbohydrates may be a serious handicap to intestinal protozoa, especially such forms that live anaerobic or semianaerobic lives. On the other hand, it is possible that a bacterial flora, altered by the high protein diet, produces metabolites toxic to protozoa, or else that it produces unfavorable physicochemical conditions, such as an unfavorable pH, or oxidation-reduction potential. In other words, the same arguments can be employed in this instance as in the case of milk or lactose diet. A discussion of this problem has been presented by Read (1950).

An indirect action, originating from host tissues rather than from bacteria, must be assumed to explain the observation (Donaldson and Otto, 1946) that rats kept on a protein-deficient diet were unable to develop the same immunity from repeated sublethal infections with *Nippostrongylus muris* as rats kept on a balanced diet. Larsh (1950) used the same diet as Donaldson and Otto (1946) and found that it reduced the natural resistance and interfered with the development of acquired resistance against *Hymenolepis nana* in mice.

It is rather curious and again probably due to indirect action that proteins in the host diet even affect certain tissue and blood parasites. It has thus been observed (Actor, 1960) that an increased number of *Leishmania donovani* develops in mice kept on a protein-free diet, while, on the other hand, rats kept on a high meat diet developed more severe acute infections with *Plasmodium berghei* than controls on a balanced diet (Ramakrishnan, 1954). DeWitt (1957a,b) found that mice maintained on a torula yeast diet, that is, a diet deficient in factor 3, vitamin E, and cystine, developed heavier infections with *Schistosoma mansoni* than mice on a complete control diet and that the worms recovered from the former infections usually had not reached sexual maturity. When mice were fed torula yeast diet supplemented with vitamin E plus cystine, normal infections developed. In view of the complicated system it would be evidently premature to speculate on the role of cystine. The effects of a diet similar to that employed by DeWitt (1957a,b) were also studied in *Plasmodium berghei* infections of mice (Coatney and Greenberg, 1961). Only during the first week was there a noticeable difference between mice on the test diet and controls on a complete diet. The former showed about 5% of their erythrocytes infected, the latter about 13%. However, later in the infection the difference disappeared almost completely. Mice exposed to cercariae of *Schistosoma mansoni* developed a more severe inflammatory skin reaction, when maintained on a high protein diet, than when the diet was low in proteins (Coutinho-Abath, 1962).

X. PARASITE PROTEINS AND CHEMOTHERAPY

There is very little information available concerning the question as to whether parasiticidal drugs attack parasite proteins or interfere with some phase of their nitrogen metabolism.

Desowitz (1960a) found that Berenil, Pentamidine, Ethidium, and Antrycide in 0.5 M solutions precipitated portions of the proteins of cell-free extracts of the blood-stream forms of several species of African trypanosomes. The drugs were tightly bound to the denatured proteins and could not be eluted with H_2O or 0.1 N HCl. Suramin and tryparsamide failed to cause denaturation. It is not clear to what extent the above observations are relevant in elucidating drug activity *in vivo* since the concentrations used surpassed by far the tissue levels that can be expected in actual chemotherapeutic trials. It is, however, interesting to note that, according to Desowitz (1960a), injection of the Berenil/protein complex into rats confers definite prophylactic properties against challenging infections with *Trypanosoma gambiense* and *Trypanosoma brucei*.

An entirely different type of activity against *Leishmania donovani* has been ascribed to the antifungal antibiotic Nystatin. Ghosh and Chatterjee (1961) state that it had profound influence on the permeability of the organism. Under its influence low-molecular-weight solutes (material absorbing at 260 mμ or free amino acids) were released quantitatively into the medium; the same held true for a fraction of high-molecular-weight solutes, such as proteins or nucleic acids. It is assumed that the mode of action of the compound is purely physical, causing cellular disorganization, since no blockage of several major metabolic pathways tested occurred.

Finally, a few observations may be summarized which do not deal strictly with chemotherapy, but fit best into the present section.

Taliaferro and Pizzi (1960) observed that ablastin inhibited protein and nucleic acid synthesis of *Trypanosoma lewisi*. If they injected ablastin-containing serum into rats 1 day after they had been inoculated with juvenile (3 day) trypanosomes, the latter transformed within 2 hours into nondividing adults. Their protein synthesis (from S^{35}-amino acids) was inhibited by 66% and their nucleic acid synthesis (from adenine-8-C^{14}) by 87%.

Proteins can serve to differentiate parasite and host enzymes which have identical catalytic properties, an approach having obvious implications for chemotherapeutic measures. Bueding (1954) isolated a given enzyme, for instance, rabbit lactic dehydrogenase, and immunized a rooster with it. The serum of this animal then strongly inhibited the mammalian enzyme but in no way interfered with the activity of the corresponding enzymes of either *Schistosoma mansoni* or *Schistosoma japonicum,* proving a definite chemical difference between vertebrate and worm enzymes. In a similar way differences were demonstrated between the phosphoglucose isomerase of schistosomes and their hosts (Bueding and Mackinnon, 1955). It is especially interesting that antiserum against the lactic dehydrogenase of *Schistosoma mansoni* did not interfere with the activity of the phosphoglucose isomerase of the same worm, and the antiserum against the latter enzyme did not affect the former enzyme. In other words, no cross-reaction could be detected, indicating that the two antisera attacked specific sites of the enzymes and not groups common to different schistosome proteins.

REFERENCES

Abderhalden, E., and Heise, R. (1909). *Z. Physiol. Chem.* **62,** 136–138.
Abou Akkada, A. R., and Howard, B. H. (1960). *Biochem. J.* **76,** 445–451.
Abou Akkada, A. R., and Howard, B. H. (1962). *Biochem. J.* **82,** 313–320.
Actor, P. (1960). *Exptl. Parasitol.* **10,** 1–20.
Addis, C. J., and Chandler, A. C. (1946). *J. Parasitol.* **32,** 581–584.
Aducco, V. (1889). *Arch. Ital. Biol.* **11,** 52–69.
Agosin, M. (1956). *Bol. Chileno Parasitol.* **11,** 46–51.
Agosin, M., Brand, T. von, Rivera, G. F., and McMahon, P. (1957). *Exptl. Parasitol.* **6,** 37–51.
Aldrich, D. V., Chandler, A. C., and Daugherty, J. W. (1954). *Exptl. Parasitol.* **3,** 173–184.

Alosi, C., and Andrini, F. (1957). *Giorn. Mal. Infettive Parassit.* 9, 38–43.

Andrews, J. S. (1938). *J. Agr. Res.* 57, 349–361.

Andrews, J. S., Kauffman, W., and Davis, R. E. (1944). *Am. J. Vet. Res.* 5, 22–29.

Angeloff, S., Galaboff, S., and Nikoloff, P. (1958). *Z. Immunitaetsforsch.* 114, 464–471.

Armer, J. M. (1944). *J. Parasitol.* 30, 131–142.

Arnaki, M., Soysal, S. S., and Stary, Z. (1957). *Klin. Wochschr.* 35, 420–421.

Arru, E., and Parriciatu, A. (1960). *Parassitologia* 2, 7–11.

Asami, K. (1956). *Keio J. Med.* 5, 169–190.

Atchley, F. O., Auernheimer, A. H., and Wasley, M. A. (1961). *J. Parasitol.* 47, 297–301.

Augustine, D. L., Nazmi, M., Helmy, M., and McGavran, E. G. (1928). *J. Parasitol.* 15, 45–51.

Baba, T., Nagata, K., and Aizawa, T. (1956). *Gunma J. Med. Sci.* 5, 283–288.

Baernstein, H. D., and Tobie, E. J. (1951). *Federation Proc.* 10, 159.

Ball, E. G., McKee, R. W., Anfinsen, C. B., Cruz, W. O., and Geiman, Q. M. (1948). *J. Biol. Chem.* 175, 547–571.

Bash-Lewinson, D., and Grossowicz, N. (1957). *Bull. Res. Council Israel* E6, 91–92.

Beaumont, A. (1948). *Compt. Rend. Soc. Biol.* 142, 1369–1371.

Becker, C. E., and Geiman, Q. M. (1954). *J. Am. Chem. Soc.* 74, 3029.

Becker, C. E., and Geiman, Q. M. (1955). *Federation Proc.* 14, 180.

Bellelli, L., and Caraffa, V. (1956). *Riv. Ital. Igiene* 16, 412–418.

Benedictov, I. I. (1962). *Med. Parazitol. i Parazitarn. Bolezni* 31, 660–664; see *Chem. Abstr.* 58, 9449 (1963).

Bênex, J., and Deschiens, R. (1960). *Bull. Soc. Pathol. Exotique* 53, 932–935.

Benhamou, E. (1947). *Ann. Med. (Paris)* 38, 225–234.

Benhamou, E., Albou, A., Destaing, F., and Pugliese, J. (1949). *Bull. Mem. Soc. Med. Hop. Paris* 65, 1091–1098.

Berger, J., and Asenjo, C. F. (1940). *Science* 91, 387–388.

Bersohn, I., and Lurie, H. I. (1953). *S. African Med. J.* 27, 950–954.

Biguet, J., Capron, A., and TranVanky, P. (1962). *Ann. Inst. Pasteur* 103, 763–777.

Bird, A. F. (1954). *Nature* 174, 362.

Bird, A. F. (1955). *Science* 121, 107.

Bird, A. F. (1956). *Exptl. Parasitol.* 5, 350–358.

Bird, A. F. (1957). *Exptl. Parasitol.* 6, 383–403.

Bird, A. F., and Rogers, W. P. (1956). *Exptl. Parasitol.* 5, 449–457.

Björkman, N., Thorsell, W., and Lienert, E. (1963). *Experientia* 19, 3.

Blacklock, D. B., Gordon, R. M., and Fine, J. (1930). *Ann. Trop. Med. Parasitol* 24, 5–54.

Bondouy, T. (1910). Thesis, University of Paris.

Boni, A., and Orsi, N. (1958). *Nuovi Ann. Igiene Microbiol.* 9, 441–444.

Bonsdorff, B. von (1939). *Acta Med. Scand.* 100, 459–482.

Bonsdorff, B. von (1948). *Blood* 3, 91–102.

Boyd, M. F., and Proske, H. O. (1941). *Am. J. Trop. Med.* 21, 245–260.

Bradin, J. L. (1953). *Exptl. Parasitol.* 2, 230–235.

Brand, T. von (1933). *Z. Vergleich. Physiol.* 18, 562–596.

Brand, T. von (1934). *Z. Vergleich. Physiol.* 21, 220–235.

Brand, T. von (1937). *J. Parasitol.* 23, 316–317.

Brand, T. von (1939). *J. Parasitol.* 25, 329–342.

Brand, T. von (1952). "Chemical Physiology of Endoparasitic Animals." Academic Press, New York.

Brand, T. von, and Bowman, I. B. R. (1961). *Exptl. Parasitol.* 11, 276–297.

Brand, T. von, McMahon, P., Tobie, E. J., Thompson, M. J., and Mosettig, E. (1959). *Exptl. Parasitol.* 8, 171–181.

Brand, T. von, and Simpson, W. F. (1945). *Proc. Soc. Exptl. Biol. Med.* **60,** 368–371.

Brand, T. von, Tobie, E. J., Kissling, R. E., and Adams, G. (1949). *J. Infect. Diseases* **85,** 1–16.

Bremner, K. C. (1961). *Austrialian J. Agr. Res.* **12,** 498–512.

Briggs, N. T., Garza, B. L., and Box, E. D. (1960). *Exptl. Parasitol.* **10,** 21–27.

Brookes, J. A., and Mohr, J. L. (1963). *J. Protozool.* **10,** 138–140.

Brown, C. H. (1949). *Exptl. Cell Res.* Suppl. 1, 351–355.

Brown, C. H. (1950). *Nature* **165,** 275.

Brown, H. W., and Cort, W. W. (1927). *J. Parasitol.* **14,** 88–90.

Brown, K. N., and Williamson, J. (1964). *Exptl. Parasitol.* **15,** 69–86.

Bruni, A. (1939). *Settimana Med.* [N.S.] **27,** 1105–1106.

Bruni, A., and Passalaqua, A. (1954). *Boll. Soc. Ital. Biol. Sper.* **30,** 789–791.

Bueding, E. (1949). *Physiol. Rev.* **29,** 195–218.

Bueding, E. (1954). *In* "Cellular Metabolism and Infections" (E. Racker, ed.), pp. 25–34. Academic Press, New York.

Bueding, E., and Charms, B. (1951). *Nature* **167,** 149.

Bueding, E., and Charms, B. (1952). *J. Biol. Chem.* **196,** 615–627.

Bueding, E., and Mackinnon, J. A. (1955). *J. Biol. Chem.* **215,** 507–513.

Bueding, E., Kmetec, E., Swartzwelder, C., Abadie, S., and Saz, H. J. (1960). *Biochem. Pharmacol.* **5,** 311–322.

Burge, W. E., and Burge, G. L. (1915). *J. Parasitol.* **1,** 179–183.

Bushnell, L. D., and Erwin, L. E. (1949). *Physiol. Zool.* **22,** 178–181.

Campbell, J. W. (1960). *Exptl. Parasitol.* **9,** 1–8.

Campbell, J. W. (1963a). *Comp. Biochem. Physiol.* **8,** 13–27.

Campbell, J. W. (1963b). *Comp. Biochem. Physiol.* **8,** 181–185.

Campbell, J. W., and Lee, T. W. (1963). *Comp. Biochem. Physiol.* **8,** 29–38.

Campbell, W. C. (1960a). *J. Parasitol.* **46,** 769–775.

Campbell, W. C. (1960b). *J. Parasitol.* **46,** 848.

Carpenter, M. F. P. (1952). Dissertation, University of Michigan [not seen, quoted in Fairbairn, D., 1960].

Causse-Vaills, C., Orfila, J., and Fabiani, M. G. (1961). *Ann. Inst. Pasteur* **100,** 232–242.

Cavier, R., and Savel, J. (1952). *Compt. Rend.* **234,** 2562–2564.

Cavier, R., and Savel, J. (1954a). *Bull. Soc. Chim. Biol.* **36,** 1631–1639.

Cavier, R., and Savel, J. (1954b). *Compt. Rend.* **238,** 2448–2450.

Champêtier, G., and Fauré-Fremiet, E. (1937). *Compt. Rend.* **204,** 1901–1903.

Chatterjee, A. N., and Ghosh, J. J. (1957). *Nature* **180,** 1425.

Chatterjee, A. N., and Ghosh, J. J. (1959). *Ann. Biochem. Exptl. Med. (Calcutta)* **19,** 37–50.

Chitwood, B. G. (1936). *Proc. Helminthol. Soc. Wash., D.C.* **3,** 39–49.

Chitwood, B. G. (1938a). *Proc. Helminthol. Soc. Wash., D.C.* **5,** 18–19.

Chitwood, B. G. (1938b). *Proc. Helminthol. Soc. Wash., D.C.* **5,** 68–75.

Coatney, G. R., and Greenberg, J. (1961). *J. Parasitol.* **47,** 601–604.

Codounis, A., and Polydorides, J. (1936). *Proc. 3rd Intern. Congr. Comp. Pathol., Athens, 1936* Vol. 2, pp. 195–202. Eleftheroudakis, Athens.

Collier, H. B. (1941). *Can. J. Res.* **B19,** 90–98.

Congiu, M., and Pirlo, F. (1956). *Arch. Ital. Sci. Med. Trop. Parassitol.* **8,** 428–433.

Cook, L., Grant, P. T., and Kermack, W. O. (1961). *Exptl. Parasitol.* **11,** 372–379.

Cooper, G. R., Rein, C. R., and Beard, J. W. (1946). *Proc. Soc. Exptl. Biol. Med.* **61,** 179–183.

Cornelius, C. E., Baker, N. F., Kaneko, J. J., and Douglas, J. R. (1962). *Am. J. Vet. Res.* **23,** 837–842.

Corradetti, A., Toschi, G., and Verolini, F. (1955). *Rend. Ist. Super. Sanita* **18,** 246–255.

Cosgrove, W. B. (1959). *Can. J. Microbiol.* **5,** 573–578.

Costello, L. C., Oya, H., and Smith, W. (1963). *Arch. Biochem. Biophys.* **103,** 345–351.

Coutinho, A., and Loureiro, P. (1960). *Anales Fac. Med. Univ. Recife* **20,** 27–49.

Coutinho-Abath, E. (1962). *Rev. Inst. Med. Trop. Sao Paulo* **4,** 230–241.

Cowperthwaite, J., Weber, M. M., Packer, L., and Hutner, S. H. (1953). *Ann. N.Y. Acad. Sci.* **56,** 972–981.

Crusz, H. (1947). *J. Parasitol.* **33,** 87–98.

Crusz, H. (1948). *J. Helminthol.* **22,** 179–198.

D'Alesandro, P. A. (1959). *J. Infect. Diseases* **105,** 76–95.

Damboviceanu, A. (1928). *Compt. Rend. Soc. Biol.* **98,** 1633–1635.

Darke, S. J. (1959). *Brit. J. Nutr.* **13,** 278–282.

Dastre, A., and Stassano, H. (1903). *Compt. Rend. Soc. Biol.* **55,** 131–132.

Daugherty, J. W. (1954). *Proc. Soc. Exptl. Biol. Med.* **85,** 288–291.

Daugherty, J. W. (1955). *Exptl. Parasitol.* **4,** 455–463.

Daugherty, J. W. (1957a). *Exptl. Parasitol.* **6,** 60–67.

Daugherty, J. W. (1957b). *Am. J. Trop. Med. Hyg.* **6,** 466–470.

Daugherty, J. W., and Foster, W. B. (1958). *Exptl. Parasitol.* **7,** 99–107.

Davenport, H. E. (1949a). *Proc. Roy. Soc.* **B136,** 255–270.

Davenport, H. E. (1949b). *Proc. Roy. Soc.* **B136,** 271–280.

Davey, D. G. (1938). *Parasitology* **30,** 278–295.

Dawson, B. (1960). *Nature* **187,** 799.

Deane, M. P., and Deane, L. M. (1961). *Rev. Inst. Med. Trop. Sao Paulo* **3,** 149–160.

Deegan, T. (1956). *Trans. Roy. Soc. Trop. Med. Hyg.* **50,** 106–107.

Deegan, T., and Maegraith, B. G. (1956a). *Ann. Trop. Med. Parasitol.* **50,** 194–211.

Deegan, T., and Maegraith, B. G. (1956b). *Ann. Trop. Med. Parasitol.* **50,** 212–222.

Degkwitz, E. (1958). *Veroeff. Inst. Meeresforsch. Bremerhaven* **5,** 14–33.

Deiana, S. (1954). *Profilassi* **27,** 214–219.

Deiana, S. (1955). *Arch. Vet. Ital.* **6,** 225–229.

Del Bono, G. (1955). *Atti Soc. Ital. Sci. Vet.* **9,** 628–631.

Dent, J. N., and Schuellein, R. J. (1950). *Physiol. Zool.* **23,** 23–27.

Deschiens, R. (1948). *Ann. Inst. Pasteur* **75,** 397–410.

Deschiens, R., and Poirier, M. (1947a). *Compt. Rend. Soc. Biol.* **141,** 988–989.

Deschiens, R., and Poirier, M. (1947b). *Compt. Rend.* **224,** 689–690.

Deschiens, R., and Poirier, M. (1949). *Bull. Soc. Pathol. Exotique* **42,** 70–75.

Deschiens, R., and Poirier, M. (1953). *Compt. Rend. Soc. Biol.* **147,** 1059–1061.

Desowitz, R. S. (1959). *Nature* **184,** 986.

Desowitz, R. S. (1960a). *Exptl. Parasitol.* **9,** 233–238.

Desowitz, R. S. (1960b). *Ann. Trop. Med. Parasitol.* **54,** 281–292.

Devine, J., and Fulton, J. D. (1941). *Ann. Trop. Med. Parasitol.* **35,** 15–22.

Devine, J., and Fulton, J. D. (1942). *Ann. Trop. Med. Parasitol.* **36,** 167–170.

DeWaele, A. (1933). *Bull. Classe Sci. Acad. Roy. Belg.* [5] **19,** 649–660 [not seen, quoted in Bueding, E., 1949].

DeWitt, W. B. (1957a). *J. Parasitol.* **43,** 119–128.

DeWitt, W. B. (1957b). *J. Parasitol.* **43,** 129–135.

Diamant, B. (1961). *Acta Physiol. Scand.* **52,** 8–22.

Dinulescu, G. (1932). *Ann. Sci. Nat. (Paris), Zool.* [10] **15,** 1–183.

Dollfus, R. P. (1942). *Arch. Mus. Natl. Hist. Nat. Paris* [6] **19,** 52–53.

Donaldson, A. W., and Otto, G. F. (1946). *Am. J. Hyg.* **44,** 384–400.

Doran, D. J. (1957). *J. Protozool.* **4,** 182–190.

Doran, D. J. (1958). *J. Protozool.* **5,** 89–93.

Drilhon, A. (1936). *Compt. Rend.* **202**, 981–982.

Drinker, C. K., Field, M. E., Heim, J. W., and Leigh, O. C. (1934). *Am. J. Physiol.* **109**, 572–586.

Driver, J. R., Gammel, J. A., and Karnosh, L. J. (1926). *J. Am. Med. Assoc.* **87**, 1821–1827.

Dunlap, J. S., Dickson, W. M., and Johnson, V. L. (1959). *Am. J. Vet. Res.* **20**, 589–591.

Ebel, J. P., and Colas, J. (1954). *Compt. Rend. Soc. Biol.* **148**, 1580–1584.

Ehrlich, I., Rijavec, M., and Kurelec, B. (1963). *Bull. Sci. Conseil Acad. RPF Yougoslavie* **8**, 133.

Eisenbrandt, L. L. (1938). *Am. J. Hyg.* **27**, 117–141.

Evans, A. S. (1953). *Exptl. Parasitol.* **2**, 417–427.

Fairbairn, D. (1957). *Exptl. Parasitol.* **6**, 491–554.

Fairbairn, D. (1960). *In* "Nematology" (J. N. Sasser and W. R. Jenkins, eds.), pp. 267–296. Univ. of North Carolina Press, Chapel Hill, North Carolina.

Fairbairn, D., Wertheim, G., Harpur, R. P., and Schiller, E. L. (1961). *Exptl. Parasitol.* **11**, 248–263.

Fairbairn, H. (1934). *Trans. Roy. Soc. Trop. Med. Hyg.* **27**, 471–490.

Fairley, N. H. (1920). *J. Pathol. Bacteriol.* **23**, 289–314.

Fauré-Fremiet, E. (1913a). *Compt. Rend. Soc. Biol.* **74**, 1407–1409.

Fauré-Fremiet, E. (1913b). *Arch. Anat. Microscop.* **15**, 435–757.

Fauré-Fremiet, E., and Filhol, J. (1937). *J. Chim. Phys.* **34**, 444–451.

Fauré-Fremiet, E., and Garrault, H. (1944). *Bull. Biol. France et Belgique* **78**, 206–214.

Fauré-Fremiet, E., Ebel, J. P., and Colas, J. (1954). *Exptl. Cell Res.* **7**, 153–168.

Faust, E. C., and Hoffman, W. A. (1934). *Puerto Rico J. Public Health Trop. Med.* **10**, 1–97.

Faust, E. S., and Tallqvist, T. W. (1907). *Arch. Exptl. Pathol. Pharmakol.* **57**, 367–385.

Feinberg, J. G., and Morgan, T. J. (1953). *Brit. J. Exptl. Pathol.* **34**, 104–118.

Fermi, C. (1910). *Zentr. Bakteriol. Parasitenk., Abt. I: Orig.* **56**, 55–85.

Fetterolf, D. W. (1907). *Univ. Penn. Med. Bull.* **20**, 94–96.

Fitzgerald, P. R. (1964). *J. Parasitol.* **50**, 42–48.

Flossner, O. (1925). *Z. Biol.* **82**, 297–301.

Flury, F. (1912). *Arch. Exptl. Pathol. Pharmakol.* **67**, 275–392.

Flury, F., and Groll, H. (1913). *Arch. Exptl. Pathol. Pharmakol.* **73**, 214–232.

Flury, F., and Leeb, F. (1926). *Klin. Wochschr.* **5**, 2054–2055.

Fox, H. M. (1953). *Nature* **171**, 162–163.

Franklin, M. C., Gordon, H. McL., and Macgregor, C. H. (1946). *J. Council Sci. Ind. Res. Australia* **19**, 46–60.

Fredericq, L. (1878). *Bull. Classe Sci. Acad. Roy. Belg.* [2] **46**, 213–228 [not seen, quoted in Bueding, E., 1949].

Freeman, R. F. H. (1962). *Comp. Biochem. Physiol.* **7**, 199–209.

Freeman, R. F. H. (1963). *Comp. Biochem. Physiol.* **10**, 253–256.

French, M. H. (1938a). *J. Comp. Pathol. Therap.* **51**, 36–41.

French, M. H. (1938b). *J. Comp. Pathol. Therap.* **51**, 42–45.

Friedheim, E. A. H., and Baer, J. G. (1933). *Biochem. Z.* **265**, 329–337.

Fuhrmann, G. (1962). *Z. Tropenmed. Parasitol.* **13**, 53–67.

Fulton, J. D., and Grant, P. T. (1956). *Biochem. J.* **63**, 274–282.

Fulton, J. D., and Spooner, D. F. (1956). *Biochem. J.* **63**, 475–481.

Fulton, J. D., and Spooner, D. F. (1959). *Exptl. Parasitol.* **8**, 137–162.

Gall, D. (1956). *J. West African Sci. Assoc.* **2**, 152–157.

Gallagher, I. H. C. (1964). *Exptl. Parasitol.* **15**, 110–117.

Gazzinelli, G., and Pellegrino, J. (1964). *J. Parasitol.* **50**, 591–592.

Ghosh, B. K., and Chatterjee, A. N. (1961). *Ann. Biochem. Exptl. Med.* **21**, 343–354.

Ghosh, B. N., and Nath, M. C. (1934). *Records Malaria Survey India* **4**, 321–325.
Ghosh, B. N., and Sinton, J. A. (1934). *Records Malaria Survey India* **4**, 43–59.
Gill, J. W., and Vogel, H. J. (1962). *Biochim. Biophys. Acta* **56**, 200–201.
Gill, J. W., and Vogel, H. J. (1963). *J. Protozool.* **10**, 148–152.
Gionta, D., and Marioni, R. (1957). *Giorn. Mal. Infettive Parassit.* **9**, 1059.
Giraldo Cardona, A. J. (1960). *Rev. Iberica Parasitol.* **20**, 425–449.
Glocklin, V. C., and Fairbairn, D. (1952). *J. Cell. Comp. Physiol.* **39**, 341–356.
Goil, M. M. (1958). *J. Helminthol.* **32**, 119–124.
Goil, M. M. (1959). *Z. Parasitenk.* **19**, 362–363.
Goil, M. M. (1961). *Z. Parasitenk.* **20**, 572–575.
Goldberg, E. (1957). *Exptl. Parasitol.* **6**, 367–382.
Gonçalves, J. M., and Yamaha, T. (1959). *Res. Trab. Congr. Intern. Doenca Chagas* Rio de Janeiro, 1959, pp. 159–160. Oficina Grafica, Universidade do Brasil, Rio de Janeiro.
Goodchild, C. G. (1961). *J. Parasitol.* **47**, 830–832.
Goodchild, C. G., and Kagan, I. G. (1961). *J. Parasitol.* **47**, 175–180.
Goodchild, C. G., and Vilar-Alvarez, C. M. (1955). *Assoc. South-Eastern Biologists Bull.* **2**, 6.
Goodchild, C. G., and Vilar-Alvarez, C. M. (1962). *J. Parasitol.* **48**, 379–383.
Goodchild, C. G., and Wells, O. C. (1957). *Exptl. Parasitol.* **6**, 575–585.
Green, N. M. (1957). *Biochem. J.* **66**, 416–419.
Grembergen, G. van (1944). *Enzymologia* **11**, 268–281.
Grembergen, G. van (1949). *Enzymologia* **13**, 241–257.
Grembergen, G. van (1954). *Nature* **174**, 35.
Grembergen, G. van, and Pennoit-DeCooman, E. (1944). *Natuurw. Tijdschr. (Belg).* **26**, 91–97.
Groman, N. B. (1951). *J. Infect. Diseases* **88**, 126–150.
Guevara Pozo, D., Monteoliva, H. M., and Escobar, C. B. (1961). *Rev. Iberica Parasitol.* **21**, 3–12.
Gurtner, H. (1948). *Z. Hyg. Infektionskrankh.* **128**, 423–439.
Gutierrez, J., and Davis, R. E. (1962). *Appl. Microbiol.* **10**, 305–308.
Hamada, K., Okazaki, T., Shukuya, R., and Kaziro, K. (1962). *J. Biochem. (Tokyo)* **52**, 290–296.
Hamada, K., Okazaki, T., Shukuya, R., and Kaziro, K. (1963a). *J. Biochem. (Tokyo)* **53**, 479–483.
Hamada, K., Okazaki, T., Shukuya, R., and Kaziro, K. (1963b). *J. Biochem. (Tokyo)* **53**, 484–488.
Hamill, J. M. (1906). *J. Physiol. (London)* **33**, 479–492.
Hankes, L. V., and Stoner, R. D. (1956). *Proc. Soc. Exptl. Biol. Med.* **91**, 443–446.
Hankes, L. V., and Stoner, R. D. (1958). *Exptl. Parasitol.* **7**, 92–98.
Hara, K. (1956). *Gunma J. Med. Sci.* **5**, 173–189.
Hara, K., Oka, S., Takagi, K., Nagata, K., and Sawada, T. (1955). *Gunma J. Med. Sci.* **4**, 291–301.
Harinasuta, C., and Maegraith, B. G. (1958). *Ann. Trop. Med. Parasitol.* **52**, 508–515.
Harned, B. K., and Nash, T. P. (1932). *J. Biol. Chem.* **97**, 443–456.
Harvey, S. C. (1949). *J. Biol. Chem.* **179**, 435–453.
Harwood, P. D., Spindler, L. A., Cross, S. X., and Cutler, J. T. (1937). *Am. J. Hyg.* **25**, 362–371.
Haskins, W. T., and Olivier, L. (1958). *J. Parasitol.* **44**, 569–573.
Haskins, W. T., and Weinstein, P. P. (1957a). *J. Parasitol.* **43**, 28–32.
Haskins, W. T., and Weinstein, P. P. (1957b). *J. Parasitol.* **43**, 19–24.

Haskins, W. T., and Weinstein, P. P. (1957c). *J. Parasitol.* **43**, 25–27.

Hegner, R. (1923). *Am. J. Hyg.* **3**, 180–200.

Hegner, R., and Eskridge, L. (1937). *J. Parasitol.* **23**, 105–106.

Hellerman, L., Bovarnick, M. R., and Porter, C. C. (1946). *Federation Proc.* **3**, 400–405.

Hill, K. R. (1948). *Trans. Roy. Soc. Trop. Med. Hyg.* **41**, 641–644.

Högberg, B., Südow, G., Thon, I. L., and Uvnäs, B. (1957a). *Acta Physiol. Scand.* **38**, 265–274.

Högberg, B., Tufvesson, G., and Uvnäs, B. (1957b). *Acta Physiol. Scand.* **38**, 135–144.

Hoeppli, R. (1927). *Arch. Schiffs-u. Tropen-Hyg.* **31**, Suppl. 3, 5–88.

Hoeppli, R., and Feng, L. C. (1931). *Chinese Med. J.* **17**, 589–598.

Hoeppli, R., and Feng, L. C. (1933). *Arch. Schiffs-u. Tropen-Hyg.* **37**, 176–182.

Holmes, E. G., and Darke, S. J. (1958). *Lancet* p. 529.

Hopkins, C. A. (1950). *J. Parasitol.* **36**, 384–390.

Hoppe, J. O., and Chapman, C. W. (1947). *J. Parasitol.* **33**, 509–516.

House, H. L. (1954). *Can. J. Zool.* **32**, 351–357.

Hsü, H. F. (1938). *Bull. Fan Mem. Inst. Biol. (Peking), Zool.* **8**, 347–366.

Huang, T. Y., and Chu, C. H. (1962). *Sheng Wu Hua Yu Shing Wu Wu Li Hsueh Pao* **2**, 286–294; see *Chem. Abstr.* **59**, 14333 (1963).

Hunter, N. W. (1957). *Trans. Am. Microscop. Soc.* **76**, 36–45.

Hurlaux, R. (1947). *Ann. Sci. Nat. (Paris), Zool.* [11] **9**, 155–226.

Ichii, S., Matsumoto, K., and Sugiura, K. (1959). *Kiseichugaku Zasshi* **8**, 19–21.

Iyori, S. (1957). *Nisshin Igaku* **44**, 436–441.

Iyori, S. (1959). *Nisshin Igaku* **46**, 759–764.

Jackson, G. J. (1962). *Exptl. Parasitol.* **12**, 25–32.

Janssens, P. G., Karcher, D., Van Sande, M., Lowenthal, A., and Ghysels, G. (1961). *Bull. Soc. Pathol. Exotique* **54**, 322–331.

Jarumilinta, R., and Maegraith, B. G. (1961a). *Ann. Trop. Med. Parasitol.* **55**, 505–517.

Jarumilinta, R., and Maegraith, B. G. (1961b). *Ann. Trop. Med. Parasitol.* **55**, 518–528.

Jaskoski, B. J. (1962). *Exptl. Parasitol.* **12**, 19–24.

Jennings, J. B. (1959). *J. Helminthol.* **33**, 197–204.

Johnson, A. E. (1962). *Exptl. Parasitol.* **12**, 168–175.

Johri, L. N., and Smyth, J. D. (1956). *Parasitology* **46**, 107–116.

Jones, E. R. (1933). *Vet. Record* **13**, 1062–1063.

Kagan, I. G., and Norman, L. (1961). *Am. J. Trop. Med. Hyg.* **10**, 727–734.

Kedrowsky, B. (1931). *Z. Zellforsch. Mikroskop. Anat.* **12**, 666–714.

Keilin, D. (1925). *Proc. Roy. Soc.* Ser. B **98**, 312–339.

Keilin, D., and Wang, Y. L. (1946). *Biochem. J.* **40**, 855–866.

Kemnitz, G. von (1916). *Z. Biol.* **67**, 129–244.

Kent, F. N. (1947). *Bull. Soc. Neuchateloise Sci. Nat.* **70**, 85–108.

Kent, N. H. (1963). *Am. J. Hyg., Monogr. Ser.* **22**, 30–45.

Kessel, J. F. (1929). *Proc. Soc. Exptl. Biol. Med.* **27**, 113–118.

Kessel, J. F., and Huang, K. K. (1926). *Proc. Soc. Exptl. Biol. Med.* **23**, 388–391.

Kidder, G. W., and Dutta, B. N. (1958). *J. Gen. Microbiol.* **18**, 621–638.

Kikuchi, G., Ramirez, J., and Barron, E. S. G. (1959). *Biochim. Biophys. Acta* **36**, 335–342.

Kirby, H. (1941). *In* "Protozoa in Biological Research" (G. N. Calkins and F. M. Summers, eds.), pp. 890–1008. Columbia Univ. Press, New York.

Kitsuki, T. (1958). *Igaku Kenkyu* **28**, 24–48.

Kmetec, E., Beaver, P. C., and Bueding, E. (1963). *Comp. Biochem. Physiol.* **9**, 115–120.

Kofoid, C. A., McNeil, E., and Kopac, M. J. (1931). *Proc. Soc. Exptl. Biol. Med.* **29**, 100–102.

Kona, E. (1957a). *Vet. Casopis* **6**, 146–150.

Kona, E. (1957b). *Sb. Cesk. Akad. Zemedel. Ved, Vet. Med.* **30,** 159–164.

Kopp, I., and Solomon, H. C. (1941). *Am. J. Med. Sci.* **202,** 861–886.

Kosmin, N. (1928). *Tr. Lab. Eksperim. Biol. Mos., Zooparka* **4,** 207–218.

Krijgsman, B. J. (1936). *Z. Vergleich. Physiol.* **23,** 663–711.

Krueger, F. (1936). *Zool. Jahrb., Abt. Allgem. Zool. Physiol.* **57,** 1–56.

Krusberg, L. R. (1960). *Phytopathology* **50,** 9–22.

Kumar, S., Kumar, A., Agarwal, K. L., and Mangalik, V. S. (1958). *J. Indian Med. Assoc.* **31,** 14–17.

Kuttler, K. L., and Marble, D. W. (1960). *Am. J. Vet. Res.* **21,** 445–448.

Kuwamura, T. (1958). *Shikoku Acta Med.* **12,** 28–57.

Lahille, A. (1915). *Bull. Mem. Soc. Med. Hop. Paris* **31,** 905–917.

Larsh, J. E. (1950). *J. Parasitol.* **36,** Suppl., 45–46.

Laser, H. (1944). *Biochem. J.* **38,** 333–338.

Launoy, L. L., and Lagodsky, H. (1936). *Compt. Rend. Soc. Biol.* **122,** 1055–1058.

Launoy, L. L., and Lagodsky, H. (1937). *Bull. Soc. Pathol. Exotique* **30,** 57–68.

Lazarus, M. (1950). *Australian J. Sci. Res.* **B3,** 245–250.

Lee, D. L. (1958). *Parasitology* **48,** 437–447.

Lee, D. L. (1962). *Parasitology* **52,** 533–538.

Lee, D. L., and Lewert, R. M. (1957). *J. Infect. Diseases* **101,** 287–294.

Leland, S. E., Drudge, J. H., and Wyant, Z. N. (1959). *Exptl. Parasitol.* **8,** 383–412.

Leland, S. E., Drudge, J. H., and Wyant, Z. N. (1960). *Am. J. Vet. Res.* **21,** 458–463.

Lemaire, G., and Ribère, R. (1935). *Compt. Rend. Soc. Biol.* **118,** 1578–1579.

Lesser, E. J. (1906). *Z. Biol.* **48,** 1–18.

Levenbook, L. (1950). *Biochem. J.* **47,** 336–346.

Lewert, R. M., and Lee, C. L. (1956). *J. Infect. Diseases* **99,** 1–14.

Lewert, R. M., and Lee, C. L. (1957). *Am. J. Trop. Med. Hyg.* **6,** 473–479.

Lewert, R. M., Lee, C. L., Mandlowitz, S., and Dusanic, D. (1959). *J. Infect. Diseases* **105,** 180–187.

Lienert, E., and Thorsell, W. (1955). *Exptl. Parasitol.* **4,** 117–122.

Lincicome, D. R. (1953). *Exptl. Parasitol.* **2,** 333–340.

Linstow, O. von (1907). *Proc. Roy. Soc. Edinburgh* **B26,** 464–472.

Linton, R. W. (1930). *J. Exptl. Med.* **52,** 103–111.

Lippi, M., and Benedetto, A. (1958). *Arch. Ital. Sci. Med. Trop. Parassitol.* **39,** 253–263.

Llewellyn, J. (1954). *Parasitology* **44,** 428–437.

Loeb, L., and Fleisher, M. S. (1910). *J. Infect. Diseases* **7,** 625–631.

Loeb, L., and Smith, A. J. (1904). *Zentr. Bakteriol. Parasitenk., Abt. I: Orig.* **37,** 93–98.

Lwoff, A. (1934). *Zentr. Bakteriol. Parasitenk., Abt. I: Orig.* **130,** 497–518.

Lwoff, M. (1933). *Ann. Inst. Pasteur* **51,** 55–116.

Lwoff, M. (1951). *In* "Biochemistry and Physiology of Protozoa" (A. Lwoff, ed.), Vol. 1, pp. 129–176. Academic Press, New York.

Lynch, D. L., and Bogitsh, J. (1962). *J. Parasitol.* **48,** 241–243.

McKee, R. W., Geiman, Q. M., and Cobbey, T. S. (1947). *Federation Proc.* **6,** 276.

Maegraith, B. G. (1948). "Pathological Processes in Malaria and Blackwater Fever." Thomas, Springfield, Illinois.

Maekawa, K., and Kushibe, M. (1956). *Compt. Rend. Soc. Biol.* **150,** 832–834.

Mandlowitz, S., Dusanic, D., and Lewert, R. M. (1960). *J. Parasitol.* **46,** 89–90.

Mannozzi-Torini, M. (1940). *Arch. Sci. Biol. (Italy)* **26,** 565–580.

Mansour, T. E. (1958). *Biochim. Biophys. Acta* **30,** 492–500.

Mansour, T. E. (1959). *J. Pharmacol. Exptl. Therap.* **126,** 212–216.

Mansour, T. E., and Mansour, J. M. (1962). *J. Biol. Chem.* **237,** 629–634.

Mansour, T. E., Lago, A. D., and Hawkins, J. L. (1957). *Federation Proc.* **16,** 319.

Marco Ahuir, R., and Bellod Garcia, G. (1958). *Rev. Clin. Espan.* **58,** 228–233.

Markowicz, W., and Bock, D. (1931). *Z. Ges. Exptl. Med.* **79,** 301–310.

Martin, C. J., and Ross, I. C. (1934). *J. Helminthol.* **12,** 137–142.

Martynowicz, T., and Seniow, A. (1956). *Zool. Poloniae* **7,** 209–217.

Mastandrea, G., Mazzetti, M., and Mele, G. (1962). *Rass. Ital. Gastroenterol.* **8,** 566–581.

Matsumoto, H. (1960). *J. Osaka City Med. Center* **9,** 245–255.

Mazzetti, M., and Mele, G. (1961). *Arch. Ital. Sci. Med. Trop. Parassitol.* **42,** 65–71.

Mazzocco, P. (1923). *Compt. Rend. Soc. Biol.* **88,** 342–343.

Mehra, N., Levine, N. D., and Reber, E. F. (1960). *J. Protozool.* **7,** 12.

Mendel, L. B., and Blood, A. F. (1910). *J. Biol. Chem.* **8,** 177–213.

Mettrick, D. F., and Telford, J. M. (1963). *J. Parasitol.* **49,** 653–656.

Milleman, R. E., and Thonard, J. C. (1959). *Exptl. Parasitol.* **8,** 129–136.

Monné, L. (1955a). *Arkiv. Zool.* [2] **7,** 559–572.

Monné, L. (1955b). *Arkiv. Zool.* [2] **9,** 93–113.

Monné, L. (1959). *Arkiv. Zool.* [2] **12,** 343–358.

Monné, L. (1960). *Arkiv. Zool.* [2] **13,** 287–298.

Monné, L. (1963). *Z. Parasitenk.* **22,** 475–483.

Monné, L., and Borg, K. (1954). *Arkiv. Zool.* [2] **6,** 555–557.

Monné, L., and Hönig, G. (1954a). *Arkiv. Zool.* [2] **7,** 251–256.

Monné, L., and Hönig, G. (1954b). *Arkiv. Zool.* [2] **7,** 257–260.

Monné, L., and Hönig, G. (1954c). *Arkiv. Zool.* [2] **7,** 261–272.

Monné, L., and Hönig, G. (1954d). *Arkiv. Zool.* [2] **6,** 559–562.

Monteoliva, M. (1961). *Rev. Iberica Parasitol.* **21,** 339–344.

Monteoliva, M., Escobar, C., and Guevara Pozo, D. (1962). *Rev. Iberica Parasitol.* **22,** 49–53.

Morris, S. (1936). *J. Morphol.* **59,** 225–263.

Morrison, D. B., and Anderson, W. A. D. (1942). *U.S. Public Health Serv., Public Health Rept.* **57,** 90–94.

Morrison, D. B., and Jeskey, H. A. (1948). *J. Natl. Malaria Soc.* **7,** 259–264.

Moulder, J. W. (1948). *J. Infect. Diseases* **83,** 33–41.

Moulder, J. W., and Evans, E. A. (1946). *J. Biol. Chem.* **164,** 145–157.

Mueller, J. F. (1929). *Z. Zellforsch. Mikroskop. Anat.* **8,** 362–403.

Myuge, S. G. (1960). *Conf. Sci. Problems Plant Prod., Budapest, 1960* pp 333–338.

Nadakal, A. M. (1960). *J. Parasitol.* **46,** 475–483.

Nadakal, A. M. (1963). *J. Sci. Ind. Res.* **22,** 401–408.

Nakajima, M. (1954). *Yokohama Med. Bull.* **5,** 10–20.

Nakamura, M., and Edwards, P. R. (1959a). *Proc. Soc. Exptl. Biol. Med.* **100,** 403–404.

Nakamura, M., and Edwards, P. R. (1959b). *Nature* **183,** 397.

Nakamura, M., and Goldstein, L. (1957). *Nature* **179,** 1134.

Neal, R. A. (1956). *Nature* **178,** 599.

Neal, R. A. (1960). *Parasitology* **50,** 531–550.

Newton, B. A. (1956). *Nature* **177,** 279–280.

Newton, B. A. (1957). *J. Gen. Microbiol.* **17,** 708–717.

Nishizaki, B. (1938). *Mitt. Med. Ges. Okayama* **50,** 1418–1423.

Nishizaki, B. (1940). *Mitt. Med. Ges. Okayama* **52,** 17–24.

Northrop, J. W. (1926). *J. Gen. Physiol.* **9,** 497–502.

Ogimoto, S. (1956). *Fukuoka Acta Med.* **47,** 1077–1091.

Ohta, T., and Nishizaki, B. (1936). *Mitt. Med. Ges. Okayama* **48,** 442–463.

Olberg, H. (1955). *Zentr. Bakteriol. Parasitenk., Abt. I: Orig.* **162,** 120–135.

Owen, D. U., and Murgatroyd, F. (1928). *Ann. Trop. Med. Parasitol.* **22,** 503–530.

Oya, H., Costello, L. C., and Smith, W. N. (1963). *J. Cell. Comp. Physiol.* **62,** 287–294.

Panijel, J. (1947). *Bull. Soc. Chim. Biol.* **29**, 1098–1106.

Panzer, T. (1911). *Z. Physiol. Chem.* **73**, 109–127.

Panzer, T. (1913). *Z. Physiol. Chem.* **86**, 33–42.

Passey, R. F., and Fairbairn, D. (1957). *Can. J. Biochem. Physiol.* **35**, 511–525.

Patrick, A. (1922). *Ann. Trop. Med. Parasitol.* **16**, 451–455.

Peanasky, R. J., and Laskowski, M. (1960). *Biochim. Biophys. Acta* **37**, 167–169.

Pennoit-DeCooman, E., and Grembergen, G. van (1942). *Verhandel. Koninkl. Vlaam. Acad. Wetenschap.*, Belg., Kl. Wetenschap. **4**, No. 6, 7–77.

Perez, D., and Bloch-Raphael, C. (1946). *Compt. Rend.* **223**, 840–842.

Picken, L. E. R., Pryor, M. G., and Swann, M. M. (1947). *Nature* **159**, 434.

Pitzus, F. (1957). *Arch. Ital. Sci. Med. Trop. Parassitol.* **38**, 383–394.

Pizzi, T., and Taliaferro, W. H. (1960). *J. Infect. Diseases* **107**, 100–107.

Pollak, J. K. (1957a). *Australian J. Sci.* **19**, 208–209.

Pollak, J. K. (1957b). *Australian J. Biol. Sci.* **10**, 465–474.

Pollak, J. K., and Fairbairn, D. (1955a). *Can. J. Biochem. Physiol.* **33**, 297–306.

Pollak, J. K., and Fairbairn, D. (1955b). *Can. J. Biochem. Physiol.* **33**, 307–316.

Popov, A., and Sorokin, P. (1962). *Izv. Tsentral. Vet. Inst. Zarazni Parasitni Bolesti, Akad. Selskostopansk. Nauki Bulgar.* **6**, 187–190; see *Chem. Abstr.* **59**, 10506 (1963).

Porter, D. A. (1935). *J. Parasitol.* **21**, 226–228.

Powell, S. J. (1959). *Am. J. Trop. Med. Hyg.* **8**, 331–336.

Pozzi, G., and Pirosky, I. (1953). *Arch. Intern. Hidatidosis* **13**, 232.

Ramakrishnan, S. P. (1954). *Indian J. Malariol.* **8**, 97–105.

Rama Rao, R., and Giri, K. V. (1952). *Indian J. Malariol.* **6**, 411–414.

Rama Rao, R., and Sirsi, M. (1958). *J. Indian Inst. Sci.* **40**, 23–30.

Ramaswamy, A. S. (1956). *J. Indian Inst. Sci.* **38**, 62–72.

Ramirez, E. A., Rivera de Sala, A., Serrano, D., and Cancio, M. (1961). *Am. J. Trop. Med. Hyg.* **10**, 530–536.

Randall, R. (1934). *Philippine J. Sci.* **53**, 97–105.

Ratcliffe, H. L. (1930). *Am. J. Hyg.* **11**, 159–167.

Rathbone, L. (1955). *Biochem. J.* **61**, 574–579.

Ratnayake, W. E. (1960). *J. Parasitol.* **46**, 22.

Read, C. P. (1950). *Rice Inst. Pamphlet* **27**, No. 2, 1–94.

Read, C. P. (1952). *Exptl. Parasitol.* **1**, 353–362.

Read, C. P., and Simmons, J. E. (1962). *J. Parasitol.* **48**, 494.

Read, C. P., Simmons, J. E., Campbell, J. W., and Rothman, A. H. (1960a). *Biol. Bull.* **119**, 120–133.

Read, C. P., Simmons, J. E., and Rothman, A. H. (1960b). *J. Parasitol.* **46**, 33–41.

Read, C. P., Rothman, A. H., and Simmons, J. E. (1963). *Ann. N.Y. Acad. Sci.* **113**, 154–205.

Reid, W. M. (1942). *J. Parasitol.* **28**, 319–340.

Rhodes, M. B., Marsh, C. L., and Kelley, G. W. (1963). *Exptl. Parasitol.* **13**, 266–272.

Ribeiro, L. P., and Villela, G. G. (1956). *Rev. Brasil. Biol.* **16**, 145–147.

Rijavec, M., Kurelec, B., and Ehrlich, I. (1962). *Biol. Glasnik (Zagreb)* **15**, 103–107.

Rimington, C., Fulton, J. D., and Sheiman, H. (1947). *Biochem. J.* **41**, 619–622.

Ristic, M., and Trager, W. (1958). *J. Protozool.* **5**, 146–148.

Rocha e Silva, M., and Grana, A. (1946a). *Arch. Surg.* **52**, 523–537.

Rocha e Silva, M., and Grana, A. (1946b). *Arch. Surg.* **52**, 713–728.

Rocha e Silva, M., Porto, A., and Andrade, S. O. (1946). *Arch. Surg.* **53**, 199–213.

Rogers, W. P. (1940). *J. Helminthol.* **18**, 53–62.

Rogers, W. P. (1941a). *J. Helminthol.* **19**, 47–58.

Rogers, W. P. (1941b). *J. Helminthol.* **19**, 87–104.

Rogers, W. P. (1942). *J. Helminthol.* **20,** 139–158.

Rogers, W. P. (1949). *Australian J. Sci. Res.* **B2,** 287–303.

Rogers, W. P. (1952). *Australian J. Sci. Res.* **B5,** 210–222.

Rogers, W. P. (1955). *Exptl. Parasitol.* **4,** 21–28.

Rogers, W. P. (1962). "The Nature of Parasitism." Academic Press, New York.

Rogers, W. P., and Lazarus, M. (1949). *Parasitology* **39,** 245–250.

Rossan, R. N. (1960). *Exptl. Parasitol.* **9,** 302–333.

Rothman, A. H., and Fisher, F. M. (1964). *J. Parasitol.* **50,** 410–414.

Roy, D. N. (1937). *Parasitology* **29,** 150–162.

Ryley, J. F. (1951). *Biochem. J.* **49,** 577–585.

Ryley, J. F. (1955a). *Biochem. J.* **59,** 353–361.

Ryley, J. F. (1955b). *Biochem. J.* **59,** 361–369.

Ryley, J. F. (1956). *Biochem. J.* **62,** 215–222.

Ryley, J. F. (1962). *Biochem. J.* **85,** 211–223.

Sadun, E. H., and Walton, B. C. (1958). *Am. J. Trop. Med. Hyg.* **7,** 500–504.

Salah, M. (1938). *Trans. Roy. Soc. Trop. Med. Hyg.* **31,** 431–436.

Salisbury, L. F., and Anderson, R. J. (1939). *J. Biol. Chem.* **129,** 505–517.

Salle, A. J., and Schmidt, C. L. A. (1928). *J. Infect. Diseases* **43,** 378–384.

Salmenkova, E. A. (1962). *Med. Parazitol. i Parazitarn. Bolezni* **31,** 664–668; see *Chem. Abstr.* **58,** 9449 (1963).

Sang, J. H. (1938). *Parasitology* **30,** 141–155.

Sanz Pêrez, B. (1956). *Clin. Lab. (Zaragoza)* **61,** 253–257.

Sassuchin, D. N. (1931). *Arch. Protistenk.* **70,** 681–686.

Savel, J. (1954). Thesis, University of Paris.

Sawada, I. (1959). *J. Nara Gakugei Univ.* **8,** 31–63.

Scheff, G. (1928). *Biochem. Z.* **200,** 309–330.

Schinazi, L. A. (1957). *Science* **125,** 695–697.

Schneider, R. (1958). *Z. Tropenmed. Parasitol.* **9,** 234–243.

Scholander, P. F. (1960). *Science* **131,** 585–590.

Schopfer, W. H. (1932). *Rev. Suisse Zool.* **39,** 59–192.

Schulte, H. (1917). *Arch. Ges. Physiol.* **166,** 1–44.

Schuurmans-Stekhoven, J. H., and Botman, T. P. J. (1932). *Z. Parasitenk.* **4,** 220–239.

Schwartz, B. (1921). *J. Parasitol.* **7,** 144–150.

Seneca, H., Sang, J. B., and Troc, O. K. (1958). *Trans. Roy. Soc. Trop. Med. Hyg.* **52,** 230–234.

Senft, A. W. (1963). *Ann. N.Y. Acad. Sci.* **113,** 272–288.

Seniow, A. (1956). *Zool. Poloniae* **7,** 35–43.

Seniow, A. (1961). *Zool. Poloniae* **11,** 37–56.

Shearer, G. D., and Stewart, J. (1933). *Univ. Cambridge, Inst. Animal Pathol., Rept. Director* **3,** 87–97.

Sherman, I. W., and Hull, R. W. (1960). *J. Protozool.* **7,** 409–416.

Shumard, R. F. (1957). *J. Parasitol.* **43,** 548–554.

Sicê, A. (1930). *Bull. Soc. Pathol. Exotique* **23,** 77–79, 222–243, and 307–331.

Simmonds, R. A. (1958). *Exptl. Parasitol.* **7,** 14–22.

Simmons, J. E. (1961). *Biol. Bull.* **121,** 535–546.

Simmons, J. E., Read, C. P., and Rothman, A. H. (1960). *J. Parasitol.* **46,** 43–50.

Sinton, J. A., and Ghosh, B. N. (1934a). *Records Malaria Survey India* **4,** 15–42.

Sinton, J. A., and Ghosh, B. N. (1934b). *Records Malaria Survey India* **4,** 205–221.

Smith, M. H. (1962). *Parasitology* **52,** 18P.

Smith, M. H. (1963). *Biochim. Biophys. Acta* **71,** 370–376.

Smith, M. H., and Lee, D. L. (1963). *Proc. Roy. Soc.* **B157,** 234–257.

Smith, M. H., and Morrison, M. (1963). *Biochim. Biophys. Acta* **71**, 364–370.

Smithers, S. R., and Walker, P. J. (1961). *Exptl. Parasitol.* **11**, 39–49.

Smorodincev, I. A., and Bebesin, K. W. (1936a). *J. Biochem.* **23**, 19–20.

Smorodincev, I. A., and Bebesin, K. W. (1936b). *J. Biochem.* **23**, 21–22.

Smorodincev, I. A., and Bebesin, K. W. (1936c). *Compt. Rend. Acad. Sci. URSS* [N.S.] **2**, 189–191.

Smorodincev, I. A., and Bebesin, K. W. (1936d). *Bull. Soc. Chim. Biol.* **18**, 1097–1105.

Smorodincev, I. A., and Pawlowa, P. I. (1936). *Ann. Parasitol. Humaine Comp.* **14**, 489–494.

Smorodincev, I. A., Bebesin, K. W., and Pawlowa, P. I. (1933). *Biochem. Z.* **261**, 176–178.

Smyth, J. D. (1954). *Quart. J. Microscop. Sci.* **95**, 139–152.

Smyth, J. D., and Clegg, J. A. (1959). *Exptl. Parasitol.* **8**, 286–323.

Spedding, C. R. W. (1954). *J. Comp. Pathol. Therap.* **64**, 5–14.

Stannard, J. N., McCoy, O. R., and Latchford, W. B. (1938). *Am. J. Hyg.* **27**, 666–682.

Stauber, L. A. (1954). *Exptl. Parasitol.* **3**, 544–568.

Steinert, M. (1958). *Exptl. Cell Res.* **15**, 431–433.

Stephenson, W. (1947a). *Parasitology* **38**, 123–127.

Stephenson, W. (1947b). *Parasitology* **38**, 128–139.

Stewart, J. (1933a). *Univ. Cambridge, Inst. Animal Pathol., Rept. Director* **3**, 58–76.

Stewart, J. (1933b). *Univ. Cambridge, Inst. Animal Pathol., Rept. Director* **3**, 77–86.

Stirewalt, M. A., and Evans, A. S. (1952). *J. Infect. Diseases* **9**, 191–197.

Stoll, N. R., Cort, W. W., and Kwei, W. S. (1927). *J. Parasitol.* **13**, 166–172.

Stoner, R. D., and Hankes, L. V. (1955). *Exptl. Parasitol.* **4**, 435–444.

Stoner, R. D., and Hankes, L. V. (1958). *Exptl. Parasitol.* **7**, 145–151.

Strangeways, W. I. (1937). *Ann. Trop. Med. Parasitol.* **31**, 387–404.

Suzuoki, Z., and Suzuoki, T. (1951). *J. Biochem. (Tokyo)* **38**, 237–254.

Symons, L. E. A. (1960a). *Australian J. Biol. Sci.* **13**, 180–187.

Symons, L. E. A. (1960b). *Australian J. Biol. Sci.* **13**, 578–583.

Symons, L. E. A. (1960c). *Australian J. Biol. Sci.* **14**, 165–171.

Symons, L. E. A., and Fairbairn, D. (1962). *Federation Proc.* **21**, 913–918.

Symons, L. E. A., and Fairbairn, D. (1963). *Exptl. Parasitol.* **13**, 284–304.

Szwejkowska, G. (1929). *Bull. Intern. Acad. Polon. Sci., Cl. Sci. Math. Nat.* **B1928**, 489–519.

Taliaferro, W. H., and Pizzi, T. (1960). *Proc. Natl. Acad. Sci. U.S.* **46**, 733–745.

Tallqvist, T. W. (1907). *Z. Klin. Med.* **61**, 427–532.

Taniguchi, M., Yamazaki, H., Hiramoto, K., and Nakajima, M. (1961). *Japan. J. Vet. Sci.* **23**, 76–83.

Tanner, C. E., and Gregory, J. (1961). *Can. J. Microbiol.* **7**, 473–481.

Tasaka, M. (1935). *Fukuoka Acta Med.* **28**, 27–28 (German Summary).

Tatchell, R. J. (1958). *Parasitology* **48**, 448–458.

Tempelis, C. H., and Lysenko, M. G. (1957). *Exptl. Parasitol.* **6**, 31–36.

Thorson, R. E. (1956a). *J. Parasitol.* **42**, 21–25.

Thorson, R. E. (1956b). *J. Parasitol.* **42**, 26–30.

Thurston, J. P. (1958). *Parasitology* **48**, 149–164.

Timms, A. R., and Bueding, E. (1959). *Brit. J. Pharmacol.* **14**, 68–73.

Tobie, E. J., Brand, T. von, and Mehlman, B. (1950). *J. Parasitol.* **36**, 48–54.

Trager, W. (1957). *J. Protozool.* **4**, 269–276.

Trager, W. (1959). *Ann. Trop. Med. Parasitol.* **53**, 473–491.

Treibs, A., Mendheim, A., and Lorenz, M. (1950). *Naturwiss.* **37**, 378–379.

Turner, J. H. (1959). *Proc. Helminthol. Soc. Wash., D.C.* **26**, 114–124.

Turner, J. H., and Wilson, G. I. (1962). *Am. J. Vet. Res.* **23**, 718–724.

Uspenskaya, A. V. (1963). *Dokl. Akad. Nauk SSSR* **151**, 1476–1478.

Uvnäs, B., Diamant, B., Högberg, B., and Thon, I. L. (1960). *Am. J. Physiol.* **199,** 575–578.

van Grembergen, G., *see* Grembergen, G. van.

Van Sande, M. (1956). *Ann. Soc. Belge Med. Trop.* **36,** 335–343.

Varleta, J., Oberhauser, E., and Weinstein, V. (1961). *Bol. Chileno Parasitol.* **16,** 62–66.

Venkatachalam, P. S., and Patwardhan, V. N. (1953). *Trans. Roy. Soc. Trop. Med. Hyg.* **47,** 169–175.

Villela, G. G., and Ribeiro, L. P. (1955a). *Rev. Brasil. Biol.* **15,** 383–390.

Villela, G. G., and Ribeiro, L. P. (1955b). *Anais Acad. Brasil. Cien.* **27,** 78–89.

Vilella, G. G., and Teixeira, J. C. (1937). *J. Lab. Clin. Med.* **22,** 567–572.

von Bonsdorff, B., *see* Bonsdorff, B. von.

von Brand, T., *see* Brand, T. von.

von Kemnitz, G., *see* Kemnitz, G. von.

von Linstow, O., *see* Linstow, O. von.

Wantland, W. W., and Johansen, E. (1954). *J. Parasitol.* **40,** 479–480.

Wardle, R. A. (1937). *In* "Manitoba Essays," 60th Anniv. Comem. Vol., Univ. Manitoba, Winnipeg, pp. 338–364. MacMillan, Toronto.

Wardle, R. A. (1937). *In* "Manitoba Essays," 60th Anniv. Commem. Vol., Univ. Manitoba,

Watson, M. R., and Silvester, N. R. (1958). *Biochem. J.* **71,** 578–584.

Weatherly, N. F., Hansen, M. F., and Moser, H. C. (1963). *Exptl. Parasitol.* **14,** 37–48.

Weimer, H. E., Voge, M., Quinn, F. A., and Redlich-Moshin, J. (1955). *Proc. Soc. Exptl. Biol. Med.* **90,** 494–496.

Weimer, H. E., Markell, E. K., and Nishihara, H. (1958). *Exptl. Parasitol.* **7,** 468–476.

Weinbren, B. M., and Coyle, T. J. (1960). *J. Comp. Pathol. Therap.* **70,** 176–181.

Weinland, E. (1901). *Z. Biol.* **42,** 55–90.

Weinland, E. (1902). *Z. Biol.* **44,** 1–15 and 45–60.

Weinland, E., and Brand, T. von (1926). *Z. Vergleich. Physiol.* **4,** 212–285.

Weinstein, P. P., and Haskins, W. T. (1955). *Exptl. Parasitol.* **4,** 226–243.

Weiss, E. D., and Ball, G. H. (1947). *Proc. Soc. Exptl. Biol. Med.* **65,** 278–283.

Wellerson, R., Doscher, G., and Kupferberg, A. B. (1959). *Ann. N.Y. Acad. Sci.* **83,** 253–258.

Wertheim, G., Zeledon, R., and Read, C. P. (1960). *J. Parasitol.* **46,** 497–499.

Wertlieb, D. M., and Guttman, H. N. (1963). *J. Protozool.* **10,** 109–112.

Wetzel, R. (1927). *Deut. Tieraerztl. Wochschr.* **36,** 719–722.

Wetzel, R. (1931). *J. Parasitol.* **18,** 40–43.

Wharton, G. W. (1938). *J. Parasitol.* **24,** Suppl., 21.

Wharton, G. W. (1941). *J. Parasitol.* **27,** 81–87.

Wildführ, G., Naumann, G., and Wilde, J. (1958). *Z. Immunitaetsforsch. Exptl. Therap.* **115,** 122–134.

Williams, P. P., Davis, R. E., Doetsch, R. N., and Gutierrez, J. (1961). *Appl. Microbiol.* **9,** 405–409.

Williamson, J., and Brown, K. N. (1964). *Exptl. Parasitol.* **15,** 44–68.

Williamson, J., and Desowitz, R. S. (1961). *Exptl. Parasitol.* **11,** 161–175.

Wilson, P. A. G., and Fairbairn, D. (1961). *J. Protozool.* **8,** 410–416.

Woodruff, A. W. (1957). *Trans. Roy. Soc. Trop. Med. Hyg.* **51,** 419–424.

Yanagisawa, T. (1955). *Japan. J. Med. Sci. Biol.* **8,** 379–390.

Yanagisawa, T., and Ishii, K. (1954). *Japan. J. Med. Sci. Biol.* **7,** 215–229.

Yasuo, S. (1961). *Folia Pharmacol. Japon.* **57,** 393–398.

Yoshimuro, S. (1930). *J. Biochem. (Tokyo)* **12,** 27–34.

Zeledon, R. (1960). *Rev. Brasil. Biol.* **20,** 409–414.

Zotta, G. (1923). *Compt. Rend. Soc. Biol.* **88,** 913–915 and 1350–1352.

Zschucke, J. (1932). *Z. Hyg. Infektionskrankh.* **114,** 464–500.

Chapter 7

NUCLEIC ACIDS

I. SOME HISTOCHEMICAL OBSERVATIONS

The vast histological literature dealing with the occurrence of nucleic acids within the nuclei of parasites is based largely on observations gained by means of the Feulgen reaction, which is considered specific for deoxyribonucleic acid (DNA). No useful purpose would be served in reviewing this literature in detail. Suffice it to say that DNA has been found quite generally within the nuclei of all parasitic species studied. The few apparent exceptions, such as the negative Feulgen reaction reported for the macrogametes of *Eimeria tenella* (Ray and Gill, 1955), may be indicative of a low DNA concentration rather than proving its complete absence. The newer methods of quantitative evaluation of histochemical evidence seem hardly to have been applied to parasites as yet. However, Baker (1961) did establish by means of microspectrophotometry of Feulgen-stained nuclei that one nucleus of *Trypanosoma evansi* contained 0.2×10^{-12}gm DNA. By means of a similar technique Govaert (1953) showed that the DNA content of the vitellarian cells of *Fasciola hepatica* varies greatly, depending on their state of development.

Of greater interest, perhaps, than the universal intranuclear occurrence of DNA is its occasional occurrence in extranuclear structures. The best known of these is the kinetoplast-blepharoplast complex of trypanosomes. Convincing histochemical evidence that this structure contains DNA has been presented for *Trypanosoma cruzi* (Pizzi and Diaz, 1954), *Trypanosoma mega* (Steinert *et al.*, 1958), *Trypanosoma lewisi,* and *Trypanosoma gambiense* (Kawamitsu, 1957), as well as for *Trypanosoma evansi* (Baker, 1961), to quote the newer evidence. Older data will be found in Bresslau and Scremin (1924) and Reichenow (1928). It is probable that in all these cases DNA occurrence is limited to the kinetoplast; at any rate Baker (1961) did not find any DNA in the region of the blepharoplast of an akinetoplastic strain of *Trypanosoma evansi.*

Ribonucleic acid (RNA) occurs in the nucleoli and quite generally dispersed throughout the cytoplasm of the cells. Histochemical evidence to this effect has for example been presented by Tsunoda and Ichikawa (1955) or Ray and Gill (1955) for chicken coccidia, and by Kawamitsu (1957) for trypanosomes. However, just as in the case of DNA the occurrence of RNA in various definite extranuclear structures is of special interest.

The chromatoid bodies of entamoebas which are encountered in varying shapes within the cysts, but also within the trophozoites, have been characterized for *Entamoeba invadens* by Barker and Deutsch (1958), Barker (1963), and Barker and Svihla (1964). Histochemical evidence (reactions to more or less specific stains, such as methyl green pyronine, observations made by fluorescence microscopy, or at least partial dissolution after treatment with ribonuclease) favors the assumption that the chromatoid bodies consist of RNA plus an unidentified protein; it is justified to consider them as a ribonucleoprotein. The substance is strongly absorbing in the ultraviolet and its appearance and quantitative variations at various stages in the life cycle of the amoebas could therefore be followed in a color-translating ultraviolet microscope (Barker and Svihla, 1964). It was found that in late trophozoites and precystic forms the material was represented by small bodies which later combined to form large crystalloids with maximum crystallization in early cysts. The crystalloids were composed of units of 200 to 300 A in diameter which were closely packed to form cubic or hexagonal patterns.

Another interesting inclusion body is the so-called bipolar body of *Strigomonas oncopelti,* which according to Newton and Horne (1957) contains RNA and protein. More recently it is assumed that this structure is not, in the strict sense of the word, formed by the flagellate itself, but that it represents an intracellular symbiont (Gill and Vogel, 1963). The so-called juxtanuclear structures of avian malaria parasites are other types of bodies (Lewert, 1952). There is some indication that they correspond functionally to a nucleolus, resembling it also by containing RNA.

Special discussion is required for the volutin granules, metachromatic inclusion bodies which are often encountered in trypanosomes, hemogregarines, and other protozoa. In trypanosomes at least they appear with regularity and in great numbers after the organisms had been exposed to vital dyes or such drugs as Antrycide, dimidium bromide, or suramin (Ormerod, 1951a; Newton, 1962a). It is possible, but has not yet been proved conclusively, that these bodies have some connection with immune phenomena developing during trypanosomal infections (Ormerod, 1958, 1959). It must be realized, however, that the term volutin has been applied to a variety of intraplasmatic granules which apparently differ considerably in their chemical constitution. Thus, the volutin granules of many phytoflagellates seem to consist of polymetaphosphate (Hutner and Provasoli, 1951). Those of the trypanosomes, on the other hand, are usually described as consisting of RNA, or at least as containing a high proportion of RNA. The evidence most often quoted is van den Berghe's (1942, 1946) observation that the granules disappear after exposure to ribonuclease. However, Ormerod (1951a, 1961) stressed the point that the ribonuclease used by van den Berghe was grossly contaminated with protease. Ormerod (1951a) found that neither protease-free ribonuclease nor trypsin removed the basophilic stain from the granules, but a combination of both enzymes did. However, on the basis of various other more or less nonspecific histochemical tests he states that there is at least strong circumstantial evidence for the presence of RNA in the granules of the trypanosomes. A similar assumption is justified for the corresponding inclusions of the extracellular stages of *Toxoplasma gondii*. Das Gupta and Kulasiri (1959) reported that their basophilia disappeared upon treatment with ribonuclease.

II. CHEMICAL OBSERVATIONS

Relatively few quantitative data concerning the nucleic acid content of parasites can be found in the literature; they refer in most cases to flagellates. Hamada (1956) found in two strains of *Trichomonas vaginalis* grown *in vitro* 3.35×10^{-8} and 1.58×10^{-8} μg DNA-P per cell and in *Trichomonas foetus* 5.48×10^{-8} μg. He observed considerably higher values when the organisms were developed in the abdominal cavity of mice: 6.79×10^{-8} μg DNA-P per cell in the case of *Trichomonas vaginalis* and 1.20×10^{-7} μg in that of *Trichomonas foetus*. Michaels and Treick (1962) found in dried *Trichomonas vaginalis* 0.3 % DNA and 20 % RNA. Newton (1964) reported variations in RNA content during the growth cycle of *Strigomonas oncopelti* with extremes of 1398 and 2186 μg RNA per 10^9 flagellates. The DNA content did not show comparable variations. It remained approximately constant with values slightly in excess of 200 μg per 10^9 organisms. The only other study deals with *Plasmodium berghei*. According to Whitfeld (1953a), one parasite contained $0.87–1.55 \times 10^{-7}$ μg RNA and $0.40–0.69 \times 10^{-1}$ μg DNA. Still less is known about the nucleic acid content of helminths. Pollak and Fairbairn (1955) found in the ovaries of *Ascaris lumbricoides* 41 mg RNA-P/100 gm tissue and 9.8 mg DNA-P, that is, the proportion between both was about the same as in rat liver. Nigon and Bovet (1955) found in one spermatid of *Parascaris equorum* 2.5×10^{-6} μg DNA, while a fertilized, but unsegmented, egg contained 290×10^{-6} μg, a remarkable but not fully explainable increase.

Chemically, the nucleic acids of parasites seem to correspond more or less to those of free-living organisms. The absorption spectrum of the *Plasmodium berghei* nucleic acids corresponded exactly to that of yeast nucleic acid (Whitfeld, 1953a). Similarly, the purine and pyrimidine bases show nothing unusual in respect to their constituents. Thus, the DNA of *Trichomonas vaginalis* contained cytosine, guanine, adenine, and thymine, while its RNA contained cytosine, guanine, adenine, and uracil (Michaels and Treick, 1962). In *Strigomonas oncopelti* adenine, guanine, cytosine, uracil, and thymine have been found (Newton, 1957); in *Trypanosoma cruzi,* adenine, thymine, cytosine, and uracil (von Brand *et al.,* 1959). In *Plasmodium berghei* adenine, guanine, cytosine, and uracil were recognized as RNA bases, while adenine, guanine, cytosine, and thymine were identified in the case of DNA (Whitfeld, 1953a).

Less is known about helminths in this respect, but some data on nucleosides and nucleotides are available. Campbell (1963) fractionated the nucleotides of *Hymenolepis diminuta.* Besides such compounds as adenosine di- and triphosphate, or nicotinamide adenosine dinucleotide and its phosphate, all of which are, in all probability, involved mainly in energy metabolism, he found cytosine, uridine, and probably guanosine nucleotides. In *Ascaris lumbricoides* the occurrence of adenosine, guanosine, uridine, and cytidine can be inferred from the finding of specific kinases for these compounds in the tissues of both female and male reproductive tracts (Entner and Gonzalez, 1961). Some further relevant data will be mentioned later in the section dealing with synthetic processes.

Nucleic acids occur combined with proteins to form nucleoproteins. The amino acid composition of the residual protein moiety has been studied so far only in the case of *Trypanosoma rhodesiense* by Williamson (1963). He found that the DNA sample contained mainly aspartic acid and glycine, but also a little arginine and traces of glutamic acid and alanine, while alanine, glutamic acid, glycine, serine, and smaller amounts of lysine and arginine were found in the RNA sample.

It has been emphasized recently that DNA base composition may be of significance in elucidating taxonomic relationships of protozoa. Schildkraut *et al.* (1962) in this respect studied several protozoan species, including parasitic flagellates *(Crithidia luciliae, Crithidia fasciculata, Strigomonas oncopelti, Leishmania tarentolae,* and *Trypanosoma lewisi)* by cesium chloride density gradient centrifugation and by determining the thermal denaturation point of the samples. The DNA of the parasitic flagellates contained from 54 to 59 % guanine plus cytosine, while in free-living ciliates the values ranged from 22 to 35%. The cesium-banded DNA of *Crithidia fasciculata* showed, besides the main component, one minor satellite band, while that of *Strigomonas oncopelti* had two minor components. It was shown subsequently (Marmur *et al.*, 1963) that in this latter case one of the minor bands represented DNA from the bipolar bodies, which, as mentioned in a previous section, may represent symbiotic organisms. The single minor band found in *Leishmania enrietti* more recently has been referred to the DNA of the kinetoplast. The DNA of the minor component apparently has a lower molecular weight than the major component (Du Buy *et al.*, 1965).

III. SYNTHETIC PROCESSES

Some parasites apparently can utilize nucleosides and nucleotides for nucleic acid synthesis. However, the evidence is sometimes only indirect. It has thus been shown by Nakamura (1957) that the addition of adenosine, guanosine, and thymidine to the medium stimulated the growth of two strains of *Entamoeba histolytica,* but not of a third one; adenylic, guanylic, thymidilic, and uridylic acids promoted the growth of all three strains. Similarly, it is at best indirect evidence when nucleic acid derivatives are added to media used in growing parasites *in vitro.* Citri (1954), for instance, used cytidilic acid and RNA as components of his semisynthetic medium for *Trypanosoma cruzi;* Berntzen (1962) employed adenylic acid and RNA in one of his media for *Hymenolepis diminuta;* Senft and Senft (1962) added deoxyadenosine, deoxycytidine, deoxyguanosine, thymidine, and 5-methylcytosine to their medium used in cultivating *Schistosoma mansoni.* These data will become meaningful only when the essentiality of the compounds employed has been demonstrated. This has not yet been done in the above and other cases (e.g., *Plasmodium hexamerium,* Nydegger and Manwell, 1962; *Neoaplectana glaseri,* Jackson, 1962). Somewhat more convincing therefore is House's (1954a,b) finding that the omission of RNA from his chemically defined medium used for developing *Pseudosarcophaga affinis in vitro* leads to decreased growth and to a decrease in the number of larvae reaching third instar.

In the case of malarial parasites rapid incorporation of inorganic phosphate into nucleic acids has been demonstrated repeatedly for various species (Clarke, 1952a,b; Whitfeld, 1953a,b). However, no critical experiments with isolated parasites have been done as yet and it is therefore not possible to state what are the simplest organic compounds that can serve for synthesis of nucleic acids. The *in vitro* cultivation of malaria parasites, even inside erythrocytes, is notoriously difficult and definite conclusions in respect to their nutritional requirements must be drawn with caution. It is, however, suggestive of limited synthetic capacity that in Anfinsen and co-workers' (1946) experience the addition of both purines and pyrimidines is necessary to insure maximal *in vitro* multiplication of *Plasmodium knowlesi.*

Much more precise information is available for some trypanosomids. *Strigomonas oncopelti* possesses rather considerable powers of synthesis. Newton (1957) demonstrated that radioactive carbon from glycine, serine, and guanine specifically labeled purines, while that of acetate, aspartate, glutamate, and uracil specifically labeled pyrimidines. However, when studied in a *p*-aminobenzoic-free medium, the flagellate required adenine for growth. (Newton, 1957). As Nathan (1958) pointed out, the biochemical deficiency indicated by this observation could not be located at the hypoxanthine-adenine conversion level, because in that case neither carboxamide (imidazole counterpart of hypoxanthine) nor carboxamidine (imidazole counterpart of adenine) should be able to substitute for adenine. Actually, the latter compound could serve successfully as substitute for adenine in the cultures. This, according to Nathan (1958), makes it probable that the purine synthesis proceeds through an imidazole derivative having a potential carboxamidine rather than a potential carboxamide group at the site destined to become the C_6 of adenine.

The synthetic functions of *Crithidia fasciculata* seem to be of the same order as those reported for *Strigomonas oncopelti.* Aaronson and Nathan (1954) demonstrated its capability of utilizing a variety of compounds (adenine, guanine, xanthine, hypoxanthine, and the respective ribosides, ribotides, and deoxyribosides) for nucleic acid synthesis. Like *Strigomonas* it was unable to utilize carboxamide, but carboxamidine could serve as substrate for nucleic acid synthesis.

Other trypanosomids have much narrower synthetic powers inasmuch as they cannot incorporate simple precursors, such as glycine or formate, into purine bases, that is, they cannot synthesize the purine nucleus. This has been shown for the culture form of *Trypanosoma mega* by Boné and Steinert (1956), and the blood-stream form of *Trypanosoma lewisi.* That of *Trypanosoma equiperdum* could synthesize nucleic acid from glycine; it did, however, preferentially use pathways involving compounds with preformed purine rings (Pizzi and Taliaferro, 1960). The culture form of *Trypanosoma cruzi* could incorporate glycine very slowly into acid-soluble adenine, while adenine was freely incorporated into acid-soluble adenine nucleotides, other adenine coenzymes, and nucleic acid purines. The synthesis of the latter compounds was not inhibited by D(−) threo-chloramphenicol, a substance interfering materially with the synthesis of acid-soluble adenine compounds (Fernandes and Castellani, 1958).

In trypanosomes, DNA is synthesized not only in the nucleus, but also in the parabasal apparatus (kinetoplast). This has been shown for crithidias and the blood-stream forms of *Trypanosoma mega* with the help of autoradiograms gained from flagellates exposed previously to tritiated thymidine (Steinert *et al.,* 1958; Steinert and Steinert, 1962). This species incorporated adenine-8-C^{14} four to five times more rapidly into adenine ribosides than into guanine ribotides, and approximately twice as rapidly into adenine deoxyribotides than guanine deoxyribotides (Boné and Steinert, 1956).

The synthetic powers of some trypanosomes are limited not only insofar as closure of the purine rings is concerned, but also in respect to the synthesis of the pyrimidine rings. This, according to Fernandes and Castellani (1959), is indicated by the failure of the culture form of *Trypanosoma cruzi* to incorporate C^{14}-orotate into nucleic acid pyrimidines.

Of parasitic ciliates, only *Opalina ranarum* has been studied to some extent. Nilova and Sukhanova (1964) observed that the organism did not form nucleic acids when incubated in a medium containing tritiated thymidine. However, after incubation in the presence of C^{14}-adenine, labeled RNA could be detected both in the nuclei and the endoplasm regardless whether the experiments were done during winter, spring or summer. On the contrary, and this is very interesting, DNA was formed from C^{14}-adenine only during the summer.

Very little is known about nucleic acid synthesis in helminths. Indeed, it seems not yet to have been determined whether or not they are able to synthesize purines and pyrimidines from simple precursors. It has been established by autoradiography (Prescott and Voge, 1959) that the cysticercoids of *Hymenolepis diminuta* take up C^{14}-adenine, which is deposited mainly at the body/tail junction and in the peripheral tissue layers of the organism. Similar experiments in principle were done by Dvorak and Jones (1963) with adults of *Hymenolepis microstoma. In vivo* the worms rapidly incorporated tritiated cytidine and thymine, the former compound giving rise to both labeled nucleoli and nuclei, while the latter was incorporated only into nuclei. The labeling was confined to regions of the worms where synthetic processes could be expected, that is, the regions of the neck, developing organs as well as in embryos. Campbell (1960a) observed that adult *Hymenolepis diminuta* readily absorbed uracil, thymine, and cytosine, but not orotic acid, 5-methyl-, or 5-hydroxymethylcytosine. Apparently indicating different ways of entry for some of the above compounds is Campbell's (1960a) observation that parasites from starved hosts take up less uracil and thymine than worms from well-fed hosts, while, on the contrary, starvation of the host increased the uptake of cytosine. In the presence of glucose parasites both from starved and fed hosts increased their uracil and thymine absorption, while no similar effect was observed with cytosine. Evidently, however, the fact that tapeworms can absorb purines and pyrimidines does not exclude the possibility that they could utilize simple precursors for their synthesis.

It has been mentioned previously that Entner and Gonzalez (1961) described four nucleoside monokinases from the reproductive tracts of *Ascaris lumbricoides*. Adenosine and guanosine monophosphate kinases were present in much larger amounts than the corresponding kinases for uridine and cytidine. It proved possible to separate and partially purify the two former enzymes. Both had quite similar properties: their pH optimum was broad (pH 7–8), both required Mg^{++} which, however, could be replaced by Mn^{++}, and ATP served as the relatively specific triphosphate donor. Both kinases were more effective with the ribonucleotides than with the corresponding deoxyribonucleotides. In addition to the monophosphate kinases, Entner and Gonzalez (1961) found a nucleotide diphosphatekinase which, in contrast to the above enzymes, was unspecific both in respect to the triphosphate donor and the nucleoside diphosphate acceptor. Another enzyme potentially available for synthetic processes is a polynucleotide phosphorylase found by Entner and Gonzalez (1959) in both male and female reproductive tracts of *Ascaris lumbricoides*. Reversal of its normal activity could be demonstrated by showing that the enzyme can incorporate cytidildiphosphate into acid-insoluble material. There was also some evidence that the system could synthesize polynucleotide from nucleoside triphosphates.

IV. DEGRADATION PROCESSES

Degradation of nucleic acids *in vivo* is initiated by nucleases which break the high molecular compounds down into smaller units (oligonucleotides), a process leading rapidly to a loss of specific biological activity. It can be assumed that such enzymes occur in parasites, but they have not yet been studied. Of possible biological importance in nucleic acid metabolism is the polynucleotide phosphorylase found by Newton (1963a) in *Strigomonas oncopelti* and in the male and female reproductive systems of *Ascaris lumbricoides* by Entner and Gonzalez (1959). The latter investigators isolated a fraction rich in RNA which readily carried out phosphorolysis of synthetic polynucleotides and catalyzed an exchange reaction between inorganic phosphate and nucleoside diphosphates. It was found that the system produced adenine diphosphate from polyadenylate and cytidildiphosphate from polycytidilate.

The degradation of pyrimidines has been studied by Campbell (1960a) for *Hymenolepis diminuta*. It was observed first that freshly isolated specimens contained about 0.6 μmole each of β-alanine and β-aminoisobutyric acid, which could have originated from uracil and thymine respectively. This assumption received support from the observation that the concentrations of these two compounds increased 5- to 20-fold upon incubation of the worms in solutions containing uracil, thymine, various dihydropyrimidines, or carbamoyl-β-amino acids. The degradation of (2 C^{14}) uracil was then studied in greater detail. It led over dihydrouracil and carbamoyl-β-alanine to the following end products: $C^{14}O_2$, α (1 C^{14}) alanine, and an organic acid which was probably succinic acid. It is possible that the process involved CO_2 fixation. Campbell (1960a) visualizes incorporation of $C^{14}O_2$ from uracil into the carboxyl group of succinic acid, followed by oxidation and decarboxylation to form pyruvic acid which in turn would give rise to carboxyl group-labeled alanine by transamination.

It has not yet been established unequivocally whether the above pathway of pyrimidine utilization occurs in other parasites besides *Hymenolepis diminuta*. However, presumptive evidence has been found in rather numerous species of cestodes, in the entoparasitic trematode *Macraspis,* as well as in the ectoparasitic fluke *Entobdella* by demonstrating that these parasites have greater or smaller amounts of β-alanine and β-aminoisobutyric acid in their tissues (Campbell, 1960b,c). A noteworthy exception is *Fasciola hepatica;* neither of the above compounds was demonstrable in its tissues. In the case of *Fascioloides magna* only β-alanine was found (Campbell, 1960c).

A common end product of purine metabolism is uric acid. Usually it is excreted in not very large amounts by some cestodes and trematodes (Schopfer, 1932; Salisbury and Anderson, 1939; Goil, 1958), but details of its formation have not yet been reported. In many mammals uric acid, or at least significant portions of the uric acid produced, is not excreted as such, but excretion takes place only after the uric acid has been further degraded to allantoin. It is possible that this, or some similar, process accounts for the fact that little or no uric acid has been found in the excreta of parasitic nematodes (Rogers, 1952). Significant in this connection is the observation by Savel (1954) that the urea-NH_3 formed by *Ascaris lumbricoides* is increased upon incubation with adenine, xanthine, and uric acid. However, no corresponding increase was observed when guanine was employed as substrate, possibly due to the lack of guanase. Savel (1954) assumes that *Ascaris* can completely degrade purines, with the exception of guanine, to ammonia, a faculty much better developed in young than old specimens. This latter observation probably explains why Rogers (1952) found only muscle adenylic acid, but not several purines and related compounds, to increase urea and ammonia production of *Ascaris* muscle. Similarly, minces prepared from large *Ascaridia galli* utilized only adenylic acid and smaller amounts of adenine, while preparations from young specimens degraded adenine, adenylic acid, xanthine, uric acid, and allantoin, with ammonia as end product. Of these compounds only uric acid and allantoin led to an increased urea production. Guanine, just as in the case of *Ascaris,* did not give rise to increased ammonia or urea production. Rogers (1952) assumes the successive action of uricooxidase, allantoinase, and allantoicase to explain the breakdown of the above compounds. The last two enzymes have not been found in *Fasciola hepatica* (Florkin and Duchateau, 1943).

V. DISTURBANCES IN THE HOST'S NUCLEIC ACID METABOLISM DURING PARASITIC INFECTIONS

The possibility that parasitic infections may interfere with the nucleic acid metabolism of the host has, as yet, hardly been considered. For example, it is not known whether the pronounced nucleic acid synthesis by malarial parasites interferes with the nucleic acid synthesis of their host cells. It has, however, been shown (Lewert, 1952) that the DNA content of chicken erythrocytes decreased during infections with *Plasmodium gallinaceum,* the decrease being most noticeable as long as the parasites were small and uninucleate. He also found indications pointing toward a nucleic acid depletion in the brain cells of infected chicken.

Histochemical evidence has been presented by Sawada *et al.* (1956) indicating that the RNA content of hepatic parenchymal cells was decreased during infections of mice with *Schistosoma japonicum.* Similarly, Hamada (1959) found by means of histochemical technique that the nucleic acids had decreased in the lungs of dogs infected with *Paragonimus westermani.*

VI. NUCLEIC ACIDS OF PARASITES AND CHEMOTHERAPY

There is good evidence for the assumption that some trypanocidal drugs exert their action by interfering with the nucleic acid metabolism of the flagellates. One of the most thoroughly investigated compounds is Antrycide. It had originally been assumed that its activity was connected with an ability to split cytoplasmic ribonucleoprotein into nucleic acid and protein (Ormerod, 1951b). However, analysis, by means of biochemical methods and using *Strigomonas oncopelti* as test object showed that interference with nucleic acid synthesis is primarily involved.

Newton (1958) observed first that Antrycide changed the usual logarithmic growth pattern of *Strigomonas* to a linear one in a peptone-glucose medium, this change being paralleled by a corresponding shift in RNA, DNA, and protein synthesis. In a peptone-free medium, however, RNA synthesis was markedly inhibited, this inhibition being nullified by *p*-aminobenzoic acid (Newton, 1964). Especially strongly inhibited was the incorporation of exogenous purines into nucleic acid and this interference was even marked at Antrycide concentrations which did not prevent the incorporation of endogenously formed purines (Newton, 1964). It was shown (Newton, 1960) that the absorption of C^{14}-adenine from the environment and its transfer to the intracellular nucleotide pool remained essentially unaffected by the drug and that synthesis of nucleotides from purine bases was still possible. The suggestion was made that the compound may hinder the polymerization of nucleotides to nucleic acid. However, a partially purified polynucleotide phosphorylase isolated from *Strigomonas* was not inhibited by the drug (Newton, 1963a).

On the basis of a study of subcellular fractions isolated from the flagellates after incubation in a medium containing glucose, C^{14}-adenine, pyrimidines, and amino acids, it was found that Antrycide interfered with the synthesis of nucleic acid by a fraction containing 70 % of the total cellular RNA. The fraction consisted essentially of particles with a sedimentation constant of 80 S; they evidently correspond to ribosomes. It appears then that the activity of Antrycide may be related to its interference with the synthesis of ribosomal nucleic acid. The available evidence suggests, furthermore, that the drug may not inhibit the function of existing ribosomes, but may prevent the formation of new functional units (Newton, 1962b, 1963a). Further analysis showed that Antrycide causes isolated ribosomes to aggregate. No change in nucleic acid or protein content was induced, but the amount of Mg^{++} was decreased. Of the two main amines associated with the ribosomes, putrescine was more readily displaced by the drug then spermidine. It was also shown that under the influence of Antrycide the bonding of ribosomal RNA to protein was significantly altered (Newton, 1963b). The ribosomal aggregation phenomenon occurred also *in vivo,* resulting during fractionation experiments in a considerable decrease in the number of particles sedimenting like ribosomes, because the aggregated particles sedimented more rapidly than normal ribosomes. It is entirely possible (Ormerod, 1962; Newton, 1962a) that the aggregated ribosomes correspond to the basophilic granules appearing, as mentioned previously, under the influence of the drug.

Antrycide is an aminoquinaldine derivative, while Homidium is a phenanthridine derivative. Its mode of action, studied by Newton (1964) differs in some respect from that of the former compound. In contrast to

Antrycide, Homidium progressively prevents, in nutritive solution, multiplication of *Strigomonas*. It inhibits DNA synthesis rather rapidly, but allows limited RNA and protein synthesis. A further difference between the two compounds is that Homidium inhibited the utilization, for nucleic acid synthesis, both of preformed purines and of purines synthesized from simple precursors, while, as mentioned above, Antrycide allowed utilization of the latter.

It was recognized early that the antitrypanosomal activity of an antibiotic, Stylomycin (previously known as Puromycin), and especially its aminonucleoside might be related to interference with nucleic acid metabolism. This was postulated on basis of the observation that purines reversed the chemotherapeutic activity of the compounds against *Trypanosoma equiperdum* (Hewitt *et al.*, 1954). It was furthermore found that adenine sulfate effectively antagonized relatively slight metabolic changes induced in the same flagellate by either Stylomycin or its aminonucleoside, when the effective compounds were circulating in the blood of the host. However, the antagonistic action of adenine sulfate was not pronounced enough to counteract completely the metabolic effects of the antibiotic *in vitro* (Agosin and von Brand, 1954). Direct evidence was then adduced for *Trypanosoma cruzi*. Fernandes and Castellani (1959) observed that the aminonucleoside of Stylomycin, but not the parent compound, strongly inhibited the incorporation of adenine-8-C^{14} into the parasite's nucleic acids. It was furthermore found (Silva *et al.*, 1959) that the same compound, while not very damaging to extracellular stages of *Trypanosoma cruzi*, induced degeneration and sometimes lysis of the *Leishmania* stages. This effect was not prevented by adenine, adenosine, or simpler compounds often used in purine nucleotide synthesis.

The nucleic acid synthesis of trypanosomes can be inhibited not only by drugs, but in certain infections also by immune mechanisms. It has thus been shown (Taliaferro and Pizzi, 1960) that the injection of ablastin-containing serum into rats inhibits the nucleic acid synthesis by *Trypanosoma lewisi* from adenine-8-C^{14} by 87%.

A definite interference with nucleic acid synthesis has also been reported for some antimalarial drugs. Clarke (1952b) first observed that 10^{-5} M quinine inhibited the incorporation of P^{32}-labeled phosphate into the DNA of *Plasmodium gallinaceum*. It was shown subsequently by Schellenberg and Coatney (1961) that the cinchona alkaloids quinine, quinidine, cinchonine, and cinchonidine all had essentially the same effect, but that the inhibition was not limited to DNA synthesis; it was found also when RNA formation was studied. On the other hand, pyrimethamine and the triazine metabolite of chlorguanide inhibited only phosphate incorporation into DNA. The pyrimethamine-induced inhibition was not reversed by folic acid, folinic acid, thymine, uracil, adenine, or related compounds. The exact point of attack of the various anti-malarials was not established, but it seems to vary with the class of compounds involved. It may be mentioned that Schellenberg and Coatney (1961) assume the inhibition of phosphate incorporation into nucleic acids by the cinchona alkaloids, chloroquine and quinacrine, to be closer related to inhibition of substrate utilization than to inhibition of nucleic acid synthesis proper. They do assume, however, that the blocking of DNA synthesis by pyrimethamine and chlorguanide may be due directly to an inhibition of synthesis.

Whether anthelmintic drugs interfere with the nucleic acid metabolism of parasites is unknown. Histological evidence indicates that Miracil attacks the nuclei of schistosomes, especially those of the reproductive tract, inhibiting mitosis (Goennert, 1947). However, biochemical studies failed to uncover interference with the nucleoprotein metabolism of the worms (Bueding et al., 1947).

REFERENCES

Aaronson, S., and Nathan, H. A. (1954). *Biochim. Biophys. Acta* **15**, 306–307.

Agosin, M., and Brand, T. von (1954). *Antibiot. Chemotherapy* **4**, 624–632.

Anfinsen, C. B., Geiman, Q. M., McKee, R. W., Ormsbee, R. A., and Ball, E. G. (1946). *J. Exptl. Med.* **84**, 607–621.

Baker, J. R. (1961). *Trans. Roy. Soc. Trop. Med. Hyg.* **55**, 518–524.

Barker, D. C. (1963). *Z. Zellforsch.* **58**, 641–659.

Barker, D. C., and Deutsch, K. (1958). *Exptl. Cell Res.* **15**, 604–639.

Barker, D. C., and Svihla, G. (1964). *J. Cell Biol.* **20**, 389–398.

Berghe, L. van den (1942). *Acta Biol. Belge* **4**, 464–467.

Berghe, L. van den (1946). *J. Parasitol.* **32**, 465–466.

Berntzen, A. K. (1962). *J. Parasitol.* **48**, 785–797.

Bonê, G. J., and Steinert, M. (1956). *Nature* **178**, 308–309.

Brand, T. von, McMahon, P., Tobie, E. J., Thompson, M. J., and Mosettig, E. (1959). *Exptl. Parasitol.* **8**, 171–181.

Bresslau, E. L., and Scremin, L. (1924). *Arch. Protistenk.* **48**, 509–515.

Bueding, E., Higashi, A., Peters, L., and Valk, A. D. (1947). *Federation Proc.* **6**, 313.

Campbell, J. W. (1960a). *Biochem. J.* **77**, 105–112.

Campbell, J. W. (1960b). *Exptl. Parasitol.* **9**, 1–8.

Campbell, J. W. (1960c). *Biol. Bull.* **119**, 75–79.

Campbell, J. W. (1963). *Comp. Biochem. Physiol.* **8**, 181–185.

Citri, N. (1954). Thesis, Hebrew University, Jerusalem.

Clarke, D. H. (1952a). *J. Exptl. Med.* **96**, 439–450.

Clarke, D. H. (1952b). *J. Exptl. Med.* **96,** 451–463.

Das Gupta, B., and Kulasiri, C. (1959). *Parasitology* **49,** 594–600.

Du Buy, H. G., Mattern, C. F. T., and Riley, F. L. (1965). *Science* **147,** 754–756.

Dvorak, J. A., and Jones, A. W. (1963). *Exptl. Parasitol.* **14,** 316–322.

Entner, N., and Gonzalez, C. (1959). *Biochem. Biophys. Res. Commun.* **1,** 333–335.

Entner, N., and Gonzalez, C. (1961). *Biochim. Biophys. Acta* **47,** 52–60.

Fernandes, J. F., and Castellani, O. (1958). *Exptl. Parasitol.* **7,** 224–235.

Fernandes, J. F., and Castellani, O. (1959). *Exptl. Parasitol.* **8,** 480–485.

Florkin, M., and Duchateau, G. (1943). *Arch. Intern. Physiol. (Paris)* **53,** 267–307.

Gill, J. W., and Vogel, H. J. (1963). *J. Protozool.* **10,** 148–152.

Goennert, R. (1947). *Naturwiss.* **34,** 347.

Goil, M. M. (1958). *J. Helminthol.* **32,** 119–124.

Govaert, J. (1953). *Compt. Rend. Soc. Biol.* **147,** 1494–1496.

Hamada, M. (1959). *Shikoku Acta Med.* **14,** 165–186.

Hamada, Y. (1956). *Med. J. Osaka Univ.* **6,** 1101–1105.

Hewitt, R. I., Gumble, A. R., Wallace, W. S., and Williams, J. H. (1954). *Antibiot. Chemotherapy* **4,** 1222–1227.

House, H. L. (1954a). *Can. J. Zool.* **32,** 331–341.

House, H. L. (1954b). *Can. J. Zool.* **32,** 358–365.

Hutner, S. H., and Provasoli, L. (1951). *In* "Biochemistry and Physiology of Protozoa." (A. Lwoff, ed.), Vol. 1, pp. 27–128. Academic Press, New York

Jackson, G. J. (1962). *Trans. N.Y. Acad. Sci.* [2] **24,** 954–965.

Kawamitsu, K. (1957). *Nagasaki Igakkai Zasshi* **32,** 1398–1403.

Lewert, R. M. (1952). *J. Infect. Diseases* **91,** 125–144.

Marmur, J., Cahoon, M. E., Shimura, Y., and Vogel, H. J. (1963). *Nature* **197,** 1228–1229.

Michaels, R. M., and Treick, R. W. (1962). *Exptl. Parasitol.* **12,** 401–417.

Nakamura, M. (1957). *Biol. Bull.* **112,** 377–382.

Nathan, H. A. (1958). *J. Protozool.* **5,** 194–195.

Newton, B. A. (1957). *J. Gen. Microbiol.* **17,** 708–717.

Newton, B. A. (1958). *J. Gen. Microbiol.* **19,** II.

Newton, B. A. (1960). *Biochem. J.* **77,** 17P.

Newton, B. A. (1962a). *Parasitology* **52,** 9P.

Newton, B. A. (1962b). *Biochem. J.* **84,** 109P–110P.

Newton, B. A. (1963a). *In* "Progress in Protozoology." (J. Ludvik *et al.,* eds.), pp. 170–172. Czech. Acad. Sci., Prague.

Newton, B. A. (1963b). *Biochem. J.* **89,** 93P–94P.

Newton, B. A. (1964). *Advan. Chemotherapy* **1,** 35–83.

Newton, B. A., and Horne, R. W. (1957). *Exptl. Cell Res.* **13,** 563–574.

Nigon, V., and Bovet, P. (1955). *Compt. Rend.* **149,** 129–130.

Nilova, V. K., and Sukhanova, K. M. (1964). *Nature* **204,** 459–460.

Nydegger, L., and Manwell, R. D. (1962). *J. Parasitol.* **48,** 142–147.

Ormerod, W. E. (1951a). *Brit. J. Pharm. Chemother.* **6,** 334–341.

Ormerod, W. E. (1951b). *Brit. J. Pharmacol.* **6,** 325–333.

Ormerod, W. E. (1958). *J. Gen. Microbiol.* **19,** 271–288.

Ormerod, W. E. (1959). *J. Gen. Microbiol.* **21,** 287–294.

Ormerod, W. E. (1961). *Trans. Roy. Soc. Trop. Med. Hyg.* **55,** 313–327.

Ormerod, W. E. (1962). *Parasitology* **52,** 9P.

Pizzi, T., and Diaz, M. (1954). *Biologica (Santiago, Chile)* **20,** 71–88.

Pizzi, T., and Taliaferro, W. H. (1960). *J. Infect. Diseases* **107,** 100–107.

Pollak, J. K., and Fairbairn, D. (1955). *Can. J. Biochem. Physiol.* **33,** 297–306.

Prescott, D. M., and Voge, M. (1959). *J. Parasitol.* **45,** 587–590.

Ray, H. N., and Gill, B. S. (1955). *Indian J. Vet. Sci. Animal Husbandry* **25,** Part I, 17–23.

Reichenow, E. (1928). *Arch. Protistenk.* **61,** 144–166.

Rogers, W. P. (1952). *Australian J. Sci. Res.* **B5,** 210–222.

Salisbury, L. F., and Anderson, R. J. (1939). *J. Biol. Chem.* **129,** 505–517.

Savel, J. (1954). Thesis, University of Paris

Sawada, T., Hara, K., Takagi, K., Nagazawa, Y., and Oka, S. (1956). *Am. J. Trop. Med. Hyg.* **5,** 847–859.

Schellenberg, K. A., and Coatney, G. R. (1961). *Biochem. Pharmacol.* **6,** 143–152.

Schildkraut, C. L., Mandel, M., Levisohn, S., Smith-Sonneborn, J. E., and Marmur, J. (1962). *Nature* **196,** 795–796.

Schopfer, W. H. (1932). *Rev. Suisse Zool.* **39,** 59–192.

Senft, A. W., and Senft, D. G. (1962). *J. Parasitol.* **48,** 551–554.

Silva, L. H. P., Yoneda, S., and Fernandes, J. F. (1959). *Exptl. Parasitol.* **8,** 486–495.

Steinert, G., Firket, H., and Steinert, M. (1958). *Exptl. Cell Res.* **15,** 632–635.

Steinert, M., and Steinert, G. (1962). *J. Protozool.* **9,** 203–211.

Taliaferro, W. H., and Pizzi, T. (1960). *Proc. Natl. Acad. Sci. U.S.* **46,** 733–745.

Tsunoda, K., and Ichikawa, O. (1955). *Govt. Expt. Sta. Animal Hyg. Expt. Rept.* **29,** pp. 73–82.

van den Berghe, L., *see* Berghe, L. van den.

von Brand, T., *see* Brand, T. von.

Whitfeld, P. R. (1953a). *Australian J. Biol. Sci.* **6,** 234–243.

Whitfeld, P. R. (1953b). *Australian J. Biol. Sci.* **6,** 591–596.

Williamson, J. (1963). *Exptl. Parasitol.* **13,** 348–366.

Chapter 8

VITAMINS

I. VITAMINS IN PARASITES

Relatively few determinations of the vitamin content of parasites have been done so far. Of the fat-soluble vitamins, only vitamin Q (ubiquinone) has received some attention (Vakirtzi-Lemonias *et al.*, 1963). It was found that *Crithidia fasciculata* and *Strigomonas oncopelti* contained 0.23 and 0.40 μmole ubiquinone/gm dry weight, respectively, and that the compounds isolated from both flagellates contained nine isoprene units.

Somewhat more data are available for water-soluble vitamins. The thiamine content of one specimen of *Plasmodium berghei* has been determined as 3.30×10^{-10} μg and that of one *Trypanosoma rhodesiense* to 7.0×10^{-10} μg (Singer, 1961). It has been mentioned previously (Chapter 1) that *Diphyllobothrium latum* readily absorbs vitamin B_{12} (cobalamine) while other helminths, with the possible exception of *Ascaris lumbricoides,* do so only much less readily. In the present connection it should be noted that the vitamin seems not to occur in *Diphyllobothrium* in the free form, as Kaipainen and Wallén (1954) had assumed. Nyberg and Gräsbeck (1957) found that absorbed vitamin B_{12} does remain an unchanged cobalamine, but that it is apparently bound to a protein. The protein-B_{12} complex, however, seems not to be very stable; it is rather readily dissociated by such treatments as heat, alcohol, or proteolytic enzymes.

Quantitative microbiological assays of some other members of the vitamin B complex were done by Chance and Dirnhuber (1949), who used *Fasciola hepatica, Moniezia benedeni, Ascaris lumbricoides,* and various stages of *Nippostrongylus muris.* They found that these worms contained thiamine, nicotinic acid, pantothenic acid, and riboflavin in amounts somewhat smaller than occurred in the liver of the respective hosts. On the other hand, more pyridoxine was found in the parasites than in the host's liver. They think that a correlation with the high rate of egg production may exist, since pyridoxine is involved in the processes leading to protein synthesis. Varying amounts of nicotinic acid and of thiamine also have been reported from the hydatid fluid (Latif and El Kordy, 1946). It does seem probable that the rumen ciliates contain vitamin B. Manusardi (1931) showed that the feeding of these ciliates to pigeons can cure beriberi, but the amounts necessary were very large. It is possible that the ciliates did not actually synthesize the vitamin, but that it was derived from ingested bacteria.

More is known about the distribution of vitamin C (ascorbic acid) among parasites than of any other vitamin. Relevant studies have in part been done only by means of histochemical methods which may not be entirely specific; some caution in their evaluation is therefore indicated. Conditions appear to be variable among parasitic protozoa. Vitamin C granules have been reported from *Trypanosoma equiperdum* (Roskin and Nastiukova, 1941). It is likely that these granules represent vitamin absorbed from the environment. It was found that their number increased upon raising the ascorbic acid level of the host's blood by injection of a vitamin solution. *Opalina,* on the other hand, was reported as being entirely devoid of vitamin C granules, whereas such granules were found throughout, but confined to, the endoplasm of *Nyctotherus cordiformis* (Smyth *et al.,* 1945).

It has been shown by means of histochemical technique that *Hymenolepis nana* contains vitamin C (Coleman, 1953). Quantitative assays (Coleman and Mizelle, 1956) yielded a value of 0.015% ascorbic acid in worms recovered from mice kept on a normal, vitamin-containing diet. It seems probable that a large part of the vitamin found in the worms was derived from the host's intestinal tract. Characteristic in this connection is the observation that infected mice kept for 63 days on a scorbutigenic diet and an additional 12 days on a scorbutigenic-succinylsulfathiozole diet showed signs of scurvy, while similarly treated uninfected specimens did not. However it should be noted that Read and Phifer in unpublished experiments, mentioned by Read and Simmons (1963), could not reproduce these results. Coleman and Mizelle (1956) believe that the tapeworms can also synthesize some ascorbic acid. They base this view on the observation that *Hymenolepis* specimens maintained *in vitro* for a period of 19 days in vitamin C-free media still contained at least minimal amounts of the vitamin.

In the few trematode species studied so far, the largest deposits of histochemically demonstrable ascorbic acid were found connected to the excretory system. In *Opistioglyphe ranae* (Smyth *et al.,* 1945) they occurred within the walls of the excretory canals and in *Fasciola hepatica* (Stephenson, 1947; Pantelouris and Hale, 1962) many vitamin C granules were found both in the walls and the lumen of the excretory canals. In this latter case a functional relationship between vitamin C and iron excretion has been assumed to explain the rather curious localization of the vitamin (Pantelouris and Hale, 1962; see also Chapter 1). In other organs of the liver fluke only relatively small amounts of ascorbic acid could be demonstrated; they were observed in myoblast clusters, in the outer layers of the testes and yolk glands, as well as in some cells of the gut epithelium. Worms kept for 10 minutes *in vitro* in a solution containing ascorbic acid showed additional deposits in the cuticle, especially its base, and in the deeper layers of parenchyma around the intestinal tract, evidently indicating that absorption took place (Pantelouris and Hale, 1962). On the other hand, in *Opistioglyphe ranae* taken from its host, no ascorbic acid was demonstrable within the gut cells (Smyth *et al.*, 1945).

Vitamin C has been found in the muscles, reproductive organs, and intestine of *Parascaris equorum*, the respective amounts being 70, 80, and 110 μg/gm fresh substance (Giroud and Rakoto-Ratsimamanga, 1936), and in the body fluid of *Ascaris lumbricoides* (Rogers, 1945). Histological studies (Hill and Smyth, 1944; Smyth *et al.*, 1945) confirmed the predominant localization within the intestinal cells in the case of *Toxocara canis*.

II. VITAMIN REQUIREMENTS OF PARASITES

The facts concerning vitamin accumulation in parasites, reviewed in the preceding section, make it probable that these compounds play a role in the economy of parasites, just as they do in the case of free-living animals. The mere fact of vitamin deposition or absorption cannot, however, be accepted as definite proof of their essentiality. More convincing evidence can be obtained by showing that certain vitamins are required for successful maintenance of parasites *in vitro* over prolonged periods of time, that is, essentially, during true cultivation. One difficulty with this approach is that the vitamin requirements of many organisms are complicated, and hence it has been almost universal practice to supplement the basal media with complex mixtures of vitamins. In very few cases only has the essentiality of a certain vitamin been established by critical experimentation. For example, the modern media used for axenic cultivation of *Entamoeba invadens, Entamoeba terrapinae,* or *Entamoeba histolytica* (Stoll, 1957; Diamond, 1960, 1961; Jackson and Stoll, 1964) contain vitamin mixtures, such as vitamin supplement NCTC 109 (McQuilkin *et al.*, 1957), but it is entirely unknown whether all components of this mixture are really required. Some vitamins undoubtedly are essential to parasitic amoebas. This seems indicated by the observation that, in nonsterile cultures, B vitamins have to be added to the overlay of diphasic culture media when egg white is substituted for whole egg in the base (Rees *et al.,* 1944), or by the observation that a vitamin mixture partially restores the growth-promoting qualities, in microcultures, of media rendered ineffective by moderate heating (Baernstein *et al.,* 1957).

Ascorbic acid seems to be required by certain trichomonads, such as *Eutrichomastix colubrorum, Trichomonas foetus, Trichomonas columbae,* or *Trichomonas gallinarum* (Cailleau, 1938, 1939a,b, 1940). It is, however, not specific. In cultures of *Trichomonas columbae* it could be replaced successfully by D-isoascorbic acid, D-glucoascorbic acid, D-glucoheptoascorbic acid, reductinic acid, and reductone (Cailleau, 1939c). This observation obviously raises the question whether in this and similar cases the main function of ascorbic acid is really that of a vitamin, i.e., whether it represents an essential microconstituent of the food, or whether its beneficial influence rests on its reducing properties. A rather clear indication that the latter interpretation rather than the former is correct, in the case of trichomonads at least, is the finding by Guthrie (1946) that thioglycollate could successfully replace ascorbic acid in cultures of *Trichomonas foetus.*

Little is known about the question whether or not trichomonads require vitamins other than ascorbic acid. Folic acid and pantothenic acid promote growth, but no potentiation between these two compounds could be detected. Thiamine, lactoflavin, nicotinic acid amide, or cobalamine are apparently not required (Rieck, 1956).

A relatively large amount of information is available for certain trypanosomids. *Crithidia fasciculata* (Cowperthwaite *et al.,* 1953; Nathan *et al.,* 1956), when grown on chemically defined medium, requires high levels of folic acid. Smaller amounts only are necessary if the so-called *Crithidia* factor is added to the cultures. This latter factor becomes indispensable when folic acid is bypassed by substituting thymine for it. Connections between *Crithidia* factor and riboflavin also exist. The normal riboflavin requirements of the organism are spared, if they have access to preformed *Crithidia* factor and low concentrations of folic acid. It can be assumed (Nathan and Funk, 1959) that folic acid plays a dual role in the metabolism of *Crithidia fasciculata.* On the one hand, it serves, as in many other organisms, to form thymine, thus being involved in DNA synthesis. On the other hand, it is a precursor of the independently functioning *Crithidia* factor. The latter seems to be widely distributed in nature. It is thus synthesized by the free-living flagellate *Ochromonas* (Nathan and Cowperthwaite, 1955) and has been isolated from human urine (Patterson *et al.,* 1955). The compound received the name biopterin and has been found to be an unconjugated pteridine: 2-amino-4-hydroxy-6-(1,2-dihydroxypropyl)-pteridine.

The requirement for biopterin is not entirely specific. Several 2-amino-4-hydroxy-6-alkyl substituted pteridines can replace it, but usually with lower efficiency (Broquist and Albrecht, 1955). Dewey *et al.* (1959) also studied the efficacy of several biopterin analogs. They uncovered several active compounds, the best one being the reaction product of 2,4,5-triamino-6-hydroxy-pyrimidine with *d*-galactose which is 2-NH_2-4-OH-6-(*d*-lyxo)-tetra-OH-butylpteridine. Dewey *et al.* (1959), on the basis of further tests with various pyrimidines, reached the conclusion that *Crithidia fasciculata* is deficient in synthesizing an appropriate pyrimidine rather than the required pteridine.

Interesting connections between *Crithidia* factor and vitamin B_{12}-like vitamins also exist (Nathan and Funk, 1959; Nathan *et al.,* 1960). When *Crithidia fasciculata* had access to folic acid as the only source for pteridines, true vitamin B_{12} alone was formed. When, however, only small amounts of folic acid were given, vitamin B_{12} was formed also, but in addition various types of pseudovitamins B_{12} were produced. Their amount increased sharply, with a concomitant drop in formation of genuine vitamin B_{12}, when thymidine was used to bypass folic acid in the presence of preformed *Crithidia* factor. It was finally observed that when only small quantities of folic acid were given and the organisms had access to 2,4,5-triamino-6-hydroxypyrimidine, no vitamin B_{12} was produced. Nathan and Funk (1959) drew the conclusion that at least one unconjugated pteridine was required for any vitamin B_{12} synthesis and that a conjugated pteridine favored synthesis of true vitamin B_{12} at the expense of the pseudovitamins. It is probable that the vitamin B_{12}-like substance isolated by Seaman and Sanders (1957) from the bodies of *Crithidia fasciculata* corresponds to one of the pseudovitamins mentioned above. It could substitute for vitamin B_{12} for *Escherichia coli, Euglena gracilis,* and the soil bacterium "Lochhead 38," but not for *Ochromonas malhamensis.*

It should be stressed that the involvement of the *Crithidia* factor in vitamin B_{12} synthesis cannot be the only function of this factor, since the flagellate can still grow under conditions where no vitamin B_{12} is synthesized. Furthermore, the *Crithidia* factor is still required for growth even when vitamin B_{12} is added to the culture medium. It is possible, but has not yet been proven that the factor is needed during some phase of the lipid metabolism of the parasite (Guttman, 1963).

It is not known whether other trypanosomids require the *Crithidia* factor for growth. It has been established that *Strigomonas oncopelti* required thiamine and nicotinamide (Newton, 1956). Not essential ingredients of the medium, but materially improving the growth rate were biotin, pyridoxin, pantothenic acid, and *p*-aminobenzoic acid. The vitamin requirements of the culture form of *Trypanosoma cruzi* appear to vary with the type of medium in which they are studied. Investigated on Boné and Parent's (1963) medium, the flagellates required only thiamine and folic acid. The medium in question contained as main organic components Bacto-tryptose, sodium stearate, and glucose. On the other hand, if the parasites were grown on Citri's (1954) semisynthetic medium, a much larger series of vitamins proved necessary: thiamine, folic acid, riboflavin, *p*-aminobenzoic acid, vitamin B_{12}, citrovorum factor, and nicotinamide. As can be expected the vitamin requirements of *Trypanosoma cruzi* grown in serum-containing undefined media, appeared less complex than those mentioned above. In fact, they appeared then to require, besides the unidentified substances present in blood serum and besides hematin, only ascorbic acid. They had this requirement in common with *Leishmania tropica,* and *Leishmania donovani,* while *Leishmania agamae* and *Leishmania ceramodactyli* may be able to grow in the absence of vitamin C (Lwoff, 1933, 1938, 1939, 1940).

The only *Leishmania* species studied so far in a chemically defined medium is *Leishmania tarentolae;* its vitamin requirements have been studied by Trager (1957a). Essential were folic acid, biotin, pantothenic acid, nicotinamide, riboflavin, thiamine, and either pyridoxine plus choline, or pyridoxal or pyridoxamine. It has already been pointed out in Chapter 5 that choline was required to form pyridoxal from pyridoxine, or that pyridoxal had a specific function in the biosynthesis of choline.

Cultivation experiments with malarial parasites have been only partially successful in elucidating vitamin requirements. This is not surprising in view of the complicated media necessary for their maintenance. Trager (1941, 1943, 1947), in his initial experiments, succeeded in keeping *Plasmodium lophurae* alive for periods up to 10 to 16 days. This relatively long survival was achieved by the addition of fresh red cells every other day, in addition to the provision of a complicated medium and proper aeration. Only one vitamin, calcium pantothenate, was considered with great probability as favoring the parasites directly. Later evidence (Trager, 1954, 1955, 1957b) indicated that calcium pantothenate was beneficial only to the host cell-parasite complex. It did not favor isolated parasites. The latter required CoA, of which pantothenic acid is an integral part. It is probable that the red cell can synthesize this compound and thus provides the parasite with the requisite amounts. Trager (1957b) has pointed out that a parallel situation may exist in respect to the folic acid group of compounds. Folic acid and *p*-aminobenzoic acid benefited the erythrocyte-parasite complex, but not the isolated parasites. Folinic acid, which in some cultures is beneficial to isolated parasites may be a step toward the hitherto unknown coenzyme form of folic acid. Malarial parasites undoubtedly utilize other vitamins as well; Trager (1957b) emphasized that the red cell-parasite complex *in vivo* requires not only pantothenate, but also ascorbic acid, thiamine, riboflavin, and biotin. It is, however, not yet known in what form these compounds must be offered to the parasites *in vitro* or in what way they exert their action.

Rather considerable success has been achieved in recent years with the cultivation of the mosquito phase of avian malaria parasites (Ball and Chao, 1957; Ball, 1964). The media required are exceedingly complex and contain a variety of vitamins. Since the latter's essentiality has not been demonstrated conclusively as yet, further discussion of this problem is omitted.

Hardly anything is known about vitamin requirements of parasitic ciliates. D'Agostino Barbaro (1953) reported that additions of vitamin A or D_3 to diluted rumen content were without influence on the survival of rumen ciliates, vitamin K seemed to have some detrimental effect, while relatively large amounts of vitamin E in the medium appeared to favor survival. He speculates that this latter effect may be due to a regulating influence on cellular proliferation, or indirectly to the antioxidant properties of vitamin K.

Only little definite information concerning vitamin requirements of parasitic helminths have come to light through cultivation experiments. Vitamin mixtures such as those used in the cultivation of mammalian cells are employed, e.g., the vitamin mixture of Eagle (1955), or those contained in McQuilkin and co-workers' (1957) NCTC 109 medium and Morgan and associates' (1950) medium 199. A critical analysis concerning the question whether all vitamins contained in these or similar mixtures are really required is difficult to carry out at the present state of our knowledge because the media commonly used in helminth cultivation contain often large proportions of such chemically undefined components as chicken embryo extract, blood serum, or yeast extract. Details concerning the actual vitamin supplements employed by various authors can be found in the following papers, and those quoted in some more detail below: for trematodes, Senft and Senft (1962); for cestodes, Mueller (1959); Berntzen (1962); for nematodes, Taylor (1960); Jackson (1962).

In some cases a beneficial influence of vitamins on survival or development has been observed. Williams *et al.* (1961) found that the addition of autoclaved yeast extract to their basal medium promoted sperm and vitellarian cell production of *Diplostomum phoxini*. They determined that vitamin B_{12}, pantothenic acid, thiamine, riboflavin, or biotin did not represent essential contributions by the yeast extract, but pyridoxine or some other form of vitamin B_6 possibly did. Taylor (1963) observed that the omission of vitamins from the medium employed by her in cultivation studies with larval *Taenia crassiceps* decreased survival of the worms. Read and Simmons (1963), summarizing unpublished experiments by Read, E. L. Schiller, and A. H. Rothman, indicate that analogs of nicotinic acid inhibited growth of *Hymenolepis diminuta in vitro* and that this inhibition could be reversed readily by nicotinic acid and nicotinamide.

It has also been known for some time that vitamins can be beneficial to parasitic nematodes. The first definite information to that effect was the observation by Weinstein and Jones (1956, 1959) that a vitamin mixture enhanced slightly the development *in vitro* of *Nippostrongylus muris*. Douvres (1962) found subsequently that larvae of *Oesophagostomum radiatum,* although developing to the fourth molt in various non-supplemented media, reached each successive stage faster when vitamins were added. Leland (1963) reported that omission of vitamins from his media used in the cultivation of *Cooperia punctata* led to smaller worms and suppressed egg production. An interesting effect of vitamin B_{12} on a parasitic nematode was noted by Weinstein (1961). He found that addition of this vitamin to cultures of third-stage larval *Nippostrongylus muris* led to the accumulation of a reddish pigment in the coelomocytes, but not in other cells, the intensity of the color becoming visible depending upon the concentration of vitamin B_{12} in the environment of the larvae.

Only in one instance have the vitamin requirements of a parasitic arthropod been investigated. House (1954) found that *Pseudosarcophaga affinis* required for development on a chemically defined medium the following vitamins: thiamine, riboflavin, calcium pantothenate, nicotinic acid, cholin chloride, and biotin. Not essential were pyridoxine, folic acid, *p*-aminobenzoic acid, and inositol. Vitamin B_{12} also was not essential, but exerted a slight beneficial action on pupation.

III.   INFLUENCE OF PARASITES
ON THE VITAMIN CONTENT OF HOST TISSUES

Infections with *Plasmodium gallinaceum* seem to reduce the thiamine level of the blood serum of chicken (Rama Rao and Sirsi, 1956a). In infections with *Plasmodium berghei,* on the other hand, an increase in thiamine content of spleen and infected erythrocytes has been observed. while no change in this respect was found in liver and kidney (Singer, 1961). *Trypanosoma rhodesiense* induced an increased thiamine content of the liver in young rats and, at least during the terminal stages of the infection, also of the spleen, while on the contrary the vitamin content of the kidney was decreased. In the blood, the thiamine level was definitely increased, the degree of the change being correlated to the severity of the parasitemia (Singer, 1959, 1961).

The riboflavin level of the blood appeared slightly increased during the prepatent period of *Plasmodium gallinaceum* infection, while it was somewhat lower than normal during the acute phase of the disease (Rama Rao and Sirsi, 1956b); qualitatively similar changes have also been reported for *p*-aminobenzoic acid (Rama Rao and Sirsi, 1956c).

Studies concerning the CoA concentration of host tissues during infections with *Plasmodium berghei* have been carried out by Singer and Trager (1956). They found the per cent concentration decreased in the liver, but, because of the organ hypertrophy, the total amount of hepatic CoA was approximately unchanged. In contrast, the per cent concentration of splenic CoA appeared unchanged, resulting, again due to organ hypertrophy, in an increased total amount of CoA in the spleen. The CoA content of the kidneys was normal, but the kidneys contained, at least in young infected animals, less free pantothenate than noninfected ones.

A relatively large amount of information is available concerning vitamin B_{12} relationships. It has been found that patients with heavy hookworm infections, but not those with light ones, had a materially decreased vitamin B_{12} level in their blood serum (Layrisse *et al.*, 1959). Especially well known are the vitamin B_{12} deficiencies induced in humans by *Diphyllobothrium latum;* some of the relevant facts have already been reviewed in Chapter 1. It is sufficient to emphasize here that severe vitamin B_{12} deficiencies are often encountered in carriers of this tapeworm, especially those developing anemia. One expression of such deficiencies is a marked lowering of the vitamin-serum level (Nyberg *et al.*, 1961; Palva, 1962). Another is that the urinary excretion of vitamin B_{12} is significantly decreased in infected patients (Kaipainen and Ohela, 1957; Palva, 1962), while on the contrary the vitamin B_{12} values of the feces are approximately normal (Kaipainen and Tötterman, 1954). It is less well known that other vitamins, besides B_{12}, also show signs of abnormal behavior in *Diphyllobothrium latum* infections. Thus, Markkanen *et al.* (1961) found in tapeworm patients a significant decrease in urinary folic acid excretion, and Markkanen (1962a,b) observed a decrease in the riboflavin, nicotinic acid, and pantothenic acid content of the blood. The last two compounds were found significantly lowered only in patients with anemia, while carriers without overt anemia showed approximately normal values.

The vitamin C content of host tissues is definitely affected in some parasitic diseases. In chickens infected with *Plasmodium gallinaceum* a hypertrophy of the adrenals has been observed (Nadel *et al.,* 1949); this was due to an actual increase in tissue and not only to an increase in tissue fluid. The glands showed a normal percentage of ascorbic acid; the latter's absolute amounts, therefore, were actually increased (Josephson *et al.,* 1949). This seems to be a clear contrast to human and simian malaria where the entire body becomes depleted of ascorbic acid (Gerdjikoff, 1939; Wozonig, 1945; Sorce and Mutolo, 1946; McKee and Geiman, 1946; McKee *et al.,* 1947). Coccidiosis of the chicken also leads to an increase in suprarenal ascorbic acid (Challey, 1960), while in rats infected with *Trypanosoma hippicum* the vitamin C content of the adrenals was found markedly reduced (Nyden, 1948).

Insofar as fat-soluble vitamins are concerned, only a few data on vitamin A have become known. A depletion in the vitamin A storage of the liver was found in chicken infected with *Eimeria tenella* and *Eimeria acervulina* and this depletion could be so pronounced as to lead to ataxia, a common symptom of vitamin A deficiency (Erasmus *et al.,* 1960). Similarly (Pande and Krishnamurty, 1959), the livers of chicken infected with *Ascaridia galli* showed an abnormal low vitamin A content. This seems to be related to the damage sustained by the intestinal epithelium; the lesions being the reason that in infected chicken only a small fraction of the carotene contained in green feed supplements is absorbed and synthesized to vitamin A. However, it may be questioned whether this is the only mechanism operating in chicken. It is at any rate worth emphasizing that the vitamin A content is lowered in chickens which are being immunized by either receiving injections of *Ascaridia galli* extracts or fed minced worms (Leutskaya, 1963).

Nothing is known concerning the question whether parasitism interferes with the storage of vitamin D. It has, however, been found that parasitic infections can modify the response of the host organism to excessive doses of vitamin D. The relevant observations have been summarized in Chapter 1, to which reference is made.

IV. INFLUENCE OF VITAMINS IN THE HOST'S DIET ON PARASITES

A relatively extensive literature exists dealing with effects of vitamin-deficient diets on various parasites. Relevant data concerning parasitic protozoa are presented in Table L. No valid generalizations are possible. Shortage of one and the same vitamin, e.g., pantothenic acid, can be detrimental to the development of one parasite, but beneficial to a second one, and finally it can be without noticeable effect on a third species. Part of the difficulty in analyzing these *in vivo* experiments, or others done

TABLE L

INFLUENCE ON PARASITIC PROTOZOA OF HOST DIET DEFICIENT IN SINGLE VITAMINS[a]

Species	Host	Fat-soluble vitamins	Water – soluble vitamins (B₂ complex)									References
		Axerophthol (A)	Thiamine (B₁)	Riboflavin	Nicotinic acid	Pantothenic acid	Folic acid	p-Aminobenzoic acid	Pyridoxine (B₆)	Ascorbic acid (C)	Biotin (H)	
Flagellates												
Giardia muris	Mouse		−	±		−			±			Scholtens (1962)
Leishmania donovani	Mouse		±	±		+			+			Actor (1960)
Trypanosoma cruzi	Rat		+			+			+			Yaeger and Miller (1960a,b,c,d)
Trypanosoma lewisi	Rat					+					+	Caldwell and Gyorgy (1943, 1947); Becker et al. (1947)
Sporozoa												
Plasmodium berghei	Rat	+										Ramakrishnan (1954); Bouisset and Ruffie (1958a,b)
Plasmodium berghei	Mouse								−			Quevauviller and Louw (1955)
Plasmodium gallinaceum	Chicken		−	−			−	−			−	Brackett et al. (1946); Rama Rao and Sirsi (1956b,c); Taylor (1957)
Plasmodium lophurae	Duck		−	−		±	+				+	Trager (1943); Seeler and Ott (1944, 1945); Seeler et al. (1944); Schinazi et al. (1950)
Plasmodium knowlesi	Monkey									−		Ball et al. (1945)
Toxoplasma gondii	Chicken		±	±		±					±	Kulasiri and Prasad (1961)

[a] KEY: + = deficiency favors parasites; − = deficiency unfavorable to parasites; ± = deficiency without marked effect on parasite.

with supplementation of the host's diet with a given vitamin, rests on the fact that usually several explanations can be advanced to account for the observed effects. Thus, in most instances it is impossible to decide definitely whether a certain response by the parasite is due to a direct or an indirect action of the vitamin tested. A few examples illustrating the point will now be considered briefly.

Becker *et al.* (1947) assume that the higher parasite counts and pro-longed multiplication period of *Trypanosoma lewisi* under the influence of a pantothenate-deficient host diet result from an indirect effect only. They assume the mechanism involved to be related primarily to a de-creased efficiency by the host in producing ablastin, which in these in-fections controls the parasite levels. An increased resistance of rodents to infection with *Trypanosoma equiperdum* is induced by deficiency of the host diet in the vitamin B complex (Reiner and Paton, 1932). On the other hand, *Trypanosoma brucei* infections could be established in pigeons fed a corresponding diet, while specimens on a full diet are normally completely refractive (Sollazzo, 1929).

The complexity of the situation is enhanced when the interaction of several vitamins is considered. Interesting in this connection are observa-tions reported for the rat parasite *Eimeria nieschulzi*. Becker and Dil-worth (1941) found that vitamin B_1 in the host's ration had a slightly depressing action on the development of this parasite, as measured by the production of oocysts. Vitamin B_6, on the contrary, had a stimulating effect, but both vitamins given together had a strong inhibitory effect. This depressing action was also observed when the vitamins were ad-ministered parenterally (Becker, 1941). Pantothenic acid in the diet stimulated the parasites and nullified the growth-inhibiting action of the two combined vitamins (Becker and Smith, 1942; Becker *et al.,* 1943). Riboflavin inhibited the parasites, but nicotinic acid did not seem to affect them (Becker, 1942). Evidently in this case no guess can be hazarded as to whether the vitamins act directly or indirectly on the parasites; analysis will have to wait until the coccidia can be grown *in vitro.*

On the other hand, it is commonly assumed that some vitamins really are required by malarial parasites. It has thus been found (Brackett *et al.,* 1946) that blood-induced infections with *Plasmodium gallinaceum* are suppressed not only in chickens on a pantothenic acid-deficient diet, but also in birds treated with analogs, for example, pantoyltauramido-4-chlorobenzene. The addition of pantothenic acid to the diet completely eliminated the activity of this and similar antagonists. The fact that pantothenate favors malarial parasites *in vitro,* perhaps only indirectly, as a constituent of the host-manufactured CoA, has been mentioned previously. Even if this were the only way in which the compound is used, it still would be justified to consider it a growth requirement of the parasites.

A direct action is also probable in the case of riboflavin; lack of it leads to abnormally low parasitemias with *Plasmodium lophurae* (Seeler and Ott, 1944), while supplementation of the host diet with riboflavin leads to higher parasite counts in the case of *Plasmodium gallinaceum* than those observed in chickens on a normal diet (Rama Rao and Sirsi, 1956b). Supplementation of the diet with high doses of thiamine (Rama Rao and Sirsi, 1956a) lead, in infections with *Plasmodium gallinaceum,* to markedly increased parasitemias and early death of the host. Of interest also are some observations on the effects of diets supplemented with *p*-aminobenzoic acid. Taylor (1957) reported that small quantities of the compound or of parahydroxybenzoic acid added separately to the ration increased the severity of *Plasmodium gallinaceum* infections, and there were indications of potentiation when both substances were given simultaneously. It is curious, however, that high concentrations of *p*-aminobenzoic acid (0.1–0.5%) in the diet did interfere with the parasites' development, the infections being even lower than those observed in chicken on vitamin-deficient diet. Parahydroxybenzoic acid had no comparable suppressive effect. Daily injections of *p*-aminobenzoic acid into old or young rats infected with *Plasmodium berghei* resulted in increased parasitemias, but the treatment was without effect if they were begun after onset of latency (Fabiani *et al.,* 1960). It is impossible to decide at the present state of our knowledge whether these various effects are due to direct or indirect actions, or perhaps a combination of both. A similar uncertainty exists concerning interpretation of the observation of McKee and Geiman (1946) that the parasitemias increase when ascorbic acid is administered to monkeys infected with *Plasmodium knowlesi,* which either spontaneously had an abnormally low ascorbic acid level in their blood plasma or had been made experimentally ascorbic acid-deficient. There are some indications that ascorbic acid increases the susceptibility of *Aedes aegypti* to infection with *Plasmodium gallinaceum,* while on the contrary pantothenate, niacin, thiamine, and biotin increased the resistance of the host to the infection (Terzian *et al.,* 1953).

The field of host/parasite vitamin relationships has been under active investigation insofar as helminths are concerned, especially during the period 1930 to 1940; in later years it has attracted fewer investigators. The effects of vitamin-deficient host diets on *Ascaridia galli* have been studied primarily by Ackert and his co-workers (Ackert, 1931, 1939; Ackert *et al.,* 1927, 1931; Ackert and Nolf, 1931; Ackert and Spindler, 1929). It was found that a lack of either vitamin A or the vitamin B complex favored the worms. More specimens remained in the chicken's intestine and, at least in the case of vitamin A deficiency, the worms grew longer than worms recovered from hosts kept on a normal, full diet. A vitamin D deficiency, on the other hand, did not influence the worms materially. Hansen *et al.* (1954) reported that supplementation of the diet with vitamin B_{12} reduced the numbers of worms, but stimulated the growth of those developing. These authors assume that the restriction in worm numbers was due to a vitamin-induced increase in host resistance and not due to a direct action on the worms. Similarly, Ackert (1939, 1942) was inclined to ascribe the effects observed by his group to changes in the host's resistance. He did point out that not every diet which breaks down the host's resistance is favorable to the parasites. Thus, mainte- nance of chickens by intramuscular injections of vitamin-free nutritive solutions, or only of glucose, led to the recovery of only few and small worms (Ackert and Whitlock, 1935; Ackert *et al.,* 1940). Sadun *et al.* (1949) also assume a lowered resistance to *Ascaridia* in order to explain their observation that the nematodes recovered from birds kept on a diet deficient in folic acid were more numerous and longer than those found in controls. They found that a purified diet containing but minimal amounts of vitamin B_{12} led to a pronounced growth retardation of the worms. Other worms seem to react in a different fashion. According to Maldonado and Asenjo (1953), neither folic acid nor vitamin B_{12} seems to have much influence on *Nippostrongylus muris,* nor does a lack of vitamin A in the diet of mice have any measurable influence on the natural or acquired resistance to *Trichinella spiralis* infections (Larsh and Gilchrist, 1950).

In other cases, however, vitamin deficiencies do lower the resistance of mammals to infection with intestinal nematodes; this is especially true when host animals are fed rations deficient in vitamin A. In some cases it has then been possible to infect normally refractive hosts. e.g., hogs with *Ascaris lumbricoides* of human origin (Hiraishi, 1927), or rats with *Parascaris equorum* (Clapham, 1933). Jones and Nolan (1942), on the other hand, failed to establish *Enterobius vermicularis* in vitamin A- deficient rats. Other workers described a lowered resistance of vitamin A-deficient normal hosts to a variety of intestinal nematodes: *Nippo- strongylus muris* (Spindler, 1933), *Toxocara canis* and *Toxascaris leonina* (Wright, 1935), *Trichinella spiralis* (McCoy, 1934), and *Strongy- loides ratti* (Lawler, 1941). A similar lowering of resistance was found in the case of *Syngamus trachea,* a parasite of the respiratory tract (Clap- ham, 1934a), but not in experiments with *Heterakis gallinae* and *Ascaris lumbricoides* (Clapham, 1933, 1934b). In general, the lowered resistance of the hosts became evident by larger numbers of worms developing and often also by a reduced immunity to superinfection. Rats, for example, are usually quite resistant to superinfection with *Trichinella,* while superinfection succeeded without difficulty in vitamin A-deficient hosts. It is generally assumed that these effects are all due to an interference with the host's protective mechanisms rather than to a stimulatory effect on the parasites. Whether the same explanation holds true for Zaiman's (1940) observation that fewer *Trichinella* larvae develop in the muscles of vitamin E-deficient rats requires further study. Lowered resistance to superinfection due to thiamine or riboflavin deficiency has also been found in the case of *Nippostrongylus muris* (Watt, 1944).

Relatively little work along similar lines has been done with trematodes. Krakower *et al.* (1944) found normal growth of *Schistosoma mansoni* in guinea pigs kept on a vitamin C-deficient diet, but the eggshells produced were abnormal being reduced to granules similar to those occurring in the vitellaria. The same authors (Krakower *et al.,* 1940) had found previously that more schistosomes developed in rats kept on a vitamin A-deficient diet than on a full diet, apparently fewer juveniles being killed in the lungs and the liver in the former instance. DeWitt's (1957) experiments of the influence of a diet deficient in factor 3, vitamin E, and cystine have been mentioned in Chapter 6.

Beaver (1937) reported that *Echinostoma revolutum* either did not develop at all or showed at least greatly retarded development in pigeons kept on a diet that in all likelihood was deficient in vitamins A and D. This result is altogether different from those reviewed above concerning nematodes, but is somewhat similar to observations on cestodes summarized below, apparently indicating that nematodes and flatworms respond in different ways to nutritional deficiencies in the host's diet. Rothschild (1939), however, did obtain full development of *Cryptocotyle lingua* in gulls deprived of vitamins.

The effect of deficient diets on the cestode *Hymenolepis diminuta* have been studied by Hager (1941), Chandler (1943), Addis (1946), and Addis and Chandler (1944, 1946). It was found that essentially deficiencies in vitamins A, D, and E had no effect on the growth of the worms, but that fewer worms became established. Thiamine-deficient diets had no effect. It was shown later, however, by means of radioactive thiamine administered parenterally to the hosts, that *Hymenolepis* can acquire this compound from the body of the host even if the latter is kept on a thiamine-free diet (Chandler *et al.,* 1950). If the complete vitamin B complex, as present in yeast, was withheld from the hosts, the worms remained stunted. This deficiency was not alleviated by the addition of nine water-soluble vitamins to the diet. The deficiency effect was especially noticeable when female, immature, or castrated male rats were used as host animals, but also became apparent in noncastrated male rats when the latter were kept for longer periods on the deficient diet (Beck, 1950).

In certain contrast to the above results are those reported by Larsh (1947), who studied the influence of alcohol in infections with *Hymenolepis nana* var. *fraterna*. He found that considerably more cysticercoids developed in mice regularly receiving alcohol than in nonalcoholic ones. This was due essentially to a reduced food intake of the former group as evidenced by the fact that a nonalcoholic, partially starved group of mice showed about the same degree of infection as the alcoholic group. It was concluded that the reduced resistance to infection was largely due to avitaminosis.

REFERENCES

Ackert, J. E. (1931). *Arch. Zool. Ital.* **16**, 1369–1379.
Ackert, J. E. (1939). *Proc. 7th World's Poultry Congr., Cleveland, Ohio, 1939* pp. 265–267.
Ackert, J. E. (1942). *J. Parasitol.* **28**, 1–24.
Ackert, J. E., and Nolf, L. O. (1931). *Am. J. Hyg.* **13**, 337–344.
Ackert, J. E., and Spindler, L. A. (1929). *Am. J. Hyg.* **9**, 292–307.
Ackert, J. E., and Whitlock, J. H. (1935). *J. Parasitol.* **21**, 428.
Ackert, J. E., Fisher, M. L., and Zimmerman, N. B. (1927). *J. Parasitol.* **13**, 219–220.
Ackert, J. E., McIlvaine, M. F., and Crawford, N. Z. (1931). *Am. J. Hyg.* **13**, 320–336.
Ackert, J. E., Whitlock, J. H., and Freeman, E. A. (1940). *J. Parasitol.* **26**, 17–32.
Actor, P. (1960). *Exptl. Parasitol.* **10**, 1–20.
Addis, C. J. (1946). *J. Parasitol.* **32**, 574–580.
Addis, C. J., and Chandler, A. C. (1944). *J. Parasitol.* **30**, 229–236.
Addis, C. J., and Chandler, A. C. (1946). *J. Parasitol.* **32**, 581–584.
Baernstein, H. D., Rees, C. W., and Bartgis, I. L. (1957). *J. Parasitol.* **43**, 143–152.
Ball, E. G., Anfinsen, C. B., Geiman, Q. M., McKee, R. W., and Ormsbee, R. A. (1945). *Science* **101**, 542–544.
Ball, G. H. (1964). *J. Parasitol.* **50**, 3–10.
Ball, G. H., and Chao, J. (1957). *J. Parasitol.* **43**, 409–412.
Beaver, P. C. (1937). *Univ. Illinois Bull.* **74**, 1–96.
Beck, J. W. (1950). Dissertation, Rice Institute, Houston, Texas [not seen, quoted in Chandler, A. C., Read, C. P., and Nicholas, H. O. (1950)].
Becker, E. R. (1941). *Proc. Soc. Exptl. Biol. Med.* **46**, 494–495.
Becker, E. R. (1942). *Proc. Iowa Acad. Sci.* **49**, 503–506.
Becker, E. R., and Dilworth, R. I. (1941). *J. Infect. Diseases* **68**, 285–290.
Becker, E. R., and Smith, L. (1942). *Iowa State Coll. J. Sci.* **16**, 443–449.
Becker, E. R., Manresa, M., and Smith, L. (1943). *Iowa State Coll. J. Sci.* **17**, 257–262.
Becker, E. R., Taylor, D. J., and Fuhrmeister, C. (1947). *Iowa State Coll. J. Sci.* **21**, 237–243.
Berntzen, A. K. (1962). *J. Parasitol.* **48**, 785–797.

Boné, G. J., and Parent, G. (1963). *J. Gen. Microbiol.* **31,** 261–266.
Bouisset, L., and Ruffie, J. (1958a). *Ann. Parasitol Humaine Comp.* **33,** 209–217.
Bouisset, L., and Ruffié, J. (1958b). *Compt. Rend. Soc. Biol.* **152,** 168–171.
Brackett, S., Waletzky, E., and Baker, M. (1946). *J. Parasitol.* **32,** 453–462.
Broquist, H. P., and Albrecht, A. M. (1955). *Proc. Soc. Exptl. Biol. Med.* **89,** 178–180.
Cailleau, R. (1938). *Compt. Rend. Soc. Biol.* **127,** 861–863.
Cailleau, R. (1939a). *Compt. Rend. Soc. Biol.* **130,** 319–320.
Cailleau, R. (1939b). *Compt. Rend. Soc. Biol.* **130,** 1089–1090.
Cailleau, R. (1939c). *Compt. Rend. Soc. Biol.* **131,** 964–966.
Cailleau, R. (1940). *Compt. Rend. Soc. Biol.* **134,** 32–34.
Caldwell, F. E., and György, P. (1943). *Proc. Soc. Exptl. Biol. Med.* **53,** 116–119.
Caldwell, F. E., and György, P. (1947). *J. Infect. Diseases* **81,** 197–208.
Challey, J. R. (1960). *J. Parasitol.* **46,** 727–731.
Chance, M. R. A., and Dirnhuber, P. (1949). *Parasitology* **39,** 300–301.
Chandler, A. C. (1943). *Am. J. Hyg.* **37,** 121–130.
Chandler, A. C., Read, C. P., and Nicholas, H. O. (1950). *J. Parasitol.* **36,** 523–535.
Citri, N. (1954). Thesis, Hebrew University, Jerusalem.
Clapham, P. A. (1933). *J. Helminthol.* **11,** 9–24.
Clapham, P. A. (1934a). *Proc. Roy. Soc.* **B115,** 18–29.
Clapham, P. A. (1934b). *J. Helminthol.* **12,** 165–176.
Coleman, R. M. (1953). *Proc. Indiana Acad. Sci.* **62,** 321–322.
Coleman, R. M., and Mizelle, J. D. (1956). *Trans. Am. Microscop. Soc.* **75,** 483–491.
Cowperthwaite, J., Weber, M. M., Packer, L., and Hutner, S. H. (1953). *Ann. N.Y. Acad. Sci.* **56,** 972–981.
D'Agostino Barbaro, A. (1953). *Riv. Biol. (Perugia)* **45,** 73–91.
Dewey, V. C., Kidder, G. W., and Butler, F. P. (1959). *Biochem. Biophys. Res. Commun.* **1,** 25–28.
DeWitt, W. B. (1950). *J. Parasitol.* **43,** 119–128.
Diamond, L. S. (1960). *J. Parasitol.* **46,** 484.
Diamond, L. S. (1961). *Science* **134,** 336–337.
Douvres, F. W. (1962). *J. Parasitol.* **48,** 314–320.
Eagle, H. (1955). *Science* **122,** 501–504.
Erasmus, J., Scott, M. L., and Levine, P. P. (1960). *Poultry Sci.* **39,** 565–572.
Fabiani, G., Orfila, J., and Bonhoure, G. (1960). *Compt. Rend. Soc. Biol.* **154,** 1441–1442.
Gerdjikoff, I. (1939). *Klin. Wochschr.* **18,** 1214–1217.
Giroud, A., and Rakoto-Ratsimamanga (1936). *Bull Soc. Chim. Biol.* **18,** 375–383.
Guthrie, R. (1946). Thesis, University of Minnesota.
Guttman, H. N. (1963). *Exptl. Parasitol.* **14,** 129–142.
Hager, A. (1941). *Iowa State Coll. J. Sci.* **15,** 127–153.
Hansen, M. F., Petri, L. H., and Ackert, J. E. (1954). *Exptl. Parasitol.* **3,** 122–127.
Hill, G. R., and Smyth, J. D. (1944). *Nature* **153,** 21.
Hiraishi, T. (1927). *Japan. Med. World* **7,** 80.
House, H. L. (1954). *Can. J. Zool.* **32,** 342–350.
Jackson, G. J. (1962). *Trans. N.Y. Acad. Sci.* [2] **24,** 954–965.
Jackson, G. J., and Stoll, N. R. (1964). *Am. J. Trop. Med. Hyg.* **13,** 520–524.
Jones, M. F., and Nolan, M. O. (1942). *Proc. Helminthol. Soc. Wash., D.C.* **9,** 63–65.
Josephson, E. S. Taylor, D. J., Greenberg, J., and Nadel, E. M. (1949). *J. Natl. Malaria Soc.* **8,** 132–136.
Kaipainen, W. J., and Ohela, K. (1957). *Ann. Med. Internae Fenniae* **46,** 49–52.
Kaipainen, W. J., and Tötterman, G. (1954). *Scand. J. Clin. Lab. Invest.* **6,** 33–35.

Kaipainen, W. J., and Wallén, S. (1954). *Scand. J. Clin. Lab. Invest.* **6**, 88–90.

Krakower, C. A., Hoffman, W. A., and Axtmayer, J. H. (1940). *Puerto Rico J. Public Health Trop. Med.* **16**, 269–391.

Krakower, C. A., Hoffman, W. A., and Axtmayer, J. H. (1944). *J. Infect. Diseases* **74**, 178–183.

Kulasiri, C., and Prasad, H. (1961). *Parasitology* **51**, 265–267.

Larsh, J. E. (1947). *J. Parasitol.* **33**, 339–344.

Larsh, J. E., and Gilchrist, H. B. (1950). *J. Elisha Mitchell Sci. Soc.* **66**, 76–83.

Latif, N., and El Kordy, M. I. (1946). *J. Roy. Egypt Med. Assoc.* **29**, 71–75.

Lawler, H. J. (1941). *Am. J. Hyg.* **34**, Sect. D, 65–72.

Layrisse, M., Blumenfeld, N., Dugarte, I., and Roche, M. (1959). *Blood* **14**, 1269–1279.

Leland, S. E. (1963). *J. Parasitol.* **49**, 600–611.

Leutskaya, Z. K. (1963). *Dokl. Akad. Nauk SSSR* **153**, 243–245.

Lwoff, M. (1933). *Ann. Inst. Pasteur* **51**, 55–116.

Lwoff, M. (1938). *Compt. Rend.* **206**, 540–542.

Lwoff, M. (1939). *Compt. Rend. Soc. Biol.* **130**. 406–408.

Lwoff, M. (1940). "Recherches sur le pouvoir de synthèse des flagellés trypanosomides," Monogr. Inst. Pasteur. Masson, Paris.

McCoy, O. R. (1934). *Am. J. Hyg.* **20**, 169–180.

McKee, R. W., and Geiman, Q. M. (1946). *Proc. Soc. Exptl. Biol. Med.* **63**, 313–315.

McKee, R. W., Cobbey, T. S., and Geiman, Q. M. (1947). *Federation Proc.* **6**, 276.

McQuilkin, W. T., Evans, V. J., and Earle, W. R. (1957). *J. Natl. Cancer Inst.* **19**, 885–907.

Maldonado, J. F., and Asenjo, C. F. (1953). *Exptl. Parasitol.* **4**, 374–379.

Manusardi, L. (1931). *Boll. Zool. Agrar. Bachicolt. Univ. Studi Milano* **4**, 140–148.

Markkanen, T. (1962a). *Acta Med. Scand.* **171**, 195–199.

Markkanen, T. (1962b). *Ann. Med. Internae Fenniae* **51**, 119–123.

Markkanen, T., Brummer, P., and Savola, P. (1961). *Acta Med. Scand.* **170**, 361–363.

Morgan, J. F., Morton, H. J., and Parker, R. C. (1950). *Proc. Soc. Exptl. Biol. Med.* **73**, 1–8.

Mueller, J. F. (1959). *J. Parasitol.* **45**, 561–573.

Nadel, E. M., Taylor, D. J., Greenberg, J., and Josephson, E. S. (1949). *J. Natl. Malaria Soc.* **8**, 70–79.

Nathan, H. A., and Cowperthwaite, J. (1955). *J. Protozool.* **2**, 37–42.

Nathan, H. A., and Funk, H. B. (1959). *Am. J. Clin. Nutr.* **7**, 375–384.

Nathan, H. A., Hutner, S. H., and Levin, H. L. (1956). *Nature* **178**, 741–742.

Nathan, H. A., Baker, H., and Frank, O. (1960). *Nature* **188**, 35–37.

Newton, B. A. (1956). *Nature* **177**, 279–280.

Nyberg, W., and Gräsbeck, R. (1957). *Scand. J. Clin. Lab. Invest.* **9**, 383–387.

Nyberg, W., Gräsbeck, R., Saarni, M., and Bonsdorff, B. von (1961). *Am. J. Clin. Nutr.* **9**, 606–612.

Nyden, S. J. (1948). *Proc. Soc. Exptl. Biol. Med.* **69**, 206–210.

Palva, I. (1962). Dissertation, University of Helsinki.

Pande, P. G., and Krishnamurty, D. (1959). *Poultry Sci.* **38**, 15–25.

Pantelouris, E. M., and Hale, P. A. (1962). *Research Vet. Sci.* **3**, 300–303.

Patterson, E. L., Broquist, H. P., Albrecht, A. M., Saltza, M. H. von, and Stokstad, E. L. R. (1955). *J. Am. Chem. Soc.* **77**, 3167–3168.

Quevauviller, M. A., and Louw, J. W. (1955). *Ann. Pharm. Franc.* **13**, 20–35.

Ramakrishnan, S. P. (1954). *Indian J. Malariol.* **8**, 107–113.

Rama Rao, R., and Sirsi, M. (1956a). *J. Indian Inst. Sci.* **38**, 108–114.

Rama Rao, R., and Sirsi, M. (1956b). *J. Indian Inst. Sci.* **38**, 186–189.

Rama Rao, R., and Sirsi, M. (1956c). *J. Indian Inst. Sci.* **38**, 224–227.

Read, C. P., and Simmons, J. E. (1963). *Physiol. Rev.* **43**, 263–305.

Rees, C. W., Bozicevich, J., Reardon, L. V., and Daft, F. S. (1944). *Am. J. Trop. Med.* **24**, 189–193.

Reiner, L., and Paton, J. B. (1932). *Proc. Soc. Exptl. Biol. Med.* **30**, 345–348.

Rieck, G. W. (1956). *Proc. 3rd Intern. Congr. Animal Prod., Cambridge, Engl., 1956* Sect. II, pp. 32–34. London.

Rogers, W. P. (1945). *Parasitology* **36**, 211–218.

Roskin, G., and Nastiukova, O. (1941). *Compt. Rend. Acad. Sci. URSS* **33**, 8 [not seen, quoted in Lwoff, M. (1951)]. *In:* Biochemistry and Physiology of Protozoa (A. Lwoff, ed.) Vol. 1, pp. 129–176. Academic Press, New York.

Rothschild, M. (1939). *Novitates Zool.* **41**, 178–180.

Sadun, E. H., Totter, J. R., and Keith, C. K. (1949). *J. Parasitol.* **35**, Suppl., 13–14.

Seaman, G. R., and Sanders, F. (1957). *Science* **125**, 398–399.

Schinazi, L. A., Drell, W., Ball, G. H., and Dunn, M. S. (1950). *Proc. Soc. Exptl. Biol. Med.* **75**, 229–234.

Scholtens, R. G. (1962). *Am. J. Vet. Res.* **23**, 1084–1088.

Seeler, A. O., and Ott, W. H. (1944). *J. Infect. Diseases* **75**, 175–178.

Seeler, A. O., and Ott, W. H. (1945). *J. Infect. Diseases* **77**, 82–84.

Seeler, A. O., Ott, W. H., and Gundel, M. E. (1944). *Proc. Soc. Exptl. Biol. Med.* **55**, 107–109.

Senft, A. W., and Senft, D. G. (1962). *J. Parasitol.* **48**, 551–554.

Singer, I. (1959). *Proc. 6th Intern. Congr. Trop. Med. Malaria 1958* Vol. **3**, pp. 67–70. Casa Portuguesa, Porto.

Singer, I. (1961). *Exptl. Parasitol.* **11**, 391–401.

Singer, I., and Trager, W. (1956). *Proc. Soc. Exptl. Biol. Med.* **91**, 315–318.

Smyth, J. D., Bingley, W. J., and Hill, G. R. (1945). *J. Exptl. Biol.* **21**, 13–16.

Sollazzo, G. (1929). *Z. Immunitaetsforsch.* **60**, 239–246.

Sorce, S., and Mutolo, V. (1946). *Boll. Soc. Ital. Biol. Sper.* **22**, 399–400.

Spindler, L. A. (1933). *J. Parasitol.* **20**, 72.

Stephenson, W. (1947). *Parasitology* **38**, 140–144.

Stoll, N. R. (1957). *Science* **126**, 1236.

Taylor, A. E. R. (1957). *Trans. Roy. Soc. Trop. Med. Hyg.* **51**, 241–247.

Taylor, A. E. R. (1960). *Exptl. Parasitol.* **9**, 113–120.

Taylor, A. E. R. (1963). *Exptl. Parasitol.* **14**, 304–310.

Terzian, A., Stahler, N., and Miller, H. (1953). *J. Immunol.* **70**, 115–123.

Trager, W. (1941). *J. Exptl. Med.* **74**, 441–461.

Trager, W. (1943). *J. Exptl. Med.* **77**, 411–420.

Trager, W. (1947). *J. Parasitol.* **33**, 345–350

Trager, W. (1954). *J. Protozool.* **1**, 231–237.

Trager, W. (1955). *In* "Some Physiological Aspects and Consequences of Parasitism." (W. H. Cole, ed.), pp. 3–14. Rutgers Univ. Press, New Brunswick, New Jersey.

Trager, W. (1957a). *J. Protozool.* **4**, 269–276.

Trager, W. (1957b). *Acta Tropica* **14**, 289–301.

Vakirtzi-Lemonias, C., Kidder, G. W., and Dewey, V. C. (1963). *Comp. Biochem. Physiol.* **8**, 331–334.

Watt, J. Y. C. (1944). *Am. J. Hyg.* **39**, 145–151.

Weinstein, P. P. (1961). *Acta Cient. Venezolana* **12**, 115–119.

Weinstein, P. P., and Jones, M. F. (1956). *J. Parasitol.* **42**, 215–236.

Weinstein, P. P., and Jones, M. F. (1959). *Ann. N.Y. Acad. Sci.* **77**, 137–162.
Williams, M. O., Hopkins, C. A., and Wyllie, M. R. (1961). *Exptl. Parasitol.* **11**, 121–127.
Wozonig, H. (1945). *Z. Immunitaetsforsch.* **105**, 411–416.
Wright, W. H. (1935). *J. Parasitol.* **21**, 433.
Yaeger, R. G., and Miller, O. N. (1960a). *Exptl. Parasitol.* **9**, 215–222.
Yaeger, R. G., and Miller, O. N. (1960b). *Exptl. Parasitol.* **10**, 227–231.
Yaeger, R. G., and Miller, O. N. (1960c). *Exptl. Parasitol.* **10**, 232–237.
Yaeger, R. G., and Miller, O. N. (1960d). *Exptl. Parasitol.* **10**, 238–244.
Zaiman, H. (1940). *J. Parasitol.* **26**, Suppl., 44.

Chapter 9

RESPIRATION

I. INTRODUCTORY REMARKS

An obvious intimate connection exists between the utilization of various substrates and the gaseous exchanges of an organism. It is therefore impossible to completely separate a discussion of biochemical sequences from that of gaseous exchanges. In this presentation, for instance, the production of CO_2 from various organic substrates or from inorganic sources, the elaboration of gases other than CO_2, the electron transport mechanisms, and the influence of inorganic ions on respiratory rates have been covered in preceding chapters. The present discussion therefore will be limited to some biological oxygen relationships and such factors influencing respiration that have not been mentioned before.

II. *IN VIVO* AND *IN VITRO* OXYGEN RELATIONSHIPS

The question of whether parasites, especially intestinal ones, lead in nature a predominantly aerobic or anaerobic life has frequently been discussed. Before it can be taken up, the oxygen tension in the surroundings of parasites, their reactions to lack of oxygen, and the factors determining their respiratory rates must be considered. Parasitic habitats can be divided roughly into environments offering no or at least only very little molecular oxygen, habitats in which a more or less plentiful supply of this gas is available, and finally one habitat in which excessively high oxygen tensions are encountered, the swim bladder of some fishes. The composition of gases secreted into the latter varies considerably from species to species but can reach the exceedingly high value of approximately 98% (Scholander and van Dam, 1953). Swim bladder parasites are protozoa, e.g., *Gaussia gadi,* or helminths, e.g., *Cystidicola.* It is, however, not known whether the swim bladders of fishes harboring these parasites belong to the group with high oxygen content.

333

Most tissue parasites undoubtedly live in environments with moderate to high oxygen tension. Worms, for instance, which inhabit the lungs of vertebrates, especially the bronchi, will have access to oxygen at almost the same pressure as free-living animals. Another habitat rich in oxygen is blood, especially the arterial blood, but even in venous blood oxygen tensions varying between about 40 and 70 mm Hg are found. Occasionally lower tensions do occur; thus, the values reported for the venous blood of fish hearts varies between only 2 and 14 mm Hg (Root, 1931; Dill *et al.*, 1932). Moderate tensions are found in such parasitic habitats as the abdominal or pleural cavities, or the urinary bladder; some data concerning these and other habitats have been tabulated by von Brand (1952). Some newer figures will be found in the papers by Davies and Bronk (1957) and Montgomery (1957). Actually there is relatively little merit in quoting many definite figures concerning oxygen tension in various parasitic habitats, since many factors have a bearing on this point and may modify it. As von Brand (1960b) has pointed out, the following ones (among, undoubtedly, others) are of importance: the size of the host, the method of oxygen supply to an organ (primarily diffusion, circulatory, or tracheal system), the state of activity (for instance, the contrast between an insect flight muscle in flight and in rest), or the temperature (which is of greater importance in the case of cold-blooded than warm-blooded hosts). Furthermore, the mere presence of parasites may materially influence the local oxygen tension, since it has been established (Campbell, 1931) that inflammatory processes lower the oxygen tension.

Parasites living in plant tissues, perhaps more so than their counterparts living in animals, regularly seem to have access to greater or smaller amounts of oxygen and it is questionable whether any plant parasites find themselves exposed to severe oxygen lack. Even in the gases of roots of plants such as mangroves, which are embedded in almost completely anaerobic soil material, relatively high percentages of oxygen are found, usually between 10 and 18%, rarely less, according to Scholander *et al.* (1955).

The bile ducts (e.g., von Brand and Weise, 1932) or the intestines of larger vertebrates (e.g., Chaigneau and Charlet-Lery, 1957) are poor in oxygen or sometimes even completely oxygen-free. But again no generalizations should be made. For instance, it is generally conceded that intestinal fermentation gases are either oxygen-free or contain but very little of that gas. On the other hand, if the oxygen tension of the intestine is measured very close to the mucosa (e.g., Rogers, 1949a) by means of microelectrodes, moderate, but biologically significant, tensions are encountered. It is evident then that an organism like *Giardia,* which fixes itself to the mucosa and is very small, will have entirely different oxygen relationships than a large roundworm like *Ascaris,* which lives within the intestinal lumen. There is no question but that the rich vascularization of the intestinal wall leads to a diffusion of oxygen toward the lumen (McIver *et al.,* 1926). However, the bacterial flora of the intestine will rapidly use up this gas, and a steep oxygen gradient will be established toward the borders of the essentially anaerobic intestinal lumen.

Conditions seem to be more variable in the intestine of invertebrates. Admittedly little definite data are available, but the biological evidence is convincing. It is thus probable that largely aerobic conditions prevail in the intestine of sandflies or tsetse flies, as can be inferred from the fact that the developmental stages of leishmanias or trypanosomes living in this habitat are definitely aerobic organisms when taken into culture. Conditions in the termite intestine, on the other hand, are probably fairly strictly anaerobic, since the termite fauna is quite sensitive to oxygen. Cleveland (1925) has demonstrated conclusively that termites can be defaunated by oxygenation. The most definite information, however, is available for the intestine of *Cryptocercus,* which harbors a fauna closely related to that found in termites. Ritter (1961), by a polarographic method sensitive to about 10^{-6} M oxygen, could not detect any in the insect's hind-gut. It is interesting that he identified reduced glutathione within the intestine and found that this compound, which apparently is decisive in controlling the level of anaerobiosis in this case, was not roach-derived, but stemmed from the parasitic protozoa, intestinal bacterial associates, or both.

Most parasites can tolerate lack of oxygen for shorter or longer periods, but their sensitivity to oxygen poisoning, or their requirements of oxygen for prolonged survival vary considerably from species to species. The older literature has been reviewed in detail by von Brand (1946, 1952); for the present discussion only some examples, derived where possible from the newer literature, will be given.

Two groups of protozoa exist which justifiably can be termed obligate anaerobes in the sense that they are readily killed by oxygen even at low tensions and that they can carry out all life processes in the absence of molecular oxygen. These are the rumen ciliates (Hungate, 1942, 1955; Sugden and Oxford, 1952; Sugden, 1953; Heald and Oxford, 1953) and the termite flagellates (Trager, 1934; Hungate, 1939). Other protozoa are less sensitive to oxygen damage, but still either can be cultivated for indefinite periods under anaerobic conditions, or—this applies actually to most experimental designs used—under conditions of near-anaerobiosis. Mention can be made here of *Entamoeba* spp.; their independence from molecular oxygen has been known since Dobell and Laidlaw's (1926) classical study and has been confirmed by many subsequent workers, recently even for axenic culture conditions (Jackson and Stoll, 1964). Similarly, although able to consume oxygen, *Trichomonas* spp. thrive better in culture under anaerobic than under aerobic conditions, and this seems even to be true for the mouth-inhabiting *Trichomonas buccalis* (Hinshaw, 1927; for other species see Cleveland, 1928a,b; Witte, 1933; Asami *et al.,* 1955; Ivey, 1961; Cavier *et al.,* 1964). Trypanosomids are more exacting in their oxygen requirements; although able to withstand lack of oxygen quite well, most investigators state that anaerobiosis prevents multiplication of the culture stages (e.g., Soule, 1925; Adler and Theodor, 1931; Ray, 1932). However, Senekjie (1941) and Weinman (1953) reported successful anaerobic cultures of *Leishmania* and *Trypanosoma,* respectively. In evaluating this question consideration should be given to the difficulties of establishing strictly anaerobic conditions in media containing hemoglobin.

Some data are also available for sporozoa. Anfinsen *et al.* (1946) found 95% oxygen unsuitable for the cultivation of *Plasmodium knowlesi;* it grew equally well in the presence of 20 and 0.37% oxygen. This species and *Plasmodium lophurae* (Trager, 1950, 1957) are best cultivated under an atmosphere of 95% air + 5% CO_2. This same mixture proved best for most mosquito stages of *Plasmodium relictum,* only older oocysts and sporozoites doing better in an atmosphere of air alone (Ball and Chao, 1961; Ball, 1964). The oocysts of coccidia, though quite resistant to lack of oxygen, require oxygen for maturation, as known since Balbiani's (1884) study, but the formation of micro- and macrogametes of *Haemoproteus columbae* does not (Marchoux and Chorine, 1932).

The parasitic worms studied so far can all be classified as facultative aerobes, most of them showing a marked tolerance to lack of oxygen, but all being able to consume oxygen if available. However, paralleling the findings discussed above for protozoa, the details of the oxygen relationships vary from species to species. In contrast to protozoa, few data on helminths are available as yet which are derived from true *in vitro* cultivation studies. Such studies have shown that the intestinal stages of tapeworms are apparently fairly strictly anaerobic. Berntzen and Mueller (1964) found optimal development in cultures of *Spirometra mansonoides* when the gas phase consisted of 90% N_2 + 10% CO_2. Oxygen concentrations of 5 to 10%, while allowing survival, prevented differentiation. *Hymenolepis nana* (Berntzen, 1962) seems to respond in essentially similar ways, best results being reported from cultures gassed with 95% N_2 + 5% CO_2. The presence of carbon dioxide seems to be essential; under an atmosphere of 100% N_2 the worms survived poorly. Oxygen at atmospheric or higher pressure did not allow survival beyond 48 hours. On the other hand, larval cestodes seem not to be as exacting. Taylor

(1963) found media equilibrated with atmospheric air optimal for larval *Taenia crassiceps;* it may be significant in this connection that Farhan *et al.* (1959) found appreciable amounts of oxygen in the fluid of *Echinococcus* cysts.

Clearly aerobic are the larval stages of many parasitic nematodes. They are customarily cultivated under an atmosphere of air or air containing carbon dioxide (e.g., Weinstein and Jones, 1956; Sawyer and Weinstein, 1963; Leland, 1963). Nevertheless, nematode larvae and adult nematodes alike can withstand anaerobic periods of varying duration, as can every parasitic worm studied in this respect. Some representative data are summarized in Table LI. These data, in contrast to those reviewed above, are not derived from culture experiments in the narrow sense of the word, but have been found in experiments dealing with survival in more or less unphysiological media. It can be expected that increasing experience with true cultivation will in the not too distant future make these data obsolete. In order to avoid, as far as possible, false conclusions only such data have been included in Table LI which, for a given species, have been reported by one author in respect to both aerobic and anaerobic survival, since a comparison of aerobic and anaerobic life spans in unphysiological media of different compositions may be misleading. A survey of Table LI shows that trematodes and nematodes are sometimes very resistant to lack of oxygen, but no clear connection with the oxygen supply of the physiological environment exists. The free-living hookworm larvae, for instance, tolerate anoxic conditions rather well, while the small nematodes of the intestine succumb rapidly. Hobson (1948) has pointed out justifiably that all data on aerobic survival are derived from experiments carried out at the oxygen tension of atmospheric air, while unquestionably the endoparasitic forms usually encounter much lower tensions in nature. It is interesting to note in this connection that the first parasitic ecdysis of *Haemonchus contortus* proceeds best in cultures with a limited supply of oxygen (Stoll, 1940) and that cercariae of *Schistosoma mansoni* emerge in normal numbers from *Australorbis glabratus* at O_2 concentrations as low as 5%. However their number is considerably reduced when the atmosphere contains only 0.7% oxygen and even more so under complete anaerobiosis (Olivier *et al.,* 1953).

The eggs of many helminths are quite resistant to lack of oxygen. This is not only of theoretical but also of practical interest since many forms can survive the anaerobic digestion practiced in many sewage disposal installations. The eggs of most helminths require oxygen, however, for full development, or for hatching if eggs with developed juvenile stages are shed. For details on the limits of anoxic periods tolerated by the eggs of nematodes, cestodes, and trematodes, which frequently are many

TABLE LI

COMPARISON OF AEROBIC AND ANAEROBIC SURVIVAL OF SOME HELMINTHS[a]

Species	Medium	Temp. (°C)	Survival time (days) Anaerobic	Survival time (days) Aerobic	References
Trematodes					
Cryptocotyle lingua, metacercariae	Modified Ringer's + glucose	Room temp.	> 4	12	Stunkard (1930)
Fasciola hepatica	Tyrode's	37	20	13	Rohrbacher (1957)
Fasciola hepatica	Tyrode's + liver extract	37	20	17	Rohrbacher (1957)
Opisthorchis felineus	Ringer's	37	18	18	Erhardt (1939)
Schistosoma mansoni	Serum ultrafiltrate	37	5	12	Ross and Bueding (1950)
Cestodes					
Bothriocephalus bipunctatus	NaCl, 1%	Room temp.	< 1	Several	Harmisch (1937)
Nematodes					
Ascaris lumbricoides	NaCl, 1%	37	9	6	Weinland (1901)
"*Ascaris mystax*"	NaCl, 1% + Na₂CO₃, 0.1%	38	6	15	Bunge (1883)
Cooperia curticei	Ringer's	37	< 1	4–12	Davey (1938)
Cooperia oncophora	Ringer's	37	< 2	4–12	Davey (1938)
Eustrongylides ignotus, larvae	NaCl, 1%	37	3	19	von Brand (1938a)
Eustrongylides ignotus, larvae	NaCl, 0.85%	20	21	Several months	von Brand and Simpson (1945)
Litomosoides carinii	Ox serum	37	< 1	7	Ross and Bueding (1950)
Nematodirus filicollis	Ringer's	37	< 2	4–12	Davey (1938)
Trichostrongylus colubriformis	Ringer's	37	< 1	4–12	Davey (1938)
Trichostrongylus vitrinus	Ringer's	37	< 1	4–12	Davey (1938)

[a] Further data on anaerobic survival of additional species in Bunge (1889); von Brand (1933); Boycott (1904); McCoy (1930); Stannard et al. (1938); Stephenson (1947); Weinland and von Brand (1926); Hunter and Vernberg (1955b). For data on plant parasitic nematodes see Van Gundy et al. (1962).

weeks, the following papers should be consulted: Bataillon (1910); Looss (1911); Fauré-Fremiet (1913); Zawadowsky (1916); Zawadowsky and Orlow (1927); Zviaginzev (1934); Dinnik and Dinnik (1937); Lucker (1935); Cram (1943); Cram and Hicks (1944); Shorb (1944); Jones *et al.* (1947); Newton *et al.* (1949); Ohtsu (1959); Reyes *et al.* (1963). In accordance with the wide spectrum of physiological oxygen relationships of various helminth species, variations in hatching requirements occur. It has, for example, been shown recently (Rogers, 1960) that eggs of *Ascaris lumbricoides, Ascaridia galli,* and *Toxocara mystax* can hatch under essentially anaerobic conditions.

Insofar as the development of eggs is concerned, it has been found that the egg of *Parascaris* ceases developing under anaerobic conditions after fertilization or, possibly, the first cleavage stages (Fauré-Fremiet, 1913; Szwejkowska, 1929; Dyrdowska, 1931), the egg of *Oxyuris equi* after reaching the gastrula stage (Schalimov, 1931), and the egg of *Enterobius vermicularis* only after attaining the tadpole stage (Zawadowsky and Schalimov, 1929; Wendt, 1936). The minimal oxygen tension required to ensure full development also varies in different species. In hookworm larvae it lies around 10 mm Hg (McCoy, 1930), while in *Ascaris* development is retarded about 50% at 30 mm Hg (Brown, 1928). The eggs of *Parascaris* do not show any sign of development at 5 mm, they develop only slowly between 10 and 80 mm, and only at oxygen tensions above 80 mm Hg is normal development possible (Kosmin, 1928). Such observations are of obvious importance in exploring the possibility of autoinvasion in helminthic diseases. Nishigori (1928) claimed to have demonstrated the anaerobic transformation of the rhabditiform larvae of *Strongyloides* into filariform larvae, but his findings were not confirmed by Lee (1930). Autoinvasion is certainly possible in this species and it must be assumed that full development can take place at quite low oxygen tensions. Suggestive in this connection is the observation of Rogers (1960) that infective larvae of *Haemonchus contortus* and *Trichostrongylus axei* exsheath readily under an atmosphere of 95% N_2 + 5% CO_2, especially when the medium contains a reducing agent such as dithionite or cysteine. Curious also is the observation of Friedl (1961) that eggs of *Fascioloides magna,* embryonated under clearly aerobic conditions, can be induced to hatch in great quantities if the air is replaced by water-pumped nitrogen.

The preceding survey has shown that relatively numerous data are available concerning the reactions of protozoa and helminths to lack of oxygen; in contrast very little information has come to light in this respect concerning parasitic arthropods. Only the larvae of *Gastrophilus* and *Cordylobia* have been studied to some extent. Both can be classified with justification among the facultative anaerobes. There is unanimity of opinion that *Gastrophilus* larvae can endure anaerobiosis for periods of several days to several weeks (von Kemnitz, 1916; Dinulescu, 1932; Blanchard and Dinulescu, 1932) and it has been reported that the third instar larva of *Cordylobia* withstands lack of oxygen for 27 hours, remaining motile for the first 22 hours (Blacklock *et al.,* 1930).

III. FACTORS INFLUENCING THE AEROBIC GASEOUS EXCHANGES

All parasites studied so far under aerobic conditions consume oxygen and produce carbon dioxide regardless of whether they lead *in vivo* a predominantly aerobic or anaerobic life. Originally (Weinland, 1901) it had been assumed that intestinal worms like *Ascaris* were not capable of consuming oxygen and the possibility of aerobic processes was conceded for eggs only. As Wright (1950) pointed out, Weinland's authority was so great as to have his views accepted for the next 30 years. It was then shown independently by Daniel (1931), Alt and Tischer (1931), and Adam (1932) that intestinal protozoa and helminths actually did consume oxygen and it became immediately clear that all the tissues of *Ascaris* and not only the eggs had this faculty (Adam, 1932; Harnisch 1935a; Krueger, 1936). Insofar as parasites living in clearly aerobic habitats are concerned, their capability of consuming oxygen had never been doubted. The first qualitative proof was the observation by Nauss and Yorke (1911) that blood containing trypanosomes rapidly assumed a dark color.

In the last 30 years many observations on respiratory rates of parasitic species have been published, making it impracticable to tabulate all. Representative newer data are shown in Tables LII and LIII for parasitic protozoa and helminths. In contrast very few data on parasitic arthropods are available. Some relevant figures have been published for *Gastrophilus* larvae by L. Levenbook (unpublished experiments quoted in Laser and Rothschild, 1949) and Lai (1956) and for the endoparasitic copepod *Mytilicola intestinalis* by Krishnaswami (1960). A survey of the data shown in Tables LII and LIII shows that considerable variations in respiratory rates occur between various species; some of the factors possibly responsible for them will be discussed below. The tables also show the variability of the respiratory quotients. This is due to the interplay of aerobic and anaerobic processes so characteristic for parasites. It is obvious that contrary to many free-living organisms, the RQ of parasites is no indication of the substances being metabolized. It is true that a comparative study in sugar-containing and sugar-free media has shown in some cases a definitely higher RQ in the former (e.g., *Litomosoides carinii* with values of 0.94 and 0.44, respectively, according to Bueding, 1949a). But even in such cases it would be unjustified to try to calculate the percentage participation of carbohydrates in the over-all metabolism.

One factor of some importance in determining the respiratory intensity of an organism is its age. It has been observed repeatedly that culture forms of parasitic protozoa show a declining rate of oxygen consumption with increasing age of the cultures. This has been shown for *Trichomonas foetus* (Riedmuller, 1936), *Trichomonas vaginalis* (Tsukahara, 1961), *Leishmania donovani* (Fulton and Joyner, 1949; Chatterjee and Ghosh, 1959), and *Trypanosoma cruzi* (von Brand *et al.,* 1946). On the other hand, however, Warren (1960) described a rather regular increase in both endogenous and glucose-stimulated respiration of *Trypanosoma cruzi* taken from cultures 4 to 12 days old. This different result is not open to ready interpretation; differences in cultural procedings, or physiological changes in the strain induced by long cultivation may be involved. This latter point especially may well be of great importance. Although not an exact parallel, because no *in vitro* cultures are involved, the case of old and young strains of pathogenic African trypanosomes may be mentioned here. Jenkins and Grainge (1956), as well as Fulton and Spooner (1957), found that freshly isolated, cyclically passed strains of *Trypanosoma rhodesiense* consumed considerably less oxygen than old strains, that is, strains which had been passed from animal to animal by blood inoculation in the laboratory. The reason behind this change is again obscure; somewhat more clarified is the case of *Trypanosoma lewisi.* Flagellates taken from young infections show a significantly smaller rate of oxygen consumption than those isolated from old ones, while the opposite relationship holds true with respect to the rates of sugar consumption (Moulder, 1947, 1948b; Zwisler and Lysenko, 1954). It appears that a shift between synthetic and energy-producing processes occurs; the young flagellates were dividing while the older ones had ceased doing so. No such change was found in the case of *Trypanosoma vivax,* which of course is far removed from *Trypanosoma lewisi* insofar as the course of the infection is concerned. *Trypanosoma vivax* isolated from young infections consumed about 2 to 3 times as much oxygen as specimens isolated from old ones, and the variations in glucose consumption paralleled those of the respiratory rates (Desowitz, 1956a).

Other examples are the malarial parasites, many species of which are well suited for a study of this question because of the synchronicity of their development. Velick's (1942) data (Fig. 10) show the marked increase taking place during the 24-hour cycle of *Plasmodium cathemerium.* Comparable data for *Plasmodium knowlesi* have been presented by Maier and Coggeshall (1941).

There are relatively few relevant data at hand for parasitic worms. Alt

TABLE LII

RATES OF OXYGEN CONSUMPTION OF SOME PARASITIC PROTOZOA AT AN OXYGEN TENSION OF APPROXIMATELY 160 MM HG [a,b]

| Species | Stage | Temp. (°C) | Oxygen consumed in the | | | | RQ in the | | References |
| | | | Absence of sugar | | Presence of sugar | | Absence of sugar | Presence of sugar | |
			mm³/10⁸ /hour	mm³/mg N/hour	mm³/10⁸ /hour	mm³/mg N/hour			
Flagellates									
Endotrypanum schaudinni	C	30	4	29	47	309			Zeledon (1960a)
Leishmania enrietti	C	30	3	36	24	251			Zeledon (1960a)
Strigomonas oncopelti	C	30		146		350–600	0.9		Ryley (1955a)
Trypanosoma congolense	B	37			136			1.0	Agosin and von Brand (1954)
Trypanosoma congolense	C	30			38			0.9	von Brand and Tobie (1959)
Trypanosoma cruzi	C	30	9	71	23	178			Zeledon (1960a)
Trypanosoma equiperdum	B	37			149				Thurston (1958a)
Trypanosoma gambiense	B	37			161			0.09	von Brand *et al.* (1953, 1955)
Trypanosoma gambiense	C	29			18			0.97	von Brand *et al.* (1955)
Trypanosoma lewisi	B	37		40	167	600		0.97	Ryley (1951)
Trypanosoma vivax	B	37			127				Desowitz (1956a)
Trichomonas batrachorum	C	37	82				1.07		Doran (1958)
Trichomonas foetus	C	37	120	176	350	350			Ryley (1955b); Doran (1957)
Trichomonas vaginalis	C	37	96		269			1.02	Read and Rothman (1955)
Sporozoa									
Plasmodium cynomolgi	Segmenters	38			47				Maier and Coggeshall (1941)
Plasmodium knowlesi	Rings	38			8				Maier and Coggeshall (1941)
Plasmodium knowlesi	3/4 grown segmenters	38			34				Maier and Coggeshall (1941)

Species	Stage				Reference
Eimeria acervulina	Oocysts, young	30	350	1.12	Wilson and Fairbairn (1961)
Eimeria acervulina	Oocysts (68 hours)	30	24	0.8	Wilson and Fairbairn (1961)
Eimeria tenella	Unsporulated oocysts	30	1660		Smith and Herrick (1944)
Eimeria tenella	Sporulated oocysts	30	44		Smith and Herrick (1944)
Ciliates					
Balantidium coli	Trophozoites	37	9.4×10^6		Agosin and von Brand (1953)

[a] Some of the papers listed also contain data on other species of protozoa, or other stages of the species listed. Additional figures will be found in the following papers: flagellates: Soule (1925); Lwoff (1934); Adler and Ashbel (1934); Riedmueller (1936); Reiner *et al.* (1936); Christophers and Fulton (1938); Willems *et al.* (1942); Moulder (1947, 1948b); von Brand and Johnson (1947); Chang (1948); Fulton and Joyner (1949); Harvey (1949); von Brand *et al.* (1950); Zwisler and Lysenko (1954); Fulton and Spooner (1956); Cosgrove (1959); Chatterjee and Ghosh (1959); Tsukahara (1961); Grant *et al.* (1961); Lehmann and Sorsoli (1962); Ryley (1962); sporozoa: Bowman *et al.* (1960); ciliates: Daniel (1931).

[b] Key: C = culture forms; B = blood-stream forms.

TABLE LIII

RATES OF OXYGEN CONSUMPTION OF SOME HELMINTHS AT AN OXYGEN TENSION OF APPROXIMATELY 160 MM HG [a]

Species	Stage	Temp. (°C)	Oxygen consumption Sugar absent (mm³/mg dry weight/hour)	Oxygen consumption Sugar present (mm³/mg dry weight/hour)	RQ Sugar absent	RQ Sugar present	References
Trematodes							
Clonorchis sinensis	Adult	37	6.5				Nagamoto and Okabe (1959)
Fasciola hepatica	Adult	37.5	1.9				van Grembergen (1949)
Gastrothylax crumenifer	Adult	37	0.3				Goil (1958)
Paragonimus westermani	Adult	37.5		2.8			Shimomura (1959)
Paramphistomum explanatum	Adult	37	1.0				Goil (1958)
Schistosoma mansoni	Pairs	37.5	6.0	8.7	1.03	1.02	Bueding (1950a)
Schistosoma japonicum	Adult	37.5		10.3			Shimomura (1959)
Cestodes							
Diphyllobothrium latum	Proglottids	37	2.7	15.0			Friedheim and Baer (1933)
Diphyllobothrium latum	Plerocercoid	22		0.67			Friedheim and Baer (1933)
Echinococcus granulosus	Scoleces	37	2.0		0.88		Agosin (1959)
Hymenolepis diminuta	Adult	37	1.2	3.0	0.51	1.02	Read (1956)
Nematodes							
Ascaridia galli	Adult	37	2.5		0.96		Rogers (1948)
Gnathostoma spinigerum	Larva	37	2.7	2.9			Oba (1959)
Gnathostoma spinigerum	Male	37	3.4				Oba (1959)
Gnathostoma spinigerum	Female	37	7.9				Oba (1959)
Heterakis spumosa	Adult	38	4.0		1.1		Lazarus (1950)
Nippostrongylus muris	Larva (1 day)	30	18.4		0.73		Rogers (1948)
Nippostrongylus muris	Adult	37	6.8		0.69		Rogers (1948)
Trichinella spiralis	Larva	37.5	2.4	2.4	1.13	1.13	Stannard et al. (1938)

[a] Some of the papers listed also contain data on other species of helminths, or other stages of the species listed. Additional figures will be found in the following papers: trematodes: Hunter and Vernberg (1955a,b); Read and Yogore (1955); Vernberg and Hunter (1959, 1961); Vernberg (1961); Goil (1961); Freeman (1962); Horstmann (1962); Becker (1964); cestodes: Alt and Tischer (1931); Harnisch (1933); von Brand and Bowman (1961); von Brand and Alling (1962); Farhan et al. (1959); nematodes: Adam (1932); von Brand (1934); Krueger (1936); von Brand (1942); Laser (1944); Bueding (1949a); Bueding and Oliver-Gonzalez (1950); Glocklin and Fairbairn (1952); Passey and Fairbairn (1955); Bair (1955); Swierstra (1956); Schwabe (1957a); Costello and Grollman (1958); Rohde (1960); Saito and Kawazoe (1961); Kawazoe (1961).

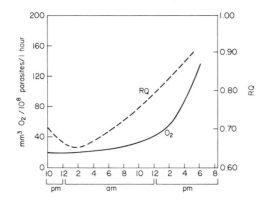

Fig. 10. Rate of oxygen consumption and respiratory quotient of *Plasmodium cathemerium* during its developmental cycle in the blood stream. (After Velick, 1942.)

and Tischer's (1931) data seem to indicate a decreasing rate of oxygen consumption along the strobila of *Moniezia,* but Friedheim and Baer's (1933) figures for *Diphyllobothrium* point in the opposite direction. It is difficult to correlate the respiratory rates of larval and adult helminths because in most cases each requires a different optimal temperature. It may be mentioned that Rogers (1948) found the respiratory rate of larval *Nippostrongylus* to decrease with age and that Schwabe (1957a) found the oxygen consumption of third stage parasitic larvae of the same worm to be considerably lower than that of the free-living larvae. Some interesting data are available for helminth eggs. According to the older experiments of Huff (1936) and Rogers (1948) on *Ascaris* and *Haemonchus* eggs, respectively, an increase in the rate of oxygen consumption occurs during development, while, in contrast, Brown (1928) had described a constant respiratory rate in the case of *Ascaris.* The more recent experiments of Passey and Fairbairn (1955) and Kawazoe (1961) have revealed a more complicated situation. The rates of oxygen consumption of the developing *Ascaris* eggs first decrease during the initial 36 hours. They then increase to reach maximal values after 10 days when the embryos have reached the vermiform stage, only to decline rapidly between days 10 to 25. This period of rapid decline is followed by a long and slower further decline, minimal values being reached after about 140 days. The low level of respiration attained by aged larvae is, of course, in full agreement with the well-known fact that mature *Ascaris* eggs remain viable for many months after having formed fully developed larvae.

Hatched larvae of *Ascaris* consume about 3 times more oxygen than embryonated eggs incubated for the same period (Kawazoe, 1961). This may be due to the increase in motility which undoubtedly occurs after hatching. Actually, however, very little concrete information is available concerning the question to what extent motility influences the respiratory rates of parasites. A rather indirect indication is the observation of Slater (1925) that electrical stimulation hastens the death of anaerobically maintained *Ascaris* specimens. It is well known that enormous differences in motility occur among parasitic protozoa; it suffices to point, on the one hand, to the vigorous motility of trypanosomes and, on the other hand, to the sluggish movements of malarial parasites or gregarines. However, it should be remembered that according to Zeuthen (1947) motility increases the metabolic rate over that of the basal metabolism at a lesser rate the smaller an organism is. It is therefore entirely possible that the influence of this factor is minimal in protozoa. On the other hand, it is true that the more or less sessile gregarinoid forms of *Leptomonas ctenocephali* consume less oxygen than the motile monadine forms (Lwoff, 1934), but whether it is really the difference in motility or some other factor that accounts for the difference in metabolic rate has not been established.

The rates of oxygen consumption of small organisms are generally higher than those of large ones, when compared on a weight basis, e.g., 240 and 285 mm^3 O_2/mg dry tissue/hour for the blood-stream forms of *Trypanosoma hippicum* (Harvey, 1949) and *Trypanosoma rhodesiense* (Christophers and Fulton, 1938), respectively, versus 8.7 and 2.4 mm^3 for *Schistosoma mansoni* (Bueding, 1950a) and *Trichinella spiralis* larvae (Stannard *et al.*, 1938). It is a well-established fact that this decline in respiration with increasing weight is not directly correlated to body weight, but in vertebrates it at least approximates the increase in body surface. In studying these relationships frequent use has been made in recent years of allometric plots, that is, plots in which weight per specimen is plotted against metabolic rate on a double logarithmic scale, the slope of the resulting line representing a measure of the power to which the body weight must be raised to describe the relationship between it and metabolic rate. Evidently two types of inquiry are possible, one concerning intraspecific relations between size and metabolism and another one dealing with interspecific comparisons.

The first intraspecific determinations on parasites were done by Krueger (1936, 1940a), who used large and small specimens of *Ascaris lumbricoides*. He found a fair proportionality between metabolism and surface when he calculated the latter according to Meeh's (1879) formula with a K value of 13.69. Much more extensive series of experiments were done by von Brand and Alling (1962) with larval and adult *Taenia taeniaeformis*. They found the aerobic metabolism, measured in terms of oxygen consumption, and the anaerobic metabolism, measured as CO_2

production, proportional to fractional powers of body weight intermediate between those characteristic for weight and surface proportionality (Fig. 11). The slopes of the regression lines were intermediate between 0.50 and 1.0 and the values obtained approximated in 3 out of 4 cases the generalized slope (0.75) calculated by Hemmingsen (1960) for poikilothermic animals.

Insofar as interspecific relationships are concerned only few data suitable for allometric plots can be found in the literature. Von Brand (1960a) plotted the data available for *Ascaris* (von Brand, 1934), *Dirofilaria* (von Brand, 1960a), *Eustrongylides* (von Brand, 1942), and *Heterakis* (Glocklin and Fairbairn, 1952) and obtained a slope of 0.62. It can be expected that this figure will change, once more species have been studied in detail. Relevant figures for other species of nematodes can be found in the papers by Rogers (1948) and Lazarus (1950) and for adult and larval trematodes in those by Goil (1958), Vernberg and Hunter (1959), and Vernberg (1963). Their data can, however, not be introduced into the above allometric plot, because the presentation of their figures is either not detailed enough or because they use different bases of reference (e.g., oxygen rates based on nitrogen content rather than on fresh weight).

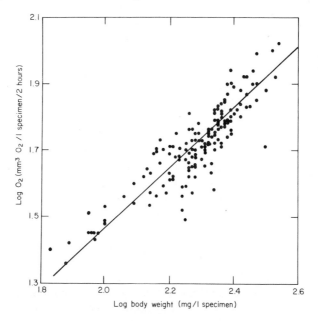

Fig. 11. Relations between weight and oxygen consumption in aerobically maintained larval *Taenia taeniaeformis*. (After von Brand and Alling, 1962; by permission of Pergamon Press.)

However, it is quite evident that here too the general relationship holds; large parasites have lower metabolic rates than small ones. To give only one example: according to Vernberg and Hunter (1959), the nitrogen content of adult *Gynaecotyla adunca* is approximately 100 times that of the cercaria, but the oxygen consumption, based on unit nitrogen, has decreased by 64%.

Another factor frequently playing a role in determining respiratory rates is the hydrogen ion concentration of the medium. As the figures of Table LIV indicate the pH range in which the respiration of parasites stays approximately unaltered, varies from species to species. Too few data are available to allow generalizations. The range is fairly narrow in blood parasites, that is, parasites living in an environment with stable hydrogen ion concentration, but it is at least equally narrow in three species of trichomonads living, respectively, in the reproductive tract, the nasal cavity, and the cecum of their hosts. The range is quite broad in *Eustrongylides* and the oocysts of *Eimeria tenella*. In both cases the impermeability of the outer coverings may be responsible rather than a failure of the respiration to respond to intracellular pH changes.

As in all cold-blooded animals, temperature is one of the most important factors determining the metabolic levels of parasites. The temperature relationships of parasites are quite varied. Some, such as *Trichinella,* complete their entire life cycle at the high temperature prevailing in homeothermic hosts. The parasites of poikilothermic hosts, on the other hand, live under more variable temperature conditions. The normal upper limit lies in most cases well below that characteristic for the environment of the first-mentioned group. Finally, there is a large group of parasites that alternates between warm- and cold-blooded hosts, and in many cases part of their life cycle is passed in the outside world. It is clear that the largest fluctuations in environmental temperature occur in this group. They are more pronounced than those to which aquatic free-living invertebrates are exposed, though probably not much more so than those encountered by some terrestrial invertebrates, for example, some insects. It may be remarked here incidentally that parasitism may change the temperature tolerance of the hosts. Vernberg and Vernberg (1963) found that the snail *Nassarius obsoleta,* parasitized by larval trematodes, is less resistant to thermal stresses than nonparasitized specimens.

The temperature fluctuations tolerated by trematodes seem to be correlated, especially insofar as the upper limits are concerned, to the temperature characteristic for the final hosts. Vernberg and Hunter (1961) found the respiratory rate of *Gynaecotyla adunca,* a bird parasite, to increase with rising temperature up to 41°C, that of the turtle parasite

TABLE LIV
Range of Hydrogen Ion Concentrations in Which the Oxygen
Consumption of Some Parasites Remains Approximately Unaltered

Species	Material	pH range	References
Flagellates			
Trichomonas foetus	Culture	6.2–6.9	Doran (1957)
Trichomonas suis	Culture	6.2–6.9	Doran (1957)
Trichomonas sp.	Culture	6.2–6.9	Doran (1957)
Trypanosoma lewisi	Blood-stream form	6.7–7.8	Moulder (1948a)
Sporozoa			
Eimeria tenella	Sporulated oocysts	4.7–8.8	Smith and Herrick (1944)
Plasmodium gallinaceum	Incubates	7.6–8.0	Silverman *et al.* (1944)
Trematodes			
Schistosoma mansoni	Adults	6.8–8.9	Bueding (1950a)
Nematodes			
Eustrongylides ignotus	Larvae	3.4–8.3	von Brand (1943)
Litomosoides carinii	Adults	6.0–7.5	Bueding (1949a)

Pleurogonius malaclemys up to 36°C, and that of the fish trematode *Saccacoelium beauforti* only up to 30°C. It is very interesting that corresponding differences occur already in larval worms, even though they are exposed to the same temperatures in one and the same species of intermediate hosts. Vernberg (1961) studied in this respect the rediae of *Himasthla quissetensis* (the adults live in sea gulls) and the sporocysts of *Zoogonus rubellus,* larvae of parasites living in the adult stage in fishes. She found that the oxygen consumption of the former larvae increased fairly regularly with temperature up to 41°C, while that of the latter began to decline above 30°C, although both larval species were isolated from *Nassarius obsoleta.*

The temperature characteristics of the oxygen consumption of parasites have been expressed in three different ways. The temperature coefficient Q_{10}, calculated from the expression

$$Q_{10} = \left(\frac{K_2}{K_1} \right)^{\frac{10}{t_2 - t_1}}$$

has often been employed (e.g., Vernberg and Hunter, 1961; Vernberg, 1961). It usually does not yield constant values over a wide range of temperatures, but has a tendency to decline with increasing temperature. An empirical curve, applicable to a variety of organisms, is the so-called "normal curve" of Krogh (1916) which originally had been established for the temperature range of 0° to 30°C, but which can for parasites profitably be extended to 37°C (von Brand, 1960c). Values obtained for parasites fit this curve rather smoothly (e.g., von Brand, 1943). Finally, frequent use has been made, especially in recent years, of Arrhenius' equation:

$$K_2 = K_1 \times e^{\dfrac{\mu}{2}\left(\dfrac{1}{T_1} - \dfrac{1}{T_2}\right)}$$

in which the symbol μ represents the energy of activation, or the temperature characteristic of the reaction involved. If the rates of oxygen consumption of parasites are plotted according to this equation for a temperature range compatible with life, usually no single straight line is obtained, but at least two bisecting lines result, as the examples shown in Fig. 12

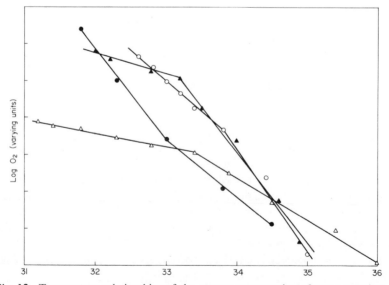

Fig. 12. Temperature relationships of the oxygen consumption of some parasites expressed according to Arrhenius' equation. Lwoff represents in his paper the temperature relationship as a straight line; a replotting of his figures showed that they fit better the two bisecting lines shown in the present figure. *Strigomonas fasciculata* (O) after Lwoff (1934); *Trypanosoma cruzi* (▲) after von Brand *et al.* (1946); *Ancylostoma caninum* (●) larvae after McCoy (1930); *Eustrongylides ignotus* (Δ) larvae after von Brand (1943).

demonstrate. With few exceptions, the temperature increment is smaller in the higher range of tolerated temperatures than in the lower one. Sometimes more than two bisecting lines are obtained, e.g., in the case of *Ascaris lumbricoides* four bisecting lines were described in the range 0.5° to 45°C (Krueger, 1940b). It is true that only one straight line was reported for *Diphyllobothrium latum* plerocercoids (Friedheim *et al.*, 1933), but these parasites were studied only in the temperature range of 20° to 37°C. The significance of bisecting lines resulting from Arrhenius' equation has given rise to a good deal of speculation. Crozier (1925) assumes that in different temperature ranges different master reactions occur, but this interpretation has not been accepted generally.

Of considerable biological importance is the response of the parasites' oxygen consumption to variations in environmental oxygen tension. It is customary in this respect — although no hard and fast lines can be drawn — to divide invertebrates into two groups. To the first group belong organisms the oxygen consumption of which remains approximately constant over a wide range of tensions; it begins to fall off only when very little oxygen is present. In the second group, on the other hand, this drop in consumption is already apparent at high tensions and the maximum oxygen consumption is frequently not reached even at tensions surpassing that of atmospheric air. It can often, though not always, be deduced from the organization of an animal to which of the two above groups it belongs. Bulky animals like actinians, which lack a circulatory system, quite generally belong to the second group simply because at moderate tensions not enough oxygen can enter the body by diffusion to satisfy the requirements of both the superficial and deeper tissue layers. On the other hand, such organisms as jellyfish have a respiration independent of the tension even if they are quite large because they contain very little living protoplasm and sufficient oxygen diffuses into the body through the surface to give all cells all the oxygen required even at relatively low tensions.

While limitation of diffusion is useful in explaining many cases, this mechanism is not sufficient to explain all variations occurring in nature. It is thus difficult to see why diffusion should limit the rate of oxygen consumption of the ciliate *Spirostomum* whose respiration has been found to depend on the environmental oxygen tension. It is similarly puzzling that the respiration of some crustaceans is independent of the tension, while in other species a distinct dependency exists, although both groups seem to contain fairly efficient oxygen-distributing mechanisms.

Parasitic protozoa and worms lack special organizational means of gathering or distributing oxygen. This is self-evident for the former, but the lack of such organs as gills or a circulatory system in the latter must be emphasized. Both groups must then rely for their oxygen supply solely on diffusion either from the body surface alone, or, in addition, on diffusion from their alimentary canal if they are blood-sucking worms. Such an endoparasitic arthropod as the *Gastrophilus* larva, on the contrary, has a tracheal system usable for the distribution of oxygen to various tissues, and endoparasitic insect larvae are known with special appendages that probably have a respiratory significance. All these latter forms cannot be considered further since nothing is known so far about their reactions to various oxygen tensions.

The few protozoan species studied in respect to their respiratory rates at various oxygen tensions belong to the group of animals with respiration independent of the tension (Table LV). This, of course, is not surprising since in such small organisms the surface/volume ratio is such as to give optimal conditions for the diffusion of oxygen into the body.

Many more data are available for helminths. Since different authors used many different oxygen tensions in their experiments, a tabular presentation is difficult. A few examples are given in Table LV and Table LVI. It is evident that some helminths, such as the ectoparasitic *Temnocephala,* and some developmental stages of trematodes, cestodes, and nematodes, have a respiration independent of the tension. They are all small organisms and diffusion appears not to limit the consumption. Into the same group belong small horse strongyle larvae, the respiration of which showed only small differences in the range 339 to 38 mm Hg, while in the case of the facultative parasite *Rhabditis strongyloides* the critical tension at which the oxygen consumption began to decline was somewhat higher than for the forms listed in Table LV, namely 58.5 mm Hg (Bair, 1955).

To the group showing a dependency of the oxygen consumption on the tension belong the relatively large worms shown in Table LVI, but also the following small and delicate worms: *Litomosoides carinii* and *Schistosoma mansoni* (Bueding, 1949b), the scoleces and brood capsules of *Echinococcus granulosus* (Farham *et al.,* 1959), the cercariae of *Himasthla quissetensis* (in contrast to the rediae of this species), and adult *Gynaecotyla adunca* (Vernberg, 1963). It is curious that in this last form, and still more pronounced in the cercariae of *Zoogonus rubellus,* certain regulatory mechanisms seem to exist, as indicated by the fact that their respiratory rate declines with declining tension down to a certain point (e.g., *Zoogonus rubellus* 23 mm Hg) remaining fairly steady upon further lowering of the environmental oxygen tension (e.g., in the above case to about 4 mm) (Vernberg, 1963).

It could be argued that at least in the larger worms belonging to this group diffusion limits the oxygen consumption. If this were so, it should

TABLE LV

RESPIRATION OF PARASITES HAVING A RESPIRATION INDEPENDENT OF THE OXYGEN TENSION

| Species | Material | Oxygen consumption at specified oxygen tension [a] in % of oxygen consumption at 160 mm Hg | | | | | | References |
		760 mm	160 mm	38 mm	15 mm	8 mm	.1 mm	
Protozoa								
Trypanosoma cruzi	Culture forms	102	100	102	54			von Brand et al. (1946)
Plasmodium knowlesi	Incubates	90	100	114			9	McKee et al. (1946)
Turbellarians								
Temnocephala spp.	Adults from *Trichodactylus*	180	100	117	92	95		Gonzalez (1949)
Temnocephala spp.	Adults from *Aegla*		100	114	95	97		Gonzalez (1949)
Trematodes								
Gynaecotyla adunca	Cercariae	124	100	85				Hunter and Vernberg (1955b)
Cestodes								
Diphyllobothrium latum	Eggs	100	100		Approx. 100			Friedheim and Baer (1933)
Nematodes								
Ascaris lumbricoides	Eggs	110	100	90	103	30		Passey and Fairbairn (1955)
Trichinella spiralis	Larvae	89	100	101		92		Stannard et al. (1938)

[a] The tensions listed are those used by most authors; some, however, used oxygen tensions differing by a few millimeters from those listed.

TABLE LVI

RESPIRATION OF PARASITES HAVING A RESPIRATION DEPENDENT ON THE TENSION

Species	Material	Oxygen consumption at specified oxygen tension [a] in % of oxygen consumption at 160 mm Hg							References
		760 mm	160 mm	80 mm	38 mm	15 mm	8 mm		
Trematodes									
Fasciola hepatica	Adults		100	68	46		27		Harnisch (1932)
Fasciola hepatica	Adults	140	100		53				van Grembergen (1949)
Himasthla quissetensis	Cercariae		100		57	30	11		Vernberg (1963)
Cestodes									
Diphyllobothrium latum	Plerocercoids	130	100		72				Friedheim and Baer (1933)
Diphyllobothrium latum	Posterior proglottids	180	100		66				Friedheim and Baer (1933)
Hymenolepis diminuta	Adults		100		65	18			Read (1956)
Triaenophorus nodulosus	Adults	133	100				21		Harnisch (1933)
Nematodes									
Ascaris lumbricoides	Adults	200	100	63	40	10			Krueger (1936)
Ascaris lumbricoides	Adults	300	100		50				Laser (1944)

[a] The tensions listed are those used by most authors; some, however, used oxygen tensions differing by a few millimeters from those listed.

be expected that this dependency would disappear, or at least be drastically reduced under conditions where the distance through which the oxygen has to diffuse in order to reach all the tissues is reduced. Such conditions are realized if minced tissues or homogenates are used. The first fact emerging from such experiments is that initially the rate of oxygen consumption at a specific oxygen tension is appreciably higher with minced material than with intact helminths. (Table LVII). During longer lasting experiments, however, the rate of the minced material sinks materially, often below that of the whole animal. This may or may not be a phenomenon of dying. At any rate, the increased initial consumption could be taken as an indication that the internal tissues could not get enough oxygen *in situ* by diffusion, and, after mincing, either paid off an oxygen debt or at least had an opportunity to oxidize at their maximal capacity.

There is, however, a second point to be considered, namely, the influence of the oxygen tension on the oxygen consumption of minced material; this is a somewhat controversial point. Harnisch (1932, 1933) maintained that minced material of *Fasciola* and *Triaenophorus* shows essentially the same dependency as the total animals, while on the contrary van Grembergen (1944, 1949) reports that the oxygen consumption of minced *Fasciola* and *Moniezia* has become independent of the tension over a wide range. Although this difference in results should be resolved by a reinvestigation, it should be remembered that Harnisch investigated the endogenous rate, while van Grembergen studied the oxygen consumption with succinate as substrate. Both Harnisch (1933) and van Grembergen *et al.* (1949) agree, however, that minced *Ascaris* still has a respiration dependent on the tension and in this case both studied the endogenous rate only. Rathbone (1955) reported that oxidation of succinate by suspensions of *Ascaris* muscle was dependent on the oxygen tension. Kmetec and Bueding (1961) finally found in studies with subcellular fractions isolated from *Ascaris* muscle that both DPNH oxidase

TABLE LVII

COMPARISON OF THE RATES OF OXYGEN CONSUMPTION
OF ENTIRE WORMS AND MINCED WORMS

Species	Period (hours)	Oxygen consumption (mm^3/gm fresh weight/hour)		References
		Entire worms	Minced worms	
Fasciola hepatica	1	94	144	Harnisch (1932)
Fasciola hepatica	0.5	350	412	van Grembergen (1949)
Ascaris lumbricoides	1	80	260	Laser (1944)

and succinic oxidase activities were strictly dependent on the oxygen tension, providing evidence that the terminal oxidase was a flavoprotein enzyme. It is then probable that the dependency of one or several key enzymes on the partial pressure of oxygen is responsible for the corresponding feature of the over-all respiration. This concept, in modern guise, is the old idea of Harnisch (1935b, 1936, 1949, 1950), who distinguished between "primary" and "secondary" aerobiosis, the former independent of, the latter dependent on, the tension; both were assumed to be mediated by different enzymes.

It is important to realize that the term "respiration dependent on oxygen tension" does not necessarily infer an inflexible relationship. Indeed it has been shown as far back as 1939 by von Buddenbrock that some invertebrates show a respiration dependent on the partial pressure only at high but not at low temperatures. The explanation seems to be that in the former case the oxygen demands of the tissues are so high that not all the tissues get enough oxygen at moderate tensions, although they do, even at low tensions, when the lowering of the temperature decreases the over-all demands of the organism. In parasites, von Brand (1947) found a similar situation both in respect to the normal and the postanaerobic respiration of larval *Eustrongylides* (Fig. 13). Another seemingly important, though largely ignored, point is that some organisms with an oxygen-tension-dependent respiration can raise their respiratory rate at

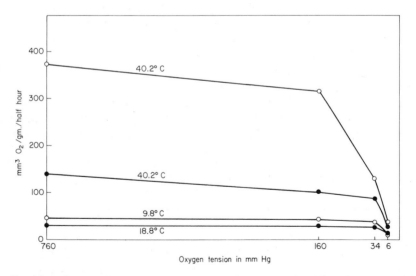

Fig. 13. Influence of temperature on the dependency of the aerobic and postanaerobic oxygen consumption of *Eustrongylides ignotus* larvae on the oxygen tension. After von Brand, (1947); (●) aerobic respiration, (O) postanaerobic respiration.

one and the same temperature and one and the same oxygen tension under certain circumstances, for instance, during digestion or during recovery from anaerobiosis. Unless one assumes rather pronounced changes in oxygen diffusion, the most plausible explanation of the phenomenon is to postulate a key role for one or more enzymes dependent on the partial pressure of oxygen (von Brand and Mehlman, 1953) in determining the over-all amount of oxygen consumed. The existence of the above relationship has not yet been established unequivocally in parasites; in fact, the relevant question has not yet been raised. However, it can be pointed out (see below) that some parasites with proved or probable dependency of their oxygen consumption on the tension are capable of repaying at least partially an oxygen debt, that is, they evidently can increase the inflow of oxygen. In a rather rigidly built organism like a nematode it is unlikely that this could be achieved by increasing the surface area available for diffusion. But since other mechanisms of changing diffusion rates can be postulated, the question would merit a thorough special study.

The response of parasites to variations in environmental oxygen tension and the tension prevailing in their actual habitat will be of decisive importance in deciding the question whether they lead *in situ* a predominantly aerobic or anaerobic life. It must be recognized, however, that deductions concerning this question are largely derived from theoretical considerations, since only few actual determinations of respiratory rates at the oxygen tensions prevailing in their immediate surroundings have been done. Insofar as small nematodes of the intestinal tract are concerned, an attempt to correlate their oxygen consumption with the oxygen tension of the habitat has been made by Rogers (1949b). As Fig. 14 indicates, the oxygen consumption of *Nippostrongylus muris* and *Nematodirus* spp. may reach 80 and 40%, respectively, of the *in vitro* rate when measured at the maximum oxygen tension occurring in their habitat. In *Haemonchus contortus,* however, the rate was much lower. It does seem clear that in these, and probably many related forms, the aerobic phase of metabolism will be of great importance within the normal surroundings. This is in accord with Davey's (1937, 1938) report that small nematodes of the intestinal tract die rapidly in the complete absence of oxygen.

A similar assumption is probably justified in the case of such bloodsuckers as *Ancylostoma* and *Necator,* which have a supplementary source of oxygen in the large amounts of blood taken up; this may be true also for *Opisthorchis felineus* (Golubeva, 1945).

An entirely different situation prevails in the case of the large intestinal worms like *Ascaris* or *Moniezia,* and similar organisms, as well as the large parasite of the bile ducts, *Fasciola.* These helminths live in the very

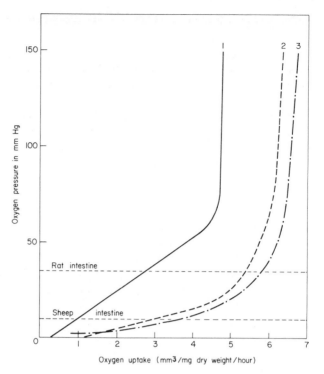

Fig. 14. Relation between the oxygen tension of the habitat and the rate of oxygen consumption of some parasitic nematodes. 1. *Haemonchus contortus;* 2. *Nematodirus* spp.; 3. *Nippostrongylus muris.* After Rogers, (1949b).

oxygen-poor intestinal or bile duct lumen, their oxygen consumption is strictly dependent upon the tension, their surface/volume ratio is such as to be quite unfavorable for the diffusion of oxygen, and their aerobic fermentations are very pronounced even at high oxygen tensions. The conclusion is hence inescapable that they lead *in vivo* a predominantly anaerobic life. A small measure of oxygen consumption will doubtless be possible in many, if not all cases; its true significance in the metabolic economy of the worms remains to be established. On the whole then it seems clear that no generalizations are possible for intestinal worms and helminths living in similar oxygen-poor habitats (von Brand, 1938b). Because parasites living side-by-side in the same habitat can be quite different in their oxygen relationships, the old controversy whether intestinal worms lead an anaerobic or aerobic life appears pointless.

Insofar as tissue helminths of vertebrates are concerned, it is convenient to make a distinction between parasites living in cysts and those inhabiting body fluids or cavities. For the former, the only definite data are those reported by Farhan *et al.* (1959) for *Echinococcus granulosus.* The cyst fluid in this instance appears to contain appreciable amounts of oxygen, and even though the oxygen consumption of scoleces and brood capsules depends on the tension, their oxygen consumption *in situ* could reach as high as 96 and 54% of the optimal rate in lung and liver cysts, respectively. A primarily aerobic life can also be assumed for larval *Eustrongylides ignotus*. Von Brand (1942) has shown that these worms accumulate an oxygen debt *in vitro* when exposed to anoxic conditions. They show, however, little signs of having done so *in vivo*, a finding compatible only with the assumption that they could get sufficient oxygen for an oxidative metabolism while living within their cysts. Evidently this particular line of reasoning must be restricted to organisms capable of accumulating an oxygen debt *in vitro*. A different type of evidence is available for the larvae of *Trichinella spiralis*. Stannard *et al.* (1938) found indications that the anaerobic metabolism is sufficient to keep the larvae alive, but that only the persistence of oxidative metabolism ensures motility. While this observation may indicate a primarily anaerobic life *in vivo*, the evidence is hardly sufficiently clear cut to permit definite conclusions, since the fact cannot be overlooked that the respiration of these larvae is independent of the tension and should allow the absorption of significant amounts even at quite low partial pressures.

Nonencysted helminths inhabiting such body fluids as blood or urine and the various body cavities will generally live under moderate to high oxygen tensions, and, in most cases, should be able to get significant amounts of oxygen. Very large parasites, such as *Ligula* or *Dioctophyme*, may represent exceptions, but have not yet been studied in this respect. It is suggestive that Smyth (1950) found that *Schistocephalus* kept *in vitro* under aerobic conditions becomes brown, although it is white in its normal habitat and stays white *in vitro* when kept under anaerobic conditions.

It has been well established that *Litomosoides carinii* depends for its survival upon an adequate supply of oxygen. It has been shown that cyanine dyes inhibit its oxygen consumption markedly (Welch *et al.*, 1947; Bueding, 1949a; Peters *et al.*, 1949) and that the worms die when the inhibition is induced *in vivo* by injecting appropriate amounts of the dyes into the hosts (Bueding, 1949a). This is a clear proof that the oxidative metabolism cannot be dispensed with, at least in this worm.

But generalizations are again not possible. The oxygen consumption of the blood-inhabiting schistosomes also is strongly inhibited by cyanines both *in vivo* and *in vitro*, but the worms are not killed even after long exposures (Bueding and Oliver-Gonzalez, 1948; Bueding *et al.*, 1947; Bueding, 1950a,b). They can apparently gain all the energy required for their vital processes from anaerobic fermentations, but it is of course possible that the small residual oxygen consumption evident under the influence of the cyanines may also be required. Under normal conditions the schistosomes consume rather large amounts of oxygen regularly, but the significance of the aerobic metabolism is in this case rather obscure. Development of the reproductive system may require the availability of oxygen.

Insofar as parasitic protozoa are concerned, it is in many cases difficult to arrive at definite views concerning their oxygen relationships *in vivo*. It has been mentioned previously that the developmental stages of Trypanosomidae in all likelihood live aerobically in nature, while the termite parasites and those of the roach *Cryptocercus* seem to be rather strict anaerobes. Protozoa, because of their small size, should encounter no difficulties in securing a maximal oxygen supply by diffusion, even at low tensions, and it can be assumed that any limiting factor must originate in the environment. Protozoa living in the intestinal lumen, for instance, will be in competition with the bacterial flora, and it can be expected that the microatmosphere will often be more or less completely depleted of oxygen, forcing them to an anaerobic metabolism (von Brand, 1946). Conditions in parasitic lesions, such as amoebic ulcers, are too obscure to allow a judgment at the present time since, as pointed out above, pathological processes sometimes have a profound influence on the local oxygen tension. Intracellular protozoa and blood parasites should normally be able to satisfy their oxygen requirements with the same facility as the host's own cells. This, however, does not imply that the parasites have a completely oxidative metabolism; on the contrary, as shown in previous chapters, the great majority of the forms studied so far is characterized by the persistence of aerobic fermentations.

IV. THE POSTANAEROBIC RESPIRATION

Many free-living invertebrates, after having been exposed to lack of oxygen, show an increased oxygen consumption lasting for a certain period when they are brought back to oxygenated surroundings. This phenomenon is known as the repayment of an oxygen debt, respiratory rebound, or respiratory overshoot, The extent to which free-living invertebrates repay an oxygen debt is very variable, ranging from a fraction of the incurred debt to a more or less pronounced overpayment (review of the literature in von Brand, 1946). The term "complete repayment of oxygen debt," which is rather frequently found, especially in the older literature, does not imply anything of fundamental importance. None of the factors determining the amount of oxygen taken up in excess of the normal aerobic rate (such as the level of anaerobic metabolism, the length of the anaerobic period, the nature of the anaerobic end products, or the question to what extent the latter are excreted or stored within the tissues) has any close quantitative connection with the amount of oxygen missed during the anoxic period (von Brand and Mehlman, 1953).

It is probably justified to assume that a respiratory rebound can occur only when end products of the anaerobic metabolism accumulate within the tissues; they seem to serve as substrates for the increased oxygen consumption. An interesting question is why organisms revert at all to an aerobic type of metabolism upon readmission of oxygen. It has been considered from the physicochemical standpoint by Zimmerman (1949). She concludes that it is probably due to differences in entropies of activation between the anaerobic and aerobic pathways, the former placing higher energy requirements on the cells than the latter.

A different question is why the postanaerobic oxygen consumption usually proceeds at a higher rate than the preanaerobic one. From the biological standpoint it can be said that in this way the anaerobic end products, which frequently are toxic, are rapidly altered to nontoxic substances, either by total oxidation or by partial resynthesis to carbohydrate. From the physicochemical standpoint the increased rate is due to an increased probability of enzyme and substrate molecules colliding if the concentration of the latter has increased. There is, however, one more general point requiring brief discussion, a point already touched upon in the preceding section: the question of the mechanism by which the surplus oxygen is secured by animals showing a dependency of their respiration on the tension. The difficulty lies in the observation that such animals increase their postanaerobic respiration at oxygen tensions at which their normal respiration is not proceeding at the maximal rate. Evidently if diffusion were the limiting factor, mechanisms changing the diffusion rate would have to be postulated; in flatworms one could think of a changed surface/volume ratio induced by muscular contraction (or relaxation). It is suggestive in this connection that Kearn (1962) showed the body surface of the monogenetic trematode *Entobdella soleae* to increase when the worm was kept under low oxygen tensions. In all cases one could speculate about a steeper oxygen gradient owing to the oxidation of the anaerobic end products; or one could, in some cases, advocate a role of the respiratory pigment in faster transport of oxygen. These, and probably other mechanisms, can well be involved, but whether they are potent enough to explain the greatly increased rate of oxygen consumption often shown during postanaerobic periods requires further study. In view of the previously mentioned finding by Rathbone (1955) and Kmetec and Bueding (1961) that *Ascaris* contains enzymes requiring high oxygen tensions for optimal functioning, it would seem possible that diffusion is not the limiting factor, but that the increase in postanaerobic rate could be explained largely on the basis of increased substrate concentration.

The question whether parasites accumulate an oxygen debt has so far not been studied for protozoa or endoparasitic arthropods, but relevant data are available for helminths. In this latter group, the same extensive variations in the repayment of the debt occur as in free-living inverte-brates. The one extreme is represented by *Litomosoides carinii* and *Schistosoma mansoni* which, according to Bueding (1949a, 1950a) do not show any sign of accumulating an oxygen debt during an anoxic period. Since in these worms practically all the anaerobically consumed carbo-hydrate is accounted for by acids excreted into the medium, it is possible that the failure to show a respiratory rebound is due to a failure of sub-strate accumulation in the tissues. It is rather remarkable that an identical situation prevails in this respect in these two worms which are quite different in their sensitivity to lack of oxygen, the former being damaged very rapidly, while the latter is quite resistant. Of intestinal flukes, *Gynaecotyla adunca* does not accumulate a measurable oxygen debt during a 24-hour anoxic period (Hunter and Vernberg, 1955b).

Ascaris is a worm that repays a small amount of an incurred oxygen debt. Originally (Adam, 1932, Harnisch, 1933) no increase in post-anaerobic oxygen consumption of entire worms had been observed, although it was found in isolated anterior ends. Later experiments by Laser (1944), however, showed that entire ascarids consume oxygen at a higher than normal rate for 2 hours after having been exposed for 18 hours to strictly anaerobic conditions. This is in line with the observation by von Brand (1937) that these worms rebuild a small amount of glycogen during a postanaerobic period. It is certain that the repayment of the oxygen debt is quite incomplete in *Ascaris* and it can again be assumed that this is connected with its well-known ability to excrete anaerobic metabolic end products.

The larvae of *Eustrongylides ignotus* repay about 30% of their oxygen debt following 16 to 18 hours' anaerobiosis (von Brand, 1942) and the respiratory quotient is exceedingly low during the initial periods of the re-payment phase (Fig. 15). This is clearly due to the retention of carbon dioxide used to rebuild the bicarbonate reserves depleted by the pre-ceding production of acidic anaerobic end products. The actual increase in oxygen consumption is marked and can in some experiments amount to about 300% during the first half hour (von Brand, 1947).

A considerably higher percentage of the incurred oxygen debt is repaid by *Hymenolepis diminuta* after 1 or 3 hours' anaerobiosis (Read, 1956), but the published data are not extensive enough to allow calculation of the percentage accurately. Finally, overpayment occurs in *Paragonimus*

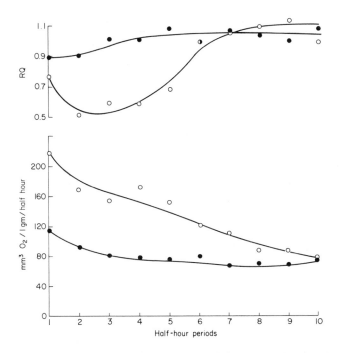

Fig. 15. Repayment of oxygen debt by *Eustrongylides ignotus* larvae. (●, Freshly isolated; O, postanaerobic 16–18 hours anaerobiosis.) After von Brand, (1942).

westermani. Read and Yogore (1955) report that this worm consumes preanaerobically 0.74 to 0.86 mm³ O_2/mg dry tissue/hour and that the rates reach, after a 30-minute anaerobiosis, values of 1.72 to 5.06 during the first and 1.58 to 2.74 during the second postanaerobic half-hour period. It would be interesting to study the repayment after longer anoxic periods; it would not be surprising if the percentage of repayment would then decline.

V. ACTION OF RESPIRATORY INHIBITORS AND STIMULANTS

Inhibitors and stimulants are powerful tools in elucidating the respiratory mechanisms, but the results of such experiments must be interpreted cautiously, especially if entire organisms are used as has been done in most parasites studied along such lines. It is clear that the oxygen consumption can be inhibited in various ways. On the one hand, the actual respiratory enzyme can be interfered with, for example, when the cytochrome system is blocked by means of cyanide. On the other hand, the over-all oxygen consumption can be cut down to various degrees depending upon the availability of alternate pathways, if a compound inhibits a certain metabolic sequence above the stage where hydrogen is activated. The African pathogenic trypanosomes are a case in point. Their oxygen consumption is reduced to a negligible fraction of the normal by various types of sulfhydryl inhibitors (von Brand *et al.,* 1950) (Fig. 16), but they do not all attack at the same point. Grant and Sargent (1960, 1961) have shown that such thiol inhibitors as *p*-chloromercuribenzoate, or organic trivalent arsenicals interfere with the normal rate of oxidation by inhibiting the L-α-glycerophosphate dehydrogenase, an integral part of the oxidase system of *Trypanosoma rhodesiense* and related forms. This enzyme is, however, not inhibited by iodoacetic acid or iodoacetamide, both potent inhibitors of the trypanosomes oxygen consumption. The activity of these compounds is explained by their interference with the glyceraldehyde-3-phosphate dehydrogenase.

A great variety of inhibitors, many different concentrations, and many different types of parasites have been used over the years. It would be impracticable to tabulate all these data; only a few recent experiments are summarized in Tables LVIII and LIX. They are sufficient to indicate a variety of responses, making it obvious that different parasites possess different respiratory mechanisms. This, of course, is in full agreement with data presented in previous chapters (cf. Chapter 6 for the distribution of the cytochromes).

In several parasites, such as the culture forms of some Trypanosomidae (Table LVII), the malarial parasites (e.g. McKee *et al.,* 1946; Bovarnick *et al.,* 1946), or such helminths as *Fasciola, Moniezia* (van Grembergen,

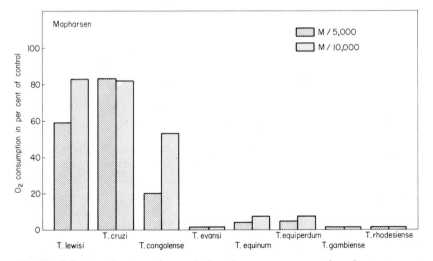

Fig. 16. Influence of an organic arsenical on the oxygen consumption of some trypanosomes. After von Brand *et al.* (1950).

TABLE LVIII

EFFECT OF SOME INHIBITORS ON THE OXYGEN CONSUMPTION OF SOME PARASITIC PROTOZOA [a]

Species	Stage	Cyanide		Azide		Indoacetate		Malonate		References
		Concentration (molar)	Inhibition (%)	Concentration (molar)	Inhibition (%)	Concentration (molar)	Inhibition (%)	Concentration (molar)	Inhibition (%)	
Flagellates										
Endotrypanum schaudinni	Culture form	10^{-4}	56	10^{-4}	24	10^{-4}	99			Zeledon (1960b)
Leishmania donovani	Culture form	10^{-3}	98	10^{-3}	40	10^{-3}	85	10^{-3}	0	Chatterjee and Ghosh (1959)
Leishmania enrietti	Culture form	10^{-4}	55	10^{-4}	37	10^{-4}	93			Zeledon (1960b)
Trichomonas foetus	Culture form	10^{-4}	11			10^{-4}	75	5×10^{-2}	2	Doran (1957)
Trichomonas gallinarum	Culture form	10^{-2}	6			10^{-3}	76	10^{-2}	$+11^{b}$	Lindblom (1961)
Trichomonas suis	Culture form	10^{-2}	$+9^{b}$			10^{-3}	61	10^{-2}	1	Lindblom (1961)
Trypanosoma cruzi	Culture form	10^{-4}	47	10^{-4}	35	10^{-4}	79			Zeledon (1960b)
Trypanosoma cruzi	Blood-stream form	10^{-4}	62			10^{-3}	30			Ryley (1956)
Trypanosoma equiperdum	Blood-stream form	10^{-3}	0			10^{-4}	82			von Brand et al. (1950); Thurston (1958a)
Trypanosoma lewisi	Blood-stream form	10^{-5}	52	10^{-3}	27	10^{-3}	81			Ryley (1951); Thurston (1958a)
Trypanosoma rhodesiense	Culture form	4.6×10^{-4}	83			10^{-3}	74			Ryley (1962)
Trypanosoma rhodesiense	Blood-stream form	4.6×10^{-4}	$+14^{b}$			10^{-3}	73			Ryley (1956)
Trypanosoma vivax	Blood-stream form	10^{-4}	2			10^{-3}	50			Ryley (1956)
Rhizopods										
Entamoeba histolytica	Culture form	10^{-3}	83			10^{-3}	26	10^{-1}	92	Takuma (1959)
Ciliates										
Balantidium coli	Culture form	4.5×10^{-4}	67					10^{-2}	42	Agosin and von Brand (1953)

[a] Data on other species of parasitic protozoa, other inhibitors, or different inhibitor concentrations will be found in some of the above papers, as well as in the following papers: trypanosomidae: von Fenyvessy and Reiner (1924, 1928); Lwoff (1934); Christophers and Fulton (1938); von Brand et al. (1946); von Brand and Johnson (1947); Moulder (1948a); von Brand and Tobie (1948); Marshall (1948); Harvey (1949); Fulton and Joyner (1949); Baernstein and Tobie (1951); Ryley (1955a); Fulton and Spooner (1956); Desowitz (1956a); Lehmann and Sorsoli (1962); trichomonads: Riedmueller (1936); Willems et al. (1942); Suzuoki and Suzuoki (1951); Read and Rothman (1955); Ryley (1955b); Read (1957); Doran (1958); Tsukahara (1961); sporozoa: Christophers and Fulton (1938); McKee et al. (1946); Bovarnick et al. (1946); Nagai (1957); Wilson and Fairbairn (1961).

[b] A plus sign preceding number indicates stimulation, rather than inhibition, of respiration.

TABLE LIX

EFFECT OF SOME INHIBITORS ON THE OXYGEN CONSUMPTION OF SOME PARASITIC HELMINTHS[a]

		Cyanide		Carbon monoxide		Azide		Iodoacetate		Malonate		
		Concentration (molar)	Inhibition (%)	Concentration (%)	Inhibition (%)	Concentration (molar)	Inhibition (%)	Concentration (molar)	Inhibition (%)	Concentration (molar)	Inhibition (%)	References
Trematodes												
Fasciola hepatica	Mince	10^{-3}	43	95	53							van Grembergen (1949)
Paramphistomum cervi	Adults	10^{-3}	+100[b]							10^{-2}	15	Lazarus (1950)
Cestodes												
Echinococcus granulosus	Scoleces	5×10^{-4}	47					10^{-3}	76	10^{-2}	7	Agosin et al. (1957)
Diphyllobothrium latum	Plerocercoids	10^{-3}	100	95	0							Friedheim and Baer (1933)
Nematodes												
Ascaridia galli	Adults	10^{-3}	62							10^{-2}	11	Rogers (1948); Massey and Rogers (1949)
Ascaris lumbricoides	Eggs, 10 days	4.6×10^{-4}	87	90	100							Passey and Fairbairn (1955)
Ascaris lumbricoides	Pieces, mince	10^{-3}	0	95	20					10^{-2}	50	Harnisch (1935a); Laser (1944); van Grembergen et al. (1949)
Eustrongylides ignotus	Larvae	3×10^{-4}	70			1.3×10^{-3}	69	10^{-3}	0			von Brand (1945)
Haemonchus contortus	Eggs	10^{-3}	68									Rogers (1948)
Heterakis spumosa	Adults	10^{-3}	50									Lazarus (1950)
Necator americanus	Larvae, free living	10^{-4}	89			10^{-2}	45					Fernando (1963)
Nematodirus spp.		10^{-3}	64									Rogers (1948)
Strongylus vulgaris	Adults	10^{-3}	15									Lazarus (1950)
Trichinella spiralis	Larvae	10^{-3}	88	10	+10[b]							Stannard et al. (1938)

[a] Some of the papers listed above also contain data on other species of helminths, or other stages of the species listed. Additional figures will be found in the following papers: Huff and Boell (1936); Wilmoth (1945); Bueding (1949a, 1950a); Bueding and Oliver-Gonzalez (1950); Hoshino and Suzuki (1956).

[b] A plus sign preceding number indicates stimulation, rather than inhibition, of respiration.

1944, 1949), or *Litomosoides* (Bueding, 1949a), the oxygen consumption is strongly inhibited by cyanide, and, where tested, by azide and carbon monoxide. Carbon monoxide inhibition, if reversed by light, indicates iron catalysis, usually referrable to the cytochrome system. Typical reversal has been found in *Ascaris* eggs (Pahl and Bachofer, 1957; Passey and Fairbairn, 1955), but in other cases, such as the malarial parasites (McKee *et al.*, 1946), reversal experiments gave equivocal results. It may be significant in this connection that a functional cytochrome system has been described for *Ascaris* eggs (in contrast to the adult worms) by Oya *et al.* (1963) and Kmetec *et al.* (1963), while no such information is available for the *Plasmodium* species. It is assumed (Moulder, 1948c) that the respiratory system of the latter contains, besides iron porphyrin proteins and pyridinoproteins, flavoproteins. This appears indicated by the observation of Bovarnick *et al.* (1946) that cresyl blue restored about 40% of the cyanide-blocked respiration of *Plasmodium lophurae*. Other artificial electron carriers, such as the often employed methylene blue, can stimulate the respiration and reverse cyanide inhibition of parasites belonging to this group, e.g., *Fasciola* or *Moniezia* (van Grembergen, 1944, 1949). This author also found a stimulation by paraphenylenediamine, a process sometimes interpreted as characteristic for the cytochrome system. However, Bueding (1949b) has pointed out that this stimulation is not specific enough to really prove the presence of a functional cytochrome system. It should also be emphasized that cyanide inhibition gives no clear indication as to the nature of the respiratory system present. In contrast to some of the organisms named above, *Litomosoides,* despite its cyanide sensitivity, does not contain a cytochrome system (Bueding and Charms, 1952).

In another group of parasites the respiration is also rather strongly inhibited by cyanide, but it is insensitive to carbon monoxide. This has been observed in the culture form of *Trypanosoma cruzi* (Baernstein and Tobie, 1951), in *Diphyllobothrium, Triaenophorus* (Friedheim and Baer, 1933) and the larvae of *Trichinella;* in the latter carbon monoxide even brought about a distinct stimulation of the respiratory rate (Stannard *et al.,* 1938). A rather pronounced respiratory stimulation under the influence of carbon monoxide has also been observed in the case of the *Gastrophilus* larva (Van de Vijver, 1964). The mechanism of these stimulations has not been elucidated definitely, and absence of carbon monoxide inhibition in these cases deserves emphasis since the *Trichinella* larvae possess a complete cytochrome system (Agosin, 1956; Goldberg, 1957); it occurs probably also in the *Gastrophilus* larvae (Van de Vijver, 1964). More readily understood is the case of *Trypanosoma cruzi* which has only a partial cytochrome system (Baernstein and Tobie, 1951; Ryley, 1956).

The oxygen consumption of *Diphyllobothrium* plerocercoids is strongly stimulated by pyocyanine which also completely reverses cyanide inhibition. In the presence of 10^{-3} M KCN and pyocyanine the respiratory rate is even 70% higher than the normal one (Friedheim *et al.*, 1933). The respiration of the *Trichinella* larvae, on the contrary, is hardly affected by methylene blue and the dye does not restore the cyanide-inhibited respiration. There is some doubt, however, whether the dye actually penetrates into the worms (Stannard *et al.*, 1938). The respiratory rate of *Trypanosoma cruzi* is strongly stimulated by methylene blue and other artificial electron carriers when succinic acid is used as substrate (Agosin and von Brand, 1955), while the response of larval *Eustrongylides* to the dye (von Brand, 1945) was essentially similar to that mentioned for *Trichinella*. A different type of stimulation is caused by dinitrophenol. This compound is an uncoupler of oxidative phosphorylation and has been found to stimulate the respiration of a variety of biological objects at low concentrations, but to be inhibitory at higher ones. It is therefore surprising that the respiration of larval *Eustrongylides* is stimulated by rather high concentrations (2×10^{-3} M to 5×10^{-4} M), according to von Brand (1945), as is that of infective larvae of *Necator americanus* (1.5×10^{-3} to 6×10^{-3} M), according to Fernando (1963). However, it must be realized that in these cases the tissue levels of the compound have not been established; it is quite possible, in view of the well-known impermeability of the nematode cuticle, that they are much lower than the environmental concentrations.

In a third group of parasites (blood-stream form of the African pathogenic trypanosomes, trichomonads, *Paramphistomum, Ascaris*) the respiration is not markedly inhibited by even fairly high concentrations of cyanide. Indeed one finds it not rarely stimulated by this compound and this latter phenomenon can be quite pronounced (Fig. 17). In *Paramphistomum,* for instance, cyanide stimulates the respiration around 100% at an oxygen tension of 160 mm. However, when the oxygen tension was raised to 760 mm only very slight stimulation took place, or even inhibition up to 30%. No activation by cyanide was observed when brei instead of intact animals was employed in the presence of methylene blue (Lazarus, 1950). In *Ascaris,* on the other hand, 10^{-2} M KCN doubled the rate of succinate oxidation by a particulate system (Rathbone, 1955). The mechanism of cyanide stimulation is not clear; it is possibly related to the carbonyl-combining property of cyanide (von Brand and Tobie, 1948) or to combination of CN with iron porphyrins, the cyanide hemochromogens having redox potentials favoring the hydrogen transport system and thus allowing increased oxidation of the substrate (Rathbone, 1955).

OXYGEN CONSUMPTION OF BLOOD FORMS 37.5°C

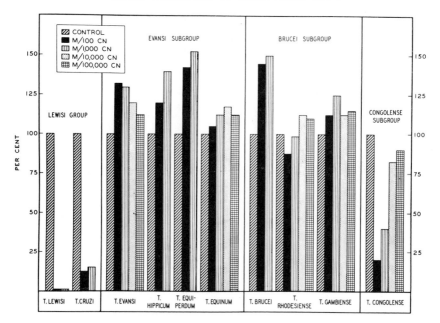

Fig. 17. Influence of cyanide on the respiration of some trypanosomes. (After von Brand and Tobie, 1948.)

It should be stressed that the above separation of parasites into three groups in respect to their reactions to respiratory inhibitors was done only for convenience sake; it does not imply identity of respiratory mechanisms within each group. Some of the differences observed between members of the first two groups have been mentioned above. A few final examples relate to the third group. While the respiration of *Trichomonas hepatica* is not stimulated, but rather inhibited by methylene blue (Willems *et al.*, 1942), that of *Ascaris* is stimulated, the stimulation being especially high (up to 1000%) in the presence of succinate. The respiration of the roundworm is slightly stimulated by paraphenylene-diamine, but not by dinitrophenol (Laser, 1944; van Grembergen *et al.*, 1949), while that of *Trichomonas* is inhibited by dinitrophenol (Willems *et al.*, 1942). It is of course known (cf. Chapter 6) that the forms having a cyanide-insensitive respiration do not have a functioning cytochrome system; their terminal respiration is, however, probably not mediated by the same mechanisms in all cases.

VI. THE CARBON DIOXIDE TRANSPORT

It has been mentioned in a preceding section that all parasites produce larger or smaller amounts of carbon dioxide as end product of their metabolism; the question arises by what mechanisms this gas is eliminated. It appears not to have been studied so far with parasitic worms and protozoa, but some relevant data for endoparasitic arthropods are available. Levenbook (1950a,b) and Levenbook and Clark (1950) studied the problem with larval *Gastrophilus*. The average carbon dioxide content of its blood was 72.4 volumes % and the carbon dioxide content of the tissues was always close to that of the blood. From 30 to 50% of the gas occurred in solution and the remainder in form of bicarbonate, while no carbamate formation could be observed. A study of the carbon dioxide dissociation curves at different temperatures revealed an adaptation to high tensions; the actual carbon dioxide tension of the blood varied between about 300 and 500 mm Hg. It was also found that the larval blood contained no carbonic anhydrase and no substance inhibiting hydration of carbon dioxide. A damaging effect on the tissues by the accumulation of that gas, however, is avoided by the strong buffer capacity of the blood which actually is better developed on both sides of its normal pH. *Gastrophilus* has this last feature in common with other insects, in contrast to what is found in other groups of animals, and this may be an adaptation to difficulties in carbon dioxide elimination inherent in the tracheal type of respiratory mechanisms.

Castella (1952) did find carbonic anhydrase in the soft tissues and to a lesser degree in the cuticle of *Gastrophilus* larvae, as well as in *Moniezia expansa, Anoplocephala magna, Fasciola hepatica, Ascaris lumbricoides,* and *Parascaris equorum.* In tapeworms the enzyme was distributed erratically along the strobila; in *Ascaris* is was most concentrated in the digestive system, being found also, however, in the genital tract and the cuticle.

VII. HOST-INDUCED VARIATIONS IN RESPIRATORY EXCHANGES OF PARASITES

It is evident that many factors which have an influence on the respiratory rates of parasites, such as temperature, pH, oxygen tension, and others, originate in the host and can exert an influence *in vivo*. It can be expected that their activities will approximate those discussed previously, when *in vitro* experiments were used for analysis. It must, however, be admitted that an *in vivo* situation is much more complicated than an *in vitro* experiment, and it is quite possible that the interaction of various factors may modify the response to one or the other of those studied *in vitro* under simplified conditions. This problem cannot be discussed profitably further because of lack of pertinent data.

More specific than the factors mentioned above are those connected with immune responses; these merit a brief special discussion. Moulder (1947, 1948b) was the first to observe that, in *Trypanosoma lewisi* infections, old specimens, that is, specimens which have ceased multiplying, have a higher rate of oxygen consumption and a higher RQ, as well as an increased sensitivity to malonate, than young, multiplying parasites; at the same time the rate of glucose utilization decreases. Moulder (1948b) suggested that these changes were due to the action of ablastin which would inhibit oxidative assimilation of glucose and concurrently would stop cell division and growth. Essentially similar results were reported by Zwisler and Lysenko (1954). These investigators observed that salicylate treatment of the rats prolonged the reproductive phase of *Trypanosoma lewisi* and that the rate of oxygen consumption of the parasites increased by approximately 50% with the appearance of ablastin.

Different results are obtained when the possible influence of immune sera on the respiratory rate of trypanosomes is studied *in vitro*. Zwisler and Lysenko (1954) found that such serum had no influence on the respiration of *Trypanosoma lewisi*. This is probably also true in other trypanosome infections, but secondary influences may bring about a reduction in the rate of oxygen consumption. Desowitz (1956b) thus found the respiratory rate of *Trypanosoma vivax* decreased considerably when studied in the sera of N'Dama cattle previously challenged with the same parasite. However, it was observed that this serum induced lysis of the trypanosomes and it must therefore be considered as very questionable whether a true respiratory inhibition was involved. Similarly, Thurston (1958b). found the oxygen consumption of *Trypanosoma brucei* reduced only by concentrations of immune serum which lysed the flagellates.

Of parasitic helminths only larval *Nippostrongylus muris* seems to have been studied in this respect. Schwabe (1957b) reported that the endogenous oxygen consumption of free-living third-stage larvae was inhibited 23 to 76% in sera of rats previously infected with the worm. Curiously, there was no difference in endogenous respiration when third-stage parasitic larvae were studied in corresponding sera, but with glucose as exogenous substrate, moderate inhibition (3 to 40%) was found. Schwabe (1957b) is of the opinion that the inhibitions observed were true inhibitions of metabolic processes and that they were not due to mechanical interference (such as blocking of the gut by antigen/antibody precipitate).

VIII. INFLUENCE OF PARASITES ON THE RESPIRATION OF THE HOST

The question whether the respiratory rate of tissues is changed from normal when the host is parasitized has been investigated repeatedly. It has thus been observed (Chatterji, 1960) that the liver of mice infected with *Trypanosoma evansi* shows an increased oxygen consumption both with glucose and succinic acid as substrates. It is assumed that the host cells are responsible for this increase, since no correlation to the degree of parasitization could be established. A similar increase in respiratory rate was observed in various tissues of hamsters infected with *Leishmania* spp. (Adler and Ashbel, 1940; Chatterji and Sen Gupta, 1959), the liver of rabbits infected with *Eimeria stiedae* (Dickson *et al.*, 1958), and, at a lower level of stimulation, in livers of rats infected with *Plasmodium berghei* (Chatterji *et al.*, 1957). To what extent the respiration of the parasites contributes to the respiratory rates of the host tissues is not clear. On the whole, the impression is gained that no significant portion of the observed rates is caused by the parasites. This, however, does not necessarily imply that the respiration of the host tissues is stimulated in the true sense of the word. It is equally possible, and has, for instance, been assumed in the case of the *Plasmodium berghei* infected livers quoted above, that an influx of metabolically active cells, such as inflammatory or hematopoetic cells, occurred. Their contribution could readily give rise to the misinterpretation that the respiratory rate of the original tissues was increased.

Similar difficulties in interpretation exist when the respiration of entire parasitized animals is compared to that of nonparasitized controls. It has been found that the oxygen consumption of trypanosome-infected rats is somewhat raised in the terminal stages of the disease (von Fenyvessy, 1926; von Brand, 1951), but, on the other hand, their basal metabolism remains essentially unchánged (Bouisset *et al.*, 1956). The relatively small rise in oxygen consumption can be related partly to an increase in body temperature of the infected animals, but may be attributable in part also to the billions of flagellates present in the blood. At any rate, it does not seem justified to assume, as Scheff and Rabati (1938) did, that the parasites kill their hosts by inducing asphyxiation through their own high oxygen demands. During the greater part of trypanosome infections both the temperature and the oxygen consumption of infected rodents stay within normal limits (Kligler *et al.*, 1929; von Brand, 1951), and even the maximal increase observed is relatively small when compared to the rates in respiration that can be induced without harm to an animal by exercise.

On the other hand, however, it is true that certain respiratory difficulties can arise during parasitic infections. The pneumonia caused by *Dic-*

tyocaulus viviparus in calves can serve as an example. Fisher and McIntyre (1960) have shown that the respiratory rate of infected animals is increased from an average of 23/minute to an average of 77/minute, while the ventilation rate increased from 25 liters/minute to 35 liters/ minute. The plasma pH remained practically unchanged, but the plasma CO_2 content was increased significantly, indicating a compensatory respiratory acidosis.

It is well known that in several parasitic infections large-scale destruction of erythrocytes occurs and that insufficient replacement leads to a diminution of the functioning hemoglobin. In malaria, for instance, destruction of red cells occurs not only at sporulation, but lysis of non-parasitized cells is also observed (Maegraith, 1954). As a consequence the resulting anemia can reach extreme degrees. In *Plasmodium falciparum* infections red cell counts as low as 0.44 million/mm³ have been observed (Carducci, 1907), and in *Plasmodium vivax* infections the count can drop to 0.56 million/mm³ (Amy, 1934), but the average in this latter infection varies between 2.2 and 4.9 million/mm³ (Fairley and Bromfield, 1933). In infections with *Babesia canis* (Maegraith *et al.*, 1957) and *Anaplasma marginale* (Rees and Hale, 1936) red cell counts below 1 million/mm³ have been observed and in those with *Haemobartonella muris* the count drops to about 2 million/mm³ (Ford and Eliot, 1928).

One of the unavoidable consequences of pronounced red cell destruction is a lowering of the oxygen-carrying capacity of the blood. The question was therefore raised, especially in the case of malaria, whether this factor could be sufficiently potent to explain the tissue anoxia which apparently lies at the root of many pathological symptoms of the disease, such as the degenerative changes observable in liver, kidneys, and other organs. The fundamental importance of tissue anoxia in malaria and related diseases, such as *Babesia* infections, has been emphasized repeatedly by Maegraith (1948, 1954, 1959) and Maegraith *et al.* (1957). It was found (Maegraith, 1956; Maegraith *et al.*, 1957) that the oxygen dissociation curves of infected blood were normal during the greater part of the infections and showed deviations only shortly prior to death. It was furthermore found that the amount of hemoglobin remaining was sufficient to satisfy, at least from a theoretical standpoint, the demands of the tissues. The question then arose whether the anoxic tissue damage could be due to a failure of the oxygen acceptance by the tissues, perhaps because of a failure of the cytochrome system.

This concept led to a study on the subcellular level, making use of mitochondria isolated from livers of mice infected with *Plasmodium berghei* or of monkeys infected with *Plasmodium knowlesi* (Riley and Deegan, 1960; Riley, 1961; Riley and Maegraith, 1962; Maegraith *et al.*, 1962). Interestingly enough, much greater changes were found in the mouse mitochondria, even though the histological liver picture is more abnormal in the *Plasmodium knowlesi* than in the *Plasmodium berghei* infection. Among the changes found in mitochondria isolated from mice infected with the latter parasite were lowered rates of succinate, glutamate, and β-hydroxybutyrate oxidation, as well as lowered P/O ratios. It was also found that both latent and Mg^{++}- stimulated ATPase activities were increased, while the dinitrophenol-stimulated activity was decreased. On the whole it appears that mitochondria isolated from infected livers showed distinct similarities, but also some differences, to mitochondria isolated from normal animals that had been "aged" *in vitro*. The observed changes can be summarized as being indicative of a loss of respiratory control and a greater dependency on cofactors than shown by normal mitochondria. There was, however, no inhibition of the oxidative enzymes proper, neither cytochrome oxidase nor substrate-specific dehydrogenases showing loss of activity, at least under optimal assay conditions. Of considerable interest also is the observation of Riley and Maegraith (1961) that the serum of malarious animals contains a factor which inhibits oxidative phosphorylation by mitochondria isolated from normal animals. On the other hand, mitochondria isolated from monkey livers infected with *Plasmodium knowlesi* (Maegraith *et al.,* 1962) showed essentially normal oxidative phosphorylation, the P/O ratios found being almost normal, as were most other parameters studied. The only definite change was a decrease in the reserve of high-energy phosphate compounds, a parallel existing in this respect to the mouse mitochondria. It is obvious that the monkey mitochondria were much less susceptible to parasite-induced changes than those from the mouse. Riley and Deegan (1960) have pointed out that in view of such observations it is uncertain whether the biochemical damage sustained by the mitochondria has a causal connection with the origin of tissue damage, such as is found in the liver. They consider it possible that the initial stimulus to liver degeneration could come from other processes, for instance, localized circulatory disturbances. If this is true the mitochondrial changes would be secondary symptoms only, rather than the primary cause of the tissue damage. However, Maegraith *et al.* (1962) have emphasized that the pathogenesis of malaria could be related to two main factors: a toxic factor damaging mitochondria and changes in blood circulation which would disrupt the oxygen supply and thus interfere with the steady state of metabolites.

Hardly anything is known concerning the question whether the respiration of parasitized invertebrates is altered. Von Brand and Files (1947) found normal respiratory rates in *Australorbis glabratus* parasitized by *Schistosoma mansoni*. Becker (1964) observed that the respiration of

Stagnicola palustris parasitized by larval trematodes was lower than normal. This is explained by decreased motility of the parasitized specimens.

REFERENCES

Adam, W. (1932). *Z. Vergleich. Physiol.* **16**, 229–251.

Adler, S., and Ashbel, R. (1934). *Arch. Zool. Ital.* **20**, 521–527.

Adler, S., and Ashbel, R. (1940). *Ann. Trop. Med. Parasitol.* **34**, 207–210.

Adler, S., and Theodor, O. (1931). *Proc. Roy. Soc.* **B108**, 453–463.

Agosin, M. (1956). *Bol. Chileno Parasitol.* **11**, 46–51.

Agosin, M. (1959). *Biologica (Santiago, Chile)* **27**, 3–32.

Agosin, M., and Brand, T. von (1953). *J. Infect. Diseases* **93**, 101–106.

Agosin, M., and Brand, T. von (1954). *Exptl. Parasitol.* **3**, 517–524.

Agosin, M., and Brand, T. von (1955). *Exptl. Parasitol.* **4**, 548–563.

Agosin, M., Brand, T. von, Rivera, G. F., and McMahon, P. (1957). *Exptl. Parasitol.* **6**, 37–51.

Alt, H. L., and Tischer, O. A. (1931). *Proc. Soc. Exptl. Biol. Med.* **29**, 222–224.

Amy, A. C. (1934). *J. Roy. Army Med. Corps* **62**, 318–329.

Anfinsen, C. B., Geiman, Q. M., McKee, R. W., Ormsbee, R. A., and Ball, E. G. (1946). *J. Exptl. Med.* **84**, 607–621.

Asami, K., Nodake, Y., and Ueno, T. (1955). *Exptl. Parasitol.* **4**, 34–39.

Baernstein, H. D., and Tobie, E. J. (1951). *Federation Proc.* **10**, 159.

Bair, T. D. (1955). *J. Parasitol.* **41**, 613–623.

Balbiani, E. G. (1884). "Leçons sur les sporozoaires." Doin, Paris.

Ball, G. H. (1964). *J. Parasitol.* **50**, 3–10.

Ball, G. H., and Chao, J. (1961). *J. Parasitol.* **47**, 787–790.

Bataillon, E. (1910). *Arch. Entwicklungsmech. Organ.* **30**, 24–44.

Becker, W. (1964). *Z. Parasitenk.* **25**, 77–102.

Berntzen, A. K. (1962). *J. Parasitol.* **48**, 785–797.

Berntzen, A. K., and Mueller, J. F. (1964). *J. Parasitol.* **50**, 705–711.

Blacklock, D. B., Gordon, R. M., and Fine, J. (1930). *Ann. Trop. Med. Parasitol.* **24**, 5–67.

Blanchard, L., and Dinulescu, G. (1932). *Compt. Rend. Soc. Biol.* **110**, 343–344.

Bouisset, L., Harant, H., and Ruffié, J. (1956). *Ann. Parasitol. Humaine Comp.* **31**, 331–349.

Bovarnick, M. R., Lindsay, A., and Hellerman, L. (1946). *J. Biol. Chem.* **163**, 523–533.

Bowman, I. B. R., Grant, P. T., and Kermack, W. O. (1960). *Exptl. Parasitol.* **9**, 131–136.

Boycott, A. E. (1904). *Trans. Epidemiol. Soc. (London)* **24**, 113–142.

Brand, T. von (1933). *Z. Vergleich. Physiol.* **18**, 562–596.

Brand, T. von (1934). *Z. Vergleich. Physiol.* **21**, 220–235.

Brand, T. von (1937). *J. Parasitol.* **23**, 316–317.

Brand, T. von (1938a). *J. Parasitol.* **24**, 445–451.

Brand, T. von (1938b). *Biodynamica* **2**, No. 41, 1–13.

Brand, T. von (1942). *Biol. Bull.* **82**, 1–13.

Brand, T. von (1943). *Biol. Bull.* **84**, 148–156.

Brand, T. von (1945). *J. Parasitol.* **31**, 381–393.

Brand, T. von (1946). "Anaerobiosis in Invertebrates," Biodynamica Monographs No. 4. Biodynamica, Normandy, Missouri.

Brand, T. von (1947). *Biol. Bull.* **92**, 162–166.

Brand, T. von (1951). *Exptl. Parasitol.* **1**, 60–65

Brand, T. von (1952). "Chemical Physiology of Endoparasitic Animals." Academic Press, New York.

Brand, T. von (1960a). *In* "Nematology" (J. N. Sasser and W. R. Jenkins, eds.), p. 233–241. Univ. of North Carolina Press, Chapel Hill, North Carolina.

Brand, T. von (1960b). *In* "Nematology" (J. N. Sasser and W. R. Jenkins, eds.), pp. 242–248. Univ. of North Carolina Press, Chapel Hill, North Carolina.

Brand, T. von (1960c). *In* "Nematology" (J. N. Sasser and W. R. Jenkins, eds.), pp. 257–266. Univ. of North Carolina Press, Chapel Hill, North Carolina.

Brand, T. von, and Alling, D. W. (1962). *Comp. Biochem. Physiol.* **5**, 141–148.

Brand, T. von, and Bowman, I. B. R. (1961). *Exptl. Parasitol.* **11**, 276–297.

Brand, T. von, and Files, V. S. (1947). *J. Parasitol.* **33**, 476–482.

Brand, T. von, and Johnson, E. M. (1947). *J. Cell. Comp. Physiol.* **29**, 33–50.

Brand, T. von, and Mehlman, B. (1953). *Biol. Bull.* **104**, 301–312.

Brand, T. von, and Simpson, W. F. (1945). *Proc. Soc. Exptl. Biol. Med.* **60**, 368–371.

Brand, T. von, and Tobie, E. J. (1948). *J. Cell. Comp. Physiol.* **31**, 49–68.

Brand, T. von, and Tobie, E. J. (1959). *J. Parasitol.* **45**, 204–208.

Brand, T. von, Johnson, E. M., and Rees, C. W. (1946). *J. Gen. Physiol.* **30**, 163–175.

Brand, T. von, and Weise, W. (1932). *Z. Vergleich. Physiol.* **18**, 339–346.

Brand, T. von, Tobie, E. J., and Mehlman, B. (1950). *J. Cell. Comp. Physiol.* **35**, 273–300.

Brand, T. von, Tobie, E. J., Mehlman, B., and Weinbach, E. C. (1953). *J. Cell. Comp. Physiol.* **41**, 1–22.

Brand, T. von, Weinbach, E. C., and Tobie, E. J. (1955). *J. Cell. Comp. Physiol.* **45**, 421–434.

Brown, H. W. (1928). *J. Parasitol.* **14**, 141–160.

Buddenbrock, W. von (1939). "Grundriss der vergleichenden Physiologie," 2nd Ed., Vol. 2. Borntraeger, Berlin.

Bueding, E. (1949a). *J. Exptl. Med.* **89**, 107–130.

Bueding, E. (1949b). *Physiol. Rev.* **29**, 195–218.

Bueding, E. (1950a). *J. Gen. Physiol.* **33**, 475–495.

Bueding, E. (1950b). *J. Parasitol.* **36**, 201–210.

Bueding, E., and Charms, B. (1952). *J. Biol. Chem.* **196**, 615–627.

Bueding, E., and Oliver-Gonzalez, J. (1948). *Proc. 4th Intern. Congr. Trop. Med. Malaria, Washington, D.C., 1948* Vol. 2, pp. 1025–1033. Government Printing Office, Washington, D.C.

Bueding, E., and Oliver-Gonzalez, J. (1950). *Brit. J. Pharmacol.* **5**, 62–64.

Bueding, E., Peters, L., and Welch, A. D. (1947). *Federation Proc.* **6**, 313.

Bunge, G. (1883). *Z. Physiol. Chem.* **8**, 48–59.

Bunge, G. (1889). *Z. Physiol. Chem.* **14**, 318–324.

Campbell, J. A. (1931). *Physiol. Rev.* **11**, 1–40.

Carducci, A. (1907). *Atti Soc. Studi Malaria* **8**, 225 [not seen, quoted in Maegraith (1948)].

Castella, E. (1952). *Anales Inst. Invest. Vet.* **4**, 344–350.

Cavier, R., Georges, P., and Savel, J. (1964). *Exptl. Parasitol.* **15**, 556–560.

Chaigneau, M., and Charlet-Lery, G. (1957). *Compt. Rend.* **245**, 2536–2538.

Chang, S. L. (1948). *J. Infect. Diseases* **82**, 109–116.

Chatterjee, A. N., and Ghosh, J. J. (1959). *Ann. Biochem. Exptl. Med.* **19**, 37–50.

Chatterji, A. (1960). *Bull. Calcutta School Trop. Med.* **8**, 119–121.

Chatterji, A., and Sen Gupta, P. C. (1959). *Bull. Calcutta School Trop. Med.* **7**, 97–99.

Chatterji, A., Mukherji, K. L., and Sen Gupta, P. C. (1957). *Bull. Calcutta School Trop. Med.* **5**, 61–62.

Christophers, S. R., and Fulton, J. D. (1938). *Ann. Trop. Med. Parasitol.* **82**, 43–75.

Cleveland, L. R. (1925). *Biol. Bull.* **48**, 309–326.

Cleveland, L. R. (1928a). *Am. J. Hyg.* **8**, 256–278.

Cleveland, L. R. (1928b). *Am. J. Hyg.* **8**, 990–1013.

Cosgrove, W. B. (1959). *Can. J. Microbiol.* **5**, 573–578.

Costello, L. C., and Grollman, S. (1958). *Exptl. Parasitol.* **7**, 319–327.

Cram, E. B. (1943). *Sewage Works J.* **15**, 1119–1138.

Cram, E. B., and Hicks, D. O. (1944). *Proc. Helminthol. Soc. Wash., D.C.* **11**, 1–9.

Crozier, W. J. (1925). *J. Gen. Physiol.* **7**, 189–216.

Daniel, G. E. (1931). *Am. J. Hyg.* **14**, 411–420.

Davey, D. G. (1937). *Nature* **140**, 645.

Davey, D. G. (1938). *J. Exptl. Biol.* **15**, 217–224.

Davies, P. W., and Bronk, D. W. (1957). *Federation Proc.* **16**, 693–696.

Desowitz, R. S. (1956a). *Exptl. Parasitol.* **5**, 250–259.

Desowitz, R. S. (1956b). *Nature* **177**, 132–133.

Dickson, W. M., Dunlap, J. S., Johnson, V. L., and Dunlap, D. (1958). *Proc. Soc. Exptl. Biol. Med.* **98**, 179–180.

Dill, D. B., Edwards, H. T., and Florkin, M. (1932). *Biol. Bull.* **62**, 23–36.

Dinnik, J. A., and Dinnik, N. N. (1937). *Med. Parazitol. i Parazitarn. Bolezni* **5**, 603–618.

Dinulescu, G. (1932). *Ann. Sci. Nat. (Paris), Zool.* **15**, 1–184.

Dobell, C., and Laidlaw, P. P. (1926). *Parasitology* **18**, 283–318.

Doran, D. J. (1957). *J. Protozool.* **4**, 182–190.

Doran, D. J. (1958). *J. Protozool.* **5**, 89–93.

Dyrdowska, M. (1931). *Compt. Rend. Soc. Biol.* **108**, 593–596.

Erhardt, A. (1939). *Arch. Schiffs- u. Tropen-Hyg.* **43**, 15–19.

Fairley, N. H., and Bromfield, R. J. (1933). *Trans. Roy. Soc. Trop. Med. Hyg.* **27**, 289–314.

Farhan, I., Schwabe, C. W., and Zobel, C. R. (1959). *Am. J. Trop. Med. Hyg.* **8**, 473–478.

Fauré-Fremiet, E. (1913). *Arch. Anat. Microscop. (Paris)* **15**, 435–757.

Fenyvessy, B. von (1926). *Biochem. Z.* **173**, 289–297.

Fenyvessy, B. von, and Reiner, L. (1924). *Z. Hyg. Infektionskrankh.* **102**, 109–119.

Fenyvessy, B. von, and Reiner, L. (1928). *Biochem. Z.* **202**, 75–80.

Fernando, M. A. (1963). *Exptl. Parasitol.* **13**, 90–97.

Fisher, E. W., and McIntyre, W. I. (1960). *J. Comp. Pathol. Therap.* **70**, 377–384.

Ford, W. W., and Eliot, C. P. (1928). *J. Exptl. Med.* **48**, 475–492.

Freeman, R. F. H. (1962). *Comp. Biochem. Physiol.* **7**, 199–209.

Friedheim, E. A. H., and Baer, J. G. (1933). *Biochem. Z.* **265**, 329–337.

Friedheim, E. A. H., Susz, B., and Baer, J. G. (1933). *Compt. Rend. Soc. Phys. Hist. Nat. Genève* **50**, 177–182 [not seen, quoted in Krueger, F. (1940b)].

Friedl, F. E. (1961). *J. Parasitol.* **47**, 770–772.

Fulton, J. D., and Joyner, L. P. (1949). *Trans. Roy. Soc. Trop. Med. Hyg.* **43**, 273–286.

Fulton, J. D., and Spooner, D. F. (1956). *Biochem. J.* **63**, 475–481.

Fulton, J. D., and Spooner, D. F. (1957). *Ann. Trop. Med. Parasitol.* **51**, 417–421.

Glocklin, V. C., and Fairbairn, D. (1952). *J. Cell. Comp. Physiol.* **39**, 341–356.

Goil, M. M. (1958). *Z. Parasitenk.* **18**, 435–440.

Goil, M. M. (1961). *Z. Parasitenk.* **20**, 568–571.

Goldberg, E. (1957). *Exptl. Parasitol.* **6**, 367–382.

Golubeva, N. A. (1945). *Med. Parazitol. i Parazitarn. Bolezni* **14**, 45–48.

Gonzalez, M. D. P. (1949). *Bol. fac. fil. cienc. letras Univ. Sao Paulo* **99** (*Zool.* No. 14), 277–324.

Grant, P. T.,nd Sargent, J. R. (1960). *Biochem. J.* **76**, 229–237.

Grant, P. T., and Sargent, J. R. (1961). *Biochem. J.* **81**, 206–214.

Grant, P. T., Sargent, J. R., and Ryley, J. F. (1961). *Biochem. J.* **81**, 200–206.

Grembergen, G. van (1944). *Enzymologia* **11**, 268–281.

Grembergen, G. van (1949). *Enzymologia* **13**, 241–257.

Grembergen, G. van, Damme, R. van, and Vercruysse, R. (1949). *Enzymologia* **13**, 325–342.

Harnisch, O. (1932). *Z. Vergleich. Physiol.* **17**, 365–386.

Harnisch, O. (1933). *Z. Vergleich. Physiol.* **19**, 310–348.

Harnisch, O. (1935a). *Z. Vergleich. Physiol.* **22**, 50–66.

Harnisch, O. (1935b). *Z. Vergleich. Physiol.* **22**, 450–465.

Harnisch, O. (1936). *Z. Vergleich. Physiol.* **23**, 391–419.

Harnisch, O. (1937). *Z. Vergleich. Physiol.* **24**, 667–686.

Harnisch, O. (1949). *Experientia* **5**, 369–370.

Harnisch, O. (1950). *Z. Vergleich. Physiol.* **32**, 482–498.

Harvey, S. C. (1949). *J. Biol. Chem.* **179**, 435–453.

Heald, P. J., and Oxford, A. E. (1953). *Biochem. J.* **53**, 506–512.

Hemmingsen, A. M. (1960). *Rept. Steno Mem. Hosp. Nord. Insulin Lab. Copenhagen* **9**, Part II, 7–110.

Hinshaw, H. C. (1927). *Univ. California (Berkeley), Publ. Zool.* **31**, 31–51.

Hobson, A. D. (1948). *Parasitology* **38**, 183–227.

Horstmann, H. J. (1962). *Z. Parasitenk.* **21**, 437–445.

Hoshino, M., and Suzuki, H. (1956). *Fukushima J. Med. Sci.* **3**, 51–56.

Huff, G. C. (1936). *J. Parasitol.* **22**, 455–463.

Huff, G. C., and Boell, E. J. (1936). *Proc. Soc. Exptl. Biol. Med.* **34**, 626–628.

Hungate, R. E. (1939). *Ecology* **20**, 230–245.

Hungate, R. E. (1942). *Biol. Bull.* **83**, 303–319.

Hungate, R. E. (1955). *In* "Biochemistry and Physiology of Protozoa" (S. Hutner and A. Lwoff, eds.), Vol. 2, pp. 159–199. Academic Press, New York

Hunter, W. S., and Vernberg, W. B. (1955a). *Exptl. Parasitol.* **4**, 54–61.

Hunter, W. S., and Vernberg, W. B. (1955b). *Exptl. Parasitol.* **4**, 427–434.

Ivey, M. H. (1961). *J. Parasitol.* **47**, 539–544.

Jackson, G. J., and Stoll, N. R. (1964). *Am. J. Trop. Med.* **13**, 520–524.

Jenkins, A. R., and Grainge, E. B. (1956). *Trans. Roy. Soc. Trop. Med. Hyg.* **50**, 481–484.

Jones, M. F., Newton, W. L., Weibel, S. R., Warren, H. B., Steinle, M. L., and Figgat, W. B. (1947). *Natl. Inst. Health Bull.* **189**, 137–172.

Kawazoe, Y. (1961). *Japan. J. Parasitol.* **10**, 26–34.

Kearn, G. C. (1962). *J. Marine Biol. Assoc. U.K.* **42**, 93–104.

Kemnitz, G. von (1916). *Z. Biol.* **67**, 129–244.

Kligler, I. J., Geiger, A., and Comaroff, R. (1929). *Ann. Trop. Med. Parasitol.* **23**, 325–335.

Kmetec, E., and Bueding, E. (1961). *J. Biol. Chem.* **236**, 584–591.

Kmetec, E., Beaver, P. C., and Bueding, E. (1963). *Comp. Biochem. Physiol.* **9**, 115–120.

Kosmin, N. P. (1928). *Z. Vergleich. Physiol.* **8**, 625–634.

Krishnaswamy, S. (1960). *Rept. Challenger Soc.* **3**, No. XII.

Krogh, A. (1916). "The Respiratory Exchange of Animals and Man." Longmans, Green, London.

Krueger, F. (1936). *Zool. Jahrb. Abt. Allgem. Zool. Physiol.* **57**, 1–56.

Krueger, F. (1940a). *Z. Wiss. Zool.* **152**, 547–570.

Krueger, F. (1940b). *Zool. Jahrb. Abt. Allgem. Zool. Physiol.* **60**, 103–128.

Lai, P. (1956). *Boll. Soc. Ital Biol. Sper.* **32**, 1588–1590.

Laser, H. (1944). *Biochem. J.* **38**, 333–338.

Laser, H., and Rothschild, L. (1949). *Biochem. J.* **45**, 598–612.

Lazarus, M. (1950). *Australian J. Sci. Res.* **B3**, 245–250.

Lee, C. U. (1930). *Arch. Schiff- u. Tropen-Hyg.* **34**, 262–274.

Lehmann, D. L., and Sorsoli, W. A. (1962). *J. Protozool.* **9**, 58–60.

Leland, S. E. (1963). *J. Parasitol.* **49**, 600–611.

Levenbook, L. (1950a). *J. Exptl. Biol.* **27**, 158–174.

Levenbook, L. (1950b). *J. Exptl. Biol.* **27**, 184–191.

Levenbook, L., and Clark, A. M. (1950). *J. Exptl. Biol.* **27**, 175–183.

Lindblom, G. P. (1961). *J. Protozool.* **8**, 139–150.

Looss, A. (1911). *Records Egypt. Govt. School Med.* **4**, 163–613.

Lucker, J. T. (1935). *Proc. Helminthol. Soc. Wash., D.C.* **2**, 54–55.

Lwoff, A. (1934). *Zentr. Bakteriol. Parasitenk., Abt. I: Orig.* **130**, 498–518.

McCoy, O. R. (1930). *Am. J. Hyg.* **11**, 413–448.

McIver, M. A., Redfield, A. C., and Benedict, E. B. (1926). *Am. J. Physiol.* **76**, 92–111.

McKee, R. W., Ormsbee, R. A., Anfinsen, C. B., Geiman, Q. M., and Ball, E. G. (1946). *J. Exptl. Med.* **84**, 569–582.

Maegraith, B. G. (1948). "Pathological Processes in Malaria and Blackwater Fever." Thomas, Springfield, Illinois.

Maegraith, B. G. (1954). *Indian J. Malariol.* **8**, 281–290.

Maegraith, B. G. (1956). *Ann. Soc. Belge Med. Trop.* **36**, 623–629.

Maegraith, B. G. (1959). *Riv. Parassitol.* **20**, 317–326.

Maegraith, B. G., Gilles, H. M., and Devakul, K. (1957). *Z. Tropenmed. Parasitol.* **8**, 485–514.

Maegraith, B. G., Riley, M. V., and Deegan, T. (1962). *Ann. Trop. Med. Parasitol.* **56**, 483–491.

Maier, J., and Coggeshall, L. T. (1941). *J. Infect. Diseases* **69**, 87–96.

Marchoux, E., and Chorine, V. (1932). *Ann. Inst. Pasteur* **49**, 75–102.

Marshall, P. B. (1948). *Brit. J. Pharmacol.* **3**, 8–14.

Massey, V., and Rogers, W. P. (1949). *Nature* **163**, 909.

Meeh, K. (1879). *Z. Biol.* **15**, 425–458.

Montgomery, H. (1957). *Federation Proc.* **16**, 697–699.

Moulder, J. W. (1947). *Science* **106**, 168–169.

Moulder, J. W. (1948a). *J. Infect. Diseases* **83**, 33–41.

Moulder, J. W. (1948b). *J. Infect. Diseases* **83**, 42–49.

Moulder, J. W. (1948c). *Ann. Rev. Microbiol.* **2**, 101–120.

Nagai, T. (1957). *Nagasaki Igakkai Zasshi* **32**, 1380–1397.

Nagamoto, T., and Okabe, K. (1959). *J. Kurume Med. Assoc.* **22**, 3757–3759.

Nauss, R. W., and Yorke, W. (1911). *Ann. Trop. Med. Parasitol.* **5**, 199–214.

Newton, W. L., Bennet, H. J., and Figgat, W. B. (1949). *Am. J. Hyg.* **49**, 166–175.

Nishigori, M. (1928). *J. Formosan Med. Assoc.* No. 276 [not seen, quoted in Lee, C. U. (1930)].

Oba, N. (1959). *J. Kurume Med. Assoc.* **22**, 2988–3005.

Ohtsu, H. (1959). *J. Chiba Med. Soc.* **35**, 281–300.

Olivier, L., Brand, T. von, and Mehlman, B. (1953). *Exptl. Parasitol.* **2**, 258–270.

Oya, H., Costello, L. C., and Smith, W. N. (1963). *J. Cell. Comp. Physiol.* **62**, 287–294.

Pahl, G., and Bachofer, C. S. (1957). *Biol. Bull.* **112**, 383–389.

Passey, R. F., and Fairbairn, D. (1955). *Can. J. Biochem. Physiol.* **33**, 1033–1046.

Peters, L., Bueding, E., Valk, A., Higashi, A., and Welch, A. D. (1949). *J. Pharmacol. Exptl. Therap.* **95**, 212–239.

Rathbone, L. (1955). *Biochem. J.* **61**, 574–579.

Ray, I. C. (1932). *Indian J. Med. Res.* **20**, 355–367.

Read, C. P. (1956). *Exptl. Parasitol.* **5**, 325–344.

Read, C. P. (1957). *J. Parasitol.* **43**, 385–394.

Read, C. P., and Rothman, A. H. (1955). *Am. J. Hyg.* **61**, 249–260.

Read, C. P., and Yogore, M. (1955). *J. Parasitol.* **41**, Suppl., 28.

Rees, C. W., and Hale, M. W. (1936). *J. Agr. Res.* **53**, 477–492.

Reiner, L., Smythe, C. V., and Pedlow, J. T. (1936). *J. Biol. Chem.* **113**, 75–88.

Reyes, W. L., Kruse, C. W., and Batson, M. St. C. (1963). *Am. J. Trop. Med. Hyg.* **12**, 46–55.

Riedmueller, L. (1936). *Zentr. Bakteriol. Parasitenk., Abt. I: Orig.* **137**, 428–433.

Riley, M. V. (1961). Dissertation, University of Liverpool.

Riley, M. V., and Deegan, T. (1960). *Biochem. J.* **76**, 41–46.

Riley, M. V., and Maegraith, B. G. (1961). *Ann. Trop. Med. Parasitol.* **55**, 489–497.

Riley, M. V., and Maegraith, B. G. (1962). *Ann. Trop. Med. Parasitol.* **56**, 473–482.

Ritter, H. (1961). *Biol. Bull.* **121**, 330–346.

Rogers, W. P. (1948). *Parasitology* **39**, 105–109.

Rogers, W. P. (1949a). *Australian J. Sci. Res.* **B2**, 157–165.

Rogers, W. P. (1949b). *Australian J. Sci. Res.* **B2**, 166–174.

Rogers, W. P. (1960). *Proc. Roy. Soc.* **B152**, 367–386.

Rohde, R. A. (1960). *Proc. Helminthol. Soc. Wash., D.C.* **27**, 160–164.

Rohrbacher, G. H. (1957). *J. Parasitol* **43**, 9–18.

Root, R. W. (1931). *Biol. Bull.* **61**, 427–456.

Ross, O. A., and Bueding, E. (1950). *Proc. Soc. Exptl. Biol. Med.* **73**, 179–182.

Ryley, J. F. (1951). *Biochem. J.* **49**, 577–585.

Ryley, J. F. (1955a). *Biochem. J.* **59**, 353–361.

Ryley, J. F. (1955b). *Biochem. J.* **59**, 361–369.

Ryley, J. F. (1956). *Biochem. J.* **62**, 215–222.

Ryley, J. F. (1962). *Biochem. J.* **85**, 211–223.

Saito, S., and Kawazoe, Y. (1961). *Japan. J. Parasitol.* **10**, 35–39.

Sawyer, T. K., and Weinstein, P. P. (1963). *J. Parasitol.* **49**, 218–224.

Schalimov, L. G. (1931). *Trudy Dinamike Razvit.* **6**, 181–196.

Scheff, G., and Rabati, F. (1938). *Biochem. Z.* **298**, 101–109.

Scholander, P. F., and Dam, L. van (1953). *Biol. Bull.* **104**, 75–86.

Scholander, P. F., Dam, L. van, and Scholander, S. I. (1955). *Am. J. Botany* **42**, 92–98.

Schwabe, C. W. (1957a). *Am. J. Hyg.* **65**, 325–337.

Schwabe, C. W. (1957b). *Am. J. Hyg.* **65**, 338–343.

Senekjie, H. A. (1941). *Am. J. Hyg.* **34**, Sect. C, 67–70.

Shimomura, M. (1959). *J. Kurume Med. Assoc.* **22**, 2435–2450.

Shorb, D. A. (1944). *J. Agr. Res.* **69**, 279–287.

Silverman, M., Ceithaml, J., Taliaferro, L. G., and Evans, E. A. (1944). *J. Infect. Diseases* **75**, 212–230.

Slater, W. K. (1925). *Biochem. J.* **19**, 604–610.

Smith, B. F., and Herrick, C. A. (1944). *J. Parasitol.* **30**, 295–302.

Smyth, J. D. (1950). *J. Parasitol.* **36**, 371–383.

Soule, M. H. (1925). *J. Infect. Diseases* **36**, 245–308.

Stannard, J. N., McCoy, O. R., and Latchford, W. B. (1938). *Am. J. Hyg.* **27**, 666–682.

Stephenson, W. (1947). *Parasitology* **38,** 116–122.

Stoll, N. R. (1940). *Growth* **4,** 383–406.

Stunkard, H. W. (1930). *J. Morphol.* **50,** 143–183.

Stunkard, H. W. (1937). *Am. Museum Novitates* **908,** 1–27

Sugden, B. (1953). *J. Gen. Microbiol.* **9,** 44–53.

Sugden, B., and Oxford, A. E. (1952). *J. Gen. Microbiol.* **7,** 145–153.

Suzuki, Z., and Suzuki, T. (1951). *J. Biochem.* **38,** 237–254.

Swierstra, D. (1956). Thesis, University of Utrecht.

Szwejkowska, G. (1929). *Bull. Intern. Acad. Polon. Sci., Cl. Sci. Math. Nat.* **B1928,** 489–519.

Takuma, I. (1959). *Endemic Diseases Bull., Nagasaki Univ.* **1,** 19–37.

Taylor, A. E. R. (1963). *Exptl. Parasitol.* **14,** 304–310.

Thurston, J. P. (1958a). *Parasitology* **48,** 165–183.

Thurston, J. P. (1958b). *Parasitology* **48,** 463–467.

Trager, W. (1934). *Biol. Bull.* **66,** 182–190.

Trager, W. (1950). *J. Exptl. Med.* **92,** 349–366.

Trager, W. (1957). *Acta Tropica* **14,** 289–301.

Tsukahara, T. (1961). *Japan. J. Microbiol.* **5,** 157–169.

Van de Vijver, G. (1964). *Exptl. Parasitol.* **15,** 97–105.

van Grembergen, G., *see* Grembergen, G. van.

Van Gundy, S. D., Stolzy, L. H., Szuszkiewicz, T. E., and Rackham, R. L. (1962). *Phytopathology* **7,** 628–632.

Velick, S. F. (1942). *Am. J. Hyg.* **35,** 152–161.

Vernberg, W. B. (1961). *Exptl. Parasitol.* **11,** 270–275.

Vernberg, W. B. (1963). *Ann. N.Y. Acad. Sci.* **113,** 261–271.

Vernberg, W. B., and Hunter, W. S. (1959). *Exptl. Parasitol.* **8,** 76–82.

Vernberg, W. B., and Hunter, W. S. (1961). *Exptl. Parasitol.* **11,** 34–38.

Vernberg, W. B., and Vernberg, F. J. (1963). *Exptl. Parasitol.* **14,** 330–332.

von Brand, T., *see* Brand, T. von.

von Buddenbrock, W., *see* Buddenbrock, W. von.

von Fenyvessy, B., *see* Fenyvessy, B. von.

von Kemnitz, G., *see* Kemnitz, G. von

Warren, L. G., (1960). *J. Parasitol.* **46,** 529–239.

Weinland, E. (1901). *Z. Biol.* **42,** 55–90.

Weinland, E., and Brand, T. von (1926). *Z. Vergleich. Physiol.* **4,** 212–285.

Weinman, D. (1953). *Ann. N.Y. Acad. Sci.* **56,** 995–1003.

Weinstein, P. P., and Jones, M. F. (1956). *J. Parasitol.* **42,** 215–236.

Welch, A. D., Peters, L., Bueding, E., Valk, A., and Higashi, A. (1947). *Science* **105,** 486–488.

Wendt, H. (1936). *Z. Kinderheilk.* **58,** 375–387.

Willems, R., Massart, L., and Peeters, G. (1942). *Naturwiss.* **30,** 169–170.

Wilmoth, J. H. (1945). *Physiol. Zool.* **18,** 60–80.

Wilson, P. A. G., and Fairbairn, D. (1961). *J. Protozool.* **8,** 410–416.

Witte, J. (1933). *Zentr. Bakteriol. Parasitenk., Abt. I: Orig.* **128,** 188–195.

Wright, W. H. (1950). *J. Parasitol.* **36,** 175–177.

Zawadowsky, M. (1916). *Compt. Rend. Soc. Biol.* **68,** 595–598.

Zawadowsky, M., and Orlow, A. P. (1927). *Trudy Lab. Eksper. Biol. Moskov, Zooparka* **3,** 99–116.

Zawadowsky, M., and Schalimov, L. G. (1929). *Trudy Lab. Eksper. Biol., Moskov, Zooparka* **5,** 1–42.

Zeledon, R. (1960a). *J. Protozool.* **7,** 146–150.

Zeledon, R. (1960b). *Rev. Biol. Trop., Univ. Costa Rica* **8**, 181–195.
Zeuthen, E. (1947). *Compt. Rend. Trav. Lab. Carlsberg., Ser. Chim.* **26**, No. 3, 17–161.
Zimmerman, J. F. (1949). *Biochim. Biophys. Acta* **3**, 198–204.
Zviaginzev, S. N. (1934). *Trudy Dinamike Razvit.* **8**, 186–202.
Zwisler, J. B., and Lysenko, M. G. (1954). *J. Parasitol.* **40**, 531–535.

AUTHOR INDEX

Numbers in *italics* refer to pages on which the complete references are listed.

Firket, H., 297, *311*
Firki, M. M., 169, *185*
Fischer, A., 15, *36,* 111, 117, *150*
Fisher, E. W., 373, *377*
Fisher, F. M., 95, *150,* 193, 194, 197, 200, *223,* 257, *293*
Fisher, M. L., 325, *328*
Fitzgerald, P. R., 275, 277, *287*
Fleisher, M. S., 250, *290*
Flössner, O., 267, *287*
Florkin, M., 306, *310,* 334, *377*
Flosi, A. Z., 30, *36*
Flury, F., 2, 3, 5, *36,* 58, 59, *74,* 101, 116, 117, *150,* 192, 193, 194, 200, 202, 204, *225,* 232, 234, 235, 238, 247, 248, 265, 266, 267, 268, 280, *287*
Fodor, O., 171, *185*
Foote, M., 33, *37,* 171, *185,* 221, *226*
Ford, W. W., 373, *377*
Forsyth, G., 49, *74*
Foster, A. O., 27, *36*
Foster, M., 45, *74*
Foster, W. B., 256, *286*
Fouquey, C., 48, 49, *74,* 202, 203, *225, 228*
Fox, H. M., 202, *225,* 239, *287*
Foy, H., 27, 28, *36*
Fraipont, J., 8, *36*
Frank, L. L., 171, *185*
Frank, O., 317, *330*
Franklin, M. C., 33, *36,* 274, *287*
Fraser, D. M., 121, *150,* 182, *185*
Fredericq, L., 253, *287*
Freeman, E. A., 326, *328*
Freeman, R. F. H., 238, 239, 241, *287,* 344, *377*
French, M. H., 158, 161, *185,* 279, *287*
Frentz, R., 222, *225*
Friedheim, E. A. H., 243, *287,* 344, 345, 351, 353, 354, 366, 367, 368, *377*
Friedl, F. E., 90, *150,* 339, *377*
Frugoni, G., 163, *184*
Fuhrmann, G., 164, *185,* 275, 279, *287*
Fuhrmeister, C., 323, 324, *328*
Fulton, J. D., 30, *36,* 44, 55, *73, 74,* 83, 85, 88, 111, 112, 113, 114, 115, 119, 121, 130, 139, 145, *149, 150,* 159, 160, 177, 180, *185,* 215, 220, *223, 225,* 242,

243, 244, 255, 260, *286, 287, 292,* 341, 343, 346, 365, *377*
Funk, H. B., 316, 317, *330*
Fuse, M., 18, *37,* 55, 68, *75*

Gaafar, S. M., 23, *34, 36*
Galaboff, S., 275, 278, *284*
Gall, D., 275, 278, *287*
Gall, E. A., 31, *36,* 159, *185*
Gallagher, C. H., 169, 172, *185*
Gallagher, I. H. C., 234, 235, *287*
Galliard, H., 177, *185*
Galysh, F. T., 168, *188*
Gammel, J. A., 279, *287*
Garrault, H., 236, *287*
Garza, B. L., 275, *285*
Gazzinelli, G., 246, *287*
Geiger, A., 88, 110, *150,* 161, *186,* 372, *378*
Geigy, R., 82, *150*
Geiling, E. M. K., 88, 120, 123, *149,* 180, *184*
Geiman, Q. M., 26, 30, 31, *38,* 44, *76,* 88, 89, 114, 121, *147, 152,* 182, *183,* 217, *223,* 235, 249, 255, 259, *284, 290,* 302, *309,* 322, 323, 325, *328, 330,* 336, 353, 364, 365, 367, *375, 379*
Genazzani, E., 14, *35,* 217, *224*
Georges, P., 336, *376*
Georgi, B. N., 33, *39*
Gerdjikoff, I., 322, *329*
Gerritsen, T., 27, *36*
Gerzeli, G., 18, 19, *36, 37,* 55, 56, 68, *74,* 119, *150,* 205, *225*
Gerzon, K., 111, 117, *154*
Gettier, A., 26, 27, *37*
Gevaudan, P., 177, *188*
Ghalioungi, P., 169, *185*
Ghosh, B. K., 178, *185,* 282, *287*
Ghosh, B. M., 220, *226*
Ghosh, B. N., 244, *288, 293*
Ghosh, J. J., 71, *73,* 85, 96, 112, 120, 124, *149,* 255, 262, 263, *285,* 341, 343, 365, *376*
Ghosh, S., 158, *187*
Ghysels, G., 164, *186,* 278, *289*
Gibbs, E., 45, 69, *72,* 80, 86, 91, 92, 94, *148*
Gilchrist, H. B., 326, *330*

SUBJECT INDEX